EAGLE Syndrome

Claudio Vicini • Paolo Zamboni
Giannicola Iannella
Editors

EAGLE Syndrome

The Many Faces of the Elongated Styloid Process

Springer

Editors

Claudio Vicini
University of Ferrara
Cona, FE, Italy

Paolo Zamboni
Vascular Diseases Center
University of Ferrara
Cona, FE, Italy

Giannicola Iannella
Department of "Organi di Senso"
University "Sapienza"
Rome, Italy

ISBN 978-3-031-92828-4 ISBN 978-3-031-92829-1 (eBook)
https://doi.org/10.1007/978-3-031-92829-1

This Springer imprint is published by the registered company Springer Nature Switzerland AG
The registered company address is: Gewerbestrasse 11, 6330 Cham, Switzerland

To all our Eagle Syndrome Patients

Foreword by Magliulo

Eagle syndrome, though relatively rare, is a condition that profoundly impacts the lives of those who experience it. Characterized by a constellation of symptoms, from sharp throat pain to difficulties in swallowing, and even radiating pain to the ear or face, Eagle syndrome can often be mistaken for other more common ailments, leading to years of misdiagnosis and suffering. The elongation of the styloid process or calcification of the stylohyoid ligament, which are at the root of this condition, can be elusive even to trained eyes, resulting in a journey filled with frustration and confusion for patients.

This book was born out of the need to shed light on Eagle syndrome—an often overlooked and under-discussed condition. Whether you are an otolaryngologist, maxillofacial surgeon, vascular surgeon, or different medical professional aiming to expand your knowledge, this book provides a comprehensive exploration of Eagle syndrome from every angle. The authors will delve into the anatomy and physiology behind the syndrome, walk through the diagnostic challenges, and examine the various treatment options that offer hope to patients. Equally important, we will hear the voices of those who have lived through this ordeal—stories of resilience, recovery, and, ultimately, healing.

By compiling current medical insights, this book seeks to fill the gap with accessible, reliable information on Eagle syndrome. It serves not only as an informative book but also as a guide for navigating the complexities of diagnosis and treatment. It is our hope that this work will contribute to a broader awareness of the condition within the medical community and provide valid support for its treatment.

I would like to express my compliments to all the authors, who have brought together in this book the leading experts in this pathology that will make this book a reference for the diagnosis and treatment of this pathology.

Enjoy your reading

Organ of Sense Department
Sapienza University of Rome
Rome, Italy

Giuseppe Magliulo

Foreword by Pelucchi

I gladly accepted the invitation from friends and colleagues to write a foreword to this book on "Eagle Syndrome."

The authors have passionately and expertly explored this topic, starting from its historical origins and moving to the complex and often challenging diagnostic and therapeutic process. I have learned that, despite the eponym, the first description of this condition was made in Italy.

A sincere thanks to the colleagues who tracked down the original text, with patience and investigative insight.

The Eagle Syndrome, which we continue to call by this name, is well described in its various and sometimes almost mysterious symptomatic manifestations. Its diagnosis is so complicated that patients—or rather, female patients, since women are overwhelmingly affected—seek help from multiple specialists, but most of the times, with no conclusive answers, constantly searching for a solution to the discomfort, torment, and often pain that seems to turn their lives into something akin to a "via Crucis."

I was taught many, too many, years ago that a diagnosis cannot be made without suspicion. I believe that the authors' intent in this text is precisely to encourage suspicion of Eagle Syndrome, especially when a set of unrelated symptoms at first glance does not find a convincing explanation. The risk of labeling these patients as "anxious," "hypochondriacs," or worse, "psychiatric," is unfortunately always present, since the psychological state of those suffering from this condition is often altered in an anxious or depressive manner, with a near-compulsive demand for surgery that could finally provide a definitive solution.

But if surgery is necessary, which type would be the most appropriate? The authors describe in detail the possible techniques and approaches, outlining their advantages, risks, and complications. They also present new robotic techniques and combined approaches that involve not only otolaryngologists but also vascular surgeons and neurosurgeons, as each patient has specific clinical, anatomical, neurological, and vascular features that must be carefully evaluated when planning the surgical approach.

In conclusion, I recall one of my first encounters with this syndrome, which had been unknown to me until then. Let's go back to the mid-1990s. We had a case with classic pain symptoms and the patient was successfully operated on, supported by the radiological findings. We presented this case at the national SIO congress with a poster we made using a newly acquired graphic design program. We had the idea to depict the patient with a cartoon where an eagle in a threatening pose was perched on his left shoulder, the affected side, of course. That poster is still displayed in the residents' classroom.

Department of Otorhinolaryngology and Audiology
University of Study of Ferrara
Ferrara, Italy

Stefano Pelucchi

Acknowledgments

This book is first of all dedicated to all our Eagle Syndrome patients, no one excluded. Their personal stories of long-lasting symptoms, difficult and delayed diagnosis, frustrations, success, and failures gave us the inspiration to write this book. Their immense gratitude was the main power for our big effort. This book was also an extraordinary teamwork of a great number of colleagues who accepted the commitment to write their own contribution with enthusiasm and competence. Thank you so much to all of them. A special mention to Alberto Caranti and Ruggero Campisi, the real and very active "connective tissue" between all the authors. Last but not least let us thank our beloved families. Their warm support during our long way from the preface to the last chapter was crucial for winning the challenge. We hope that we will be able to transmit to our readers our curiosity and passion for this rare, neglected, mysterious, challenging but exciting syndrome.

Introduction

Head or neck pain (migraine, tension headache, orofacial neuralgia, etc.) is among the most common complaints in daily practice of many medical branches (general practitioners, neurologists, ENTs, oral surgeons, etc.). Cerebrovascular events, mainly arterial but also venous, in western countries are so prevalent to be considered a real social problem. Finally, Dizziness and Tinnitus are well-recognized dilemma for patients and doctors as well. The "fil rouge" connecting in the background this wide range of so different clinical situations? In a very few number of cases of all the mentioned clinical conditions, the unexpected and underestimated cause is considered a "pathologically" elongated styloid process producing a significant mechanical conflict with cranial nerves, major vessels (carotid artery or jugular vein), and pharyngeal wall. This is a rare, not exceptional, but possible occurrence, which must be considered, demonstrated, or ruled out. Especially because among many etiologies defined as idiopathic or difficult to treat, elongated styloid may offer to the surgeon a well-defined target to manipulate for controlling the symptoms or preventing the possible complications. Unfortunately the personal experience of the authors is that the average number of different consultations reported by most of the patients before to have a correct diagnosis is of more than ten with a diagnostic delay of more than 5 years. The meaning of this not unusual story is that the symptomatic elongated styloid process described in 1927 by Wyatt Eagle skips the diagnosis in a remarkable number of consultations. Why does it happen? In our opinion, for many different and not strictly related explanations. Eagle Syndrome, the eponymous designation originating from the pioneer who first described into detail the clinical picture last century, is a newborn in the wide panorama of the human diseases. No comparison with trigeminal neuralgia, Temporo-Mandibular Joint (TMJ) dysfunction, etc. It's even more true for the most recently described jugular variant, which was depicted for the first time by the Ferrara Group in 2019. This clinical entity was probably not included in the programs of the medical studies of many of the most aged doctors still active in the practice. Also the most common Eagle Syndrome, the so-called classical variant, doesn't exceed a short mention in the medical textbooks or a quick comment in the lessons during the courses of medicine or residency in otolaryngology or neurology. This basically produces a very low level of knowledge and awareness in the medical community which increases the risk of underdiagnosis. On the other hand, ES is a rare entity of unusual occurrence in the daily practice of most General Practitioners (GPs), neurologists, Ear, Nose, Throat (ENTs), oral surgeons, and vascular surgeons. For that reason the occasional experience on the field can't fill the gap between the poor academic information and the need to recognize a defined etiology among many different possibilities in the busy clinics of the modern practice, in which most of the clinicians probably doesn't encounter more than one or two Eagle Syndrome (ES) in their complete career. Insufficient theoretical information and sporadic practice together are at high risk of underdiagnosis. Again, most of the complaints of many ES patients, irrespective of the variant, are absolutely not specific. The profile of distribution of ES pain is the same for the idiopathic or primary glossopharyngeal neuralgia, and a Transient Ischemic Attack of the Carotidal variant is clinically identical to any other Transient Ischemic Attack (TIA) with different etiology. The complex of symptoms and signs reported by most of the Jugular Eagle patients are really difficult to be related to the styloid process in combination to the C1 lateral body. The key for the diagnosis is to include ES into the differential diagnosis of a wide range of different clinical conditions and to not overlook this diagnostic option during the diagnostic process. Two more issues related to patients and doctors which contribute to an increased level of difficulties in ES diagnostic and therapeutical management. After a very frequent long history of missed diagnosis many ES patients tend to develop a neurotic profile for the prolonged frustration. Referring physicians risk underestimating the clear anatomical relevance of an elongated styloid process and may be reluctant to trust a patient whose anxiety is a reactive response to a longstanding, unexplained illness. Regrettably, the global literature, with 476 PubMed results and a sharp increase in annual contributions since 2010, primarily consists of individual or limited case reports, with scant comprehensive overviews and no dedicated monograph. This fragmented clinical expertise and scientific output likely mirrors the overall low awareness and knowledge of the syndrome within the medical community, spanning general practitioners, ENT specialists, neurologists, and oral surgeons. The primary objective of this book is to critically review the extensive but scattered literature worldwide, striving to construct a robust and credible database of available scientific evidence. A comprehensive discussion on the diagnosis and treatment of this pathology will be provided. We aim also to share our group's expertise in managing Eagle syndrome patients, both diagnostically and therapeutically. Our clinical experience predominantly encompasses the intricate carotid and jugular sub-types, which tend to be more unconventional and challenging to treat. The intended audience for this book

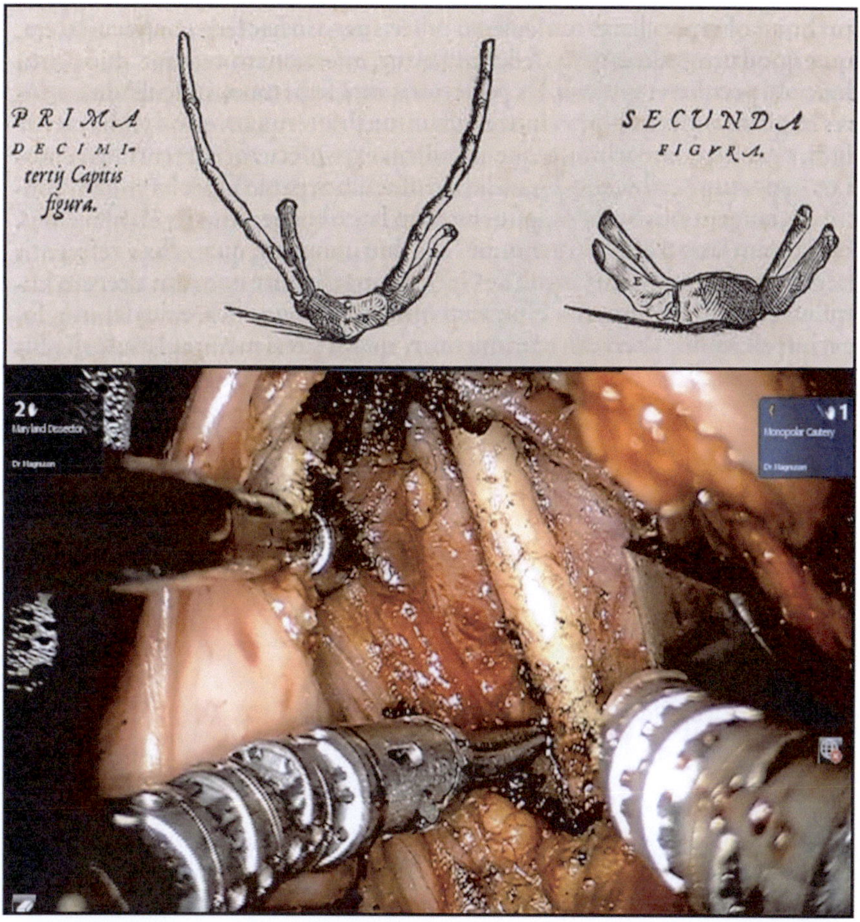

Fig. 1 In the upper anatomical drawing the ossification of the stylo-hyoid ligament as perfectly illustrated in the historical book "De Humani Corporis Fabrica" by Andreas Vesalius, published in 1543. In the lower surgical snapshot, a robotic styloidectomy carried out in 2024 is reported. About 500 years of history for a not yet completely understood disease

includes primarily ENT and head & neck surgeons, neurologists, neurosurgeons, oral surgeons, and pain specialists. Additionally, our surgical proficiency covers various forms of open styloidectomies, alongside the latest options in trans-oral approaches, such as 3D endoscopic and robotic techniques (Fig. 1).

FORLI, Italy
Ferrara, Italy
Roma, Italy

Claudio Vicini
Paolo Zamboni
Giannicola Iannella

Contents

Historical Perspective

1

Elio Maria Cunsolo, Ruggero Campisi, Alberto Caranti, Stefano Pelucchi, and Claudio Vicini

1.1 Introduction

The historical notes concerning the development of knowledge about what is currently defined by the eponym "Eagle syndrome," after the surname of Watt Eagle who played a primary role in the nosographic definition of this pathology, reveal an ancient and noble cognitive path, written by scholars and clinicians of great value. In this treatise, we will follow a chronological path, from the first anatomical description of the stylohyoid ligament to Eagle's publications, selecting the most relevant contributions, which, as far as possible, will be examined and shown in their original editorial form.

1.1.1 The First Anatomical Description

The first anatomical description, dated 1652, of the ossification of the stylohyoid ligament is attributed to Domenico Marchetti (Dominicus de Marchettis) [1]. Domenico Marchetti (1626–1688) was an anatomist, physician, and surgeon at the University of Padua (Fig. 1.1).

E. M. Cunsolo (✉)
Policlinico di Modena, Modena, MO, Italy

R. Campisi · A. Caranti · C. Vicini
University of Ferrara, Cona, FE, Italy
e-mail: claudio@claudiovicini.com

S. Pelucchi
ENT & Audiology Unit, Department of Neurosciences, University Hospital of Ferrara, Cona, FE, Italy
e-mail: stefano.pelucchi@unife.it

C. Vicini et al. (eds.), *EAGLE Syndrome*,
https://doi.org/10.1007/978-3-031-92829-1_1

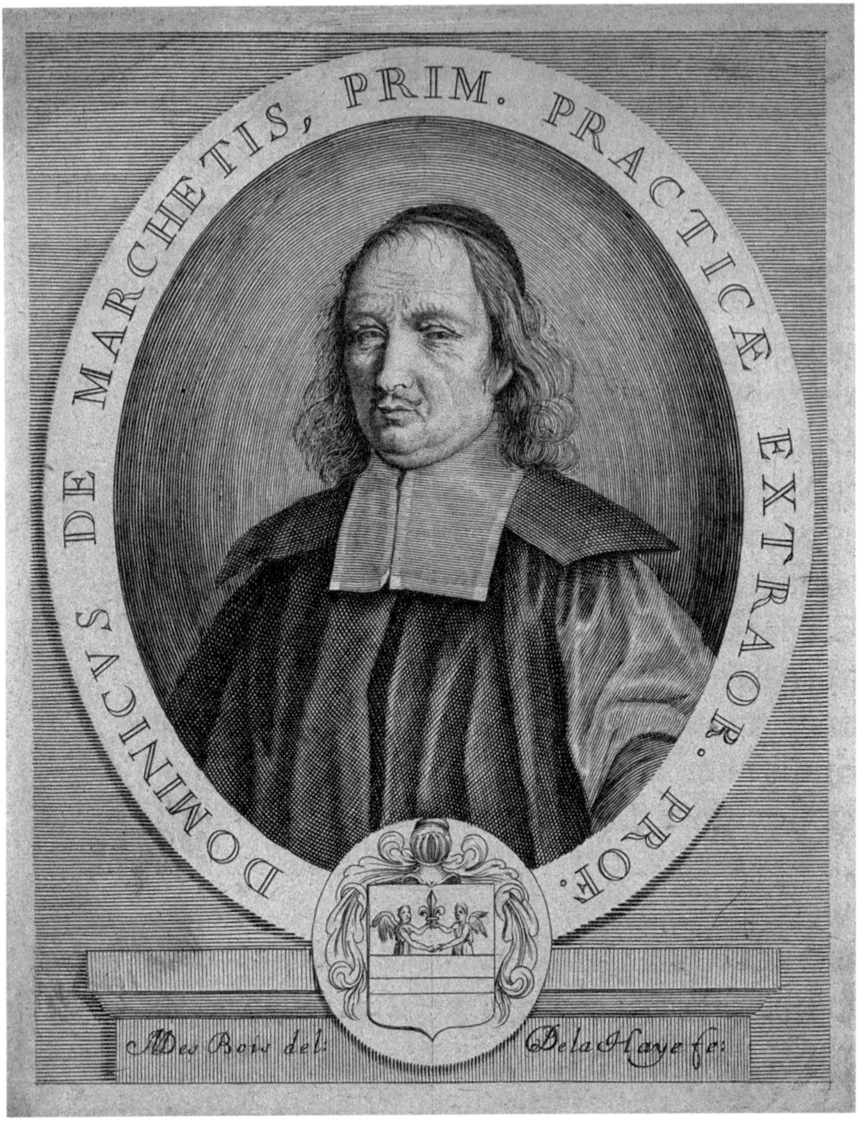

Fig. 1.1 Dominicus de Marchettis. Line engraving by C. de La Haye, 1682, after M. Desbois

He was a student of Johannes Wesling (1598–1649), a German anatomist and botanist who worked primarily in the Republic of Venice (Fig. 1.2).

Johannes Wesling's most important work was the *Syntagma anatomicum, publicis dissectionibus, in auditorum usum, diligenter aptatum* (Padua, 1641), one of the most successful anatomy manuals of its century, which had a series of translations and editions, with the second edition of 1647 being richly illustrated [2] (Fig. 1.3).

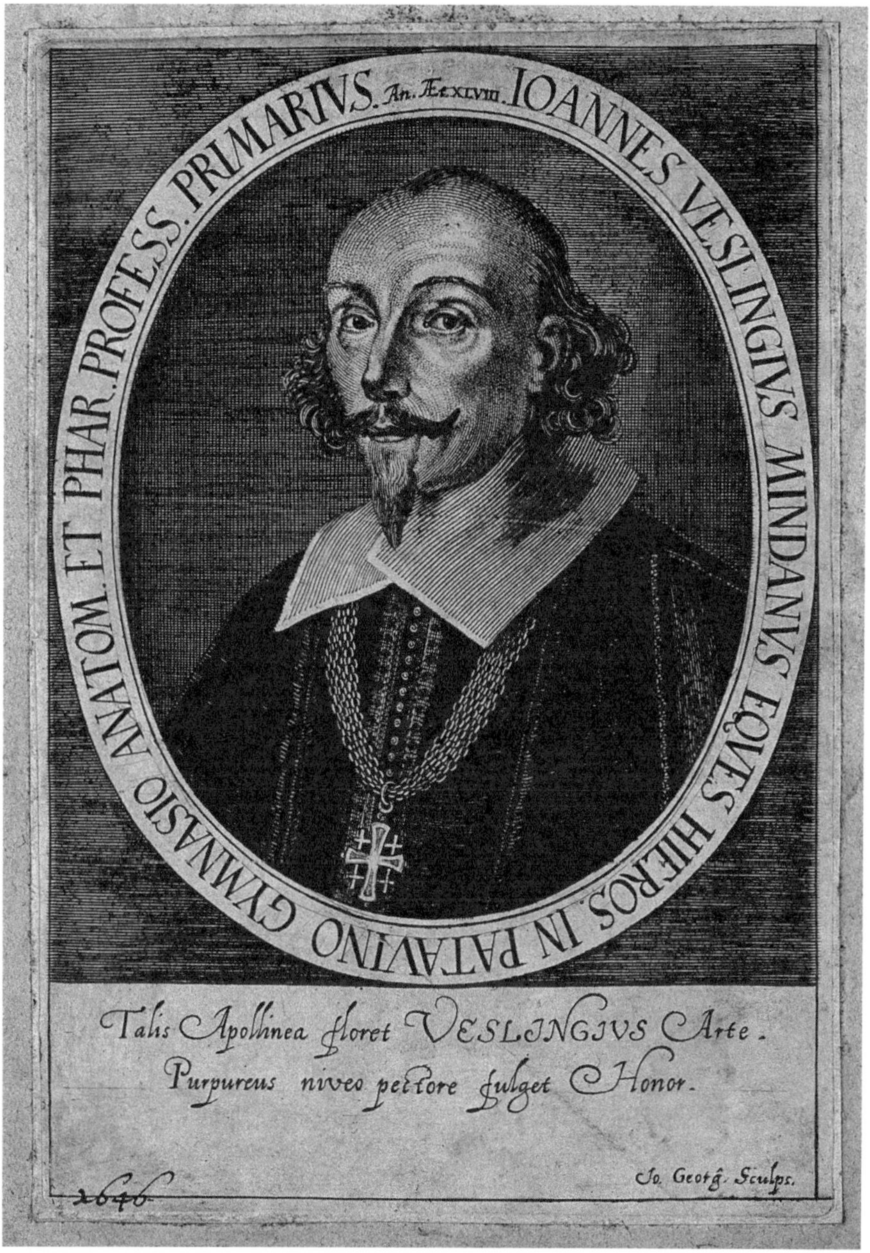
IOANNES VESLINGIVS MINDANVS EQVES HIEROS. IN PATAVINO GYMNASIO ANATOM. ET PHAR. PROFESS. PRIMARIVS. An. Æt. XLVIII.
Talis Apollinea floret VESLINGIVS Arte.
Purpureus niveo pectore fulget Honor.
Jo. Georg. Sculps.
1646

Fig. 1.2 Johann Vesling. Line engraving by J. Georgi, 1647

Domenico Marchetti belonged to a noble Paduan family. His father, Pietro, and his brother, Antonio, were anatomists, surgeons, and physicians of great and widely recognized prestige and value. His father, Pietro (1589–1673), was one of the most

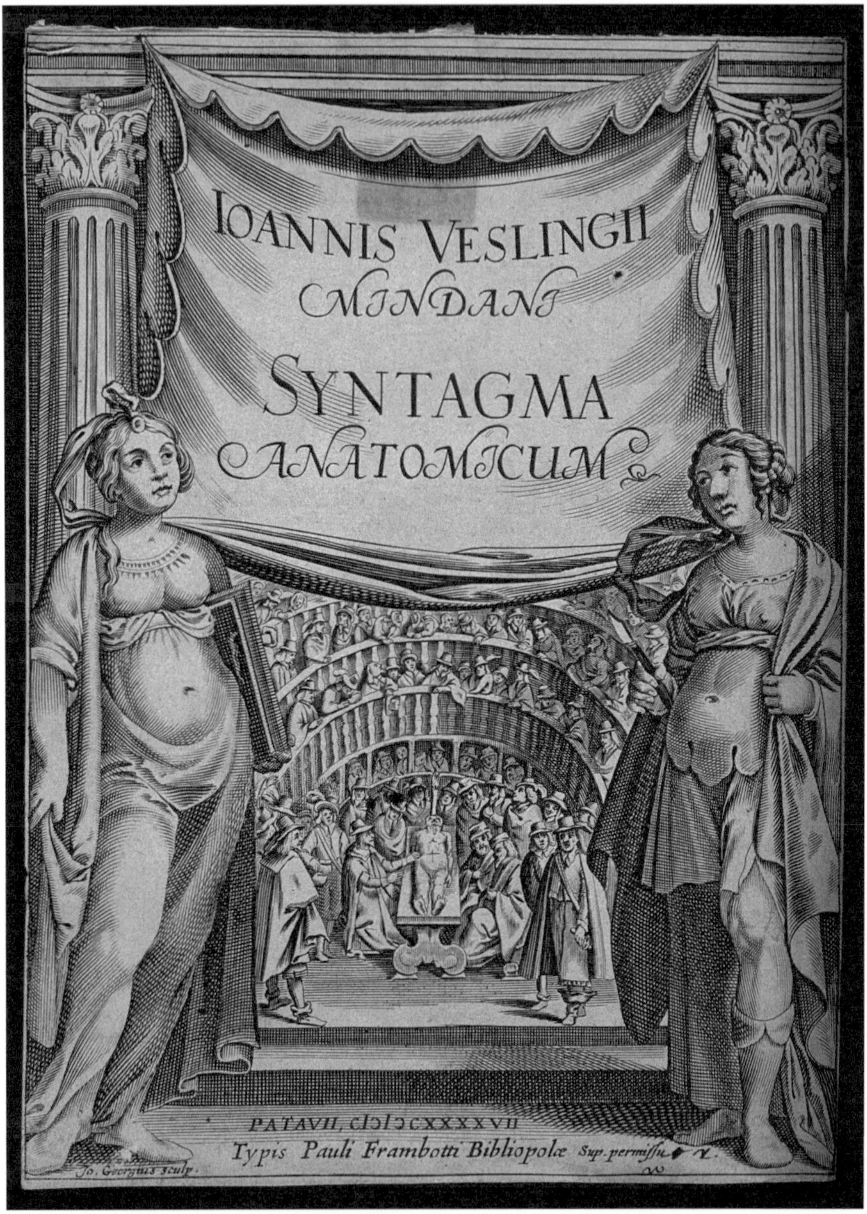

Fig. 1.3 Vesling's Syntagma anatomicum: beyond, the anatomy theatre of the University of Padua. Engraving by Giovanni Georgi, 1647

famous anatomists and surgeons of his time, proudly Venetian, as can be deduced from the "Lion of Saint Mark" hanging from his rich collar (Fig. 1.4).

He distinguished himself, in particular, as a true pioneer in the "neurosurgical" therapy of gunshot wounds [3] (Fig. 1.5).

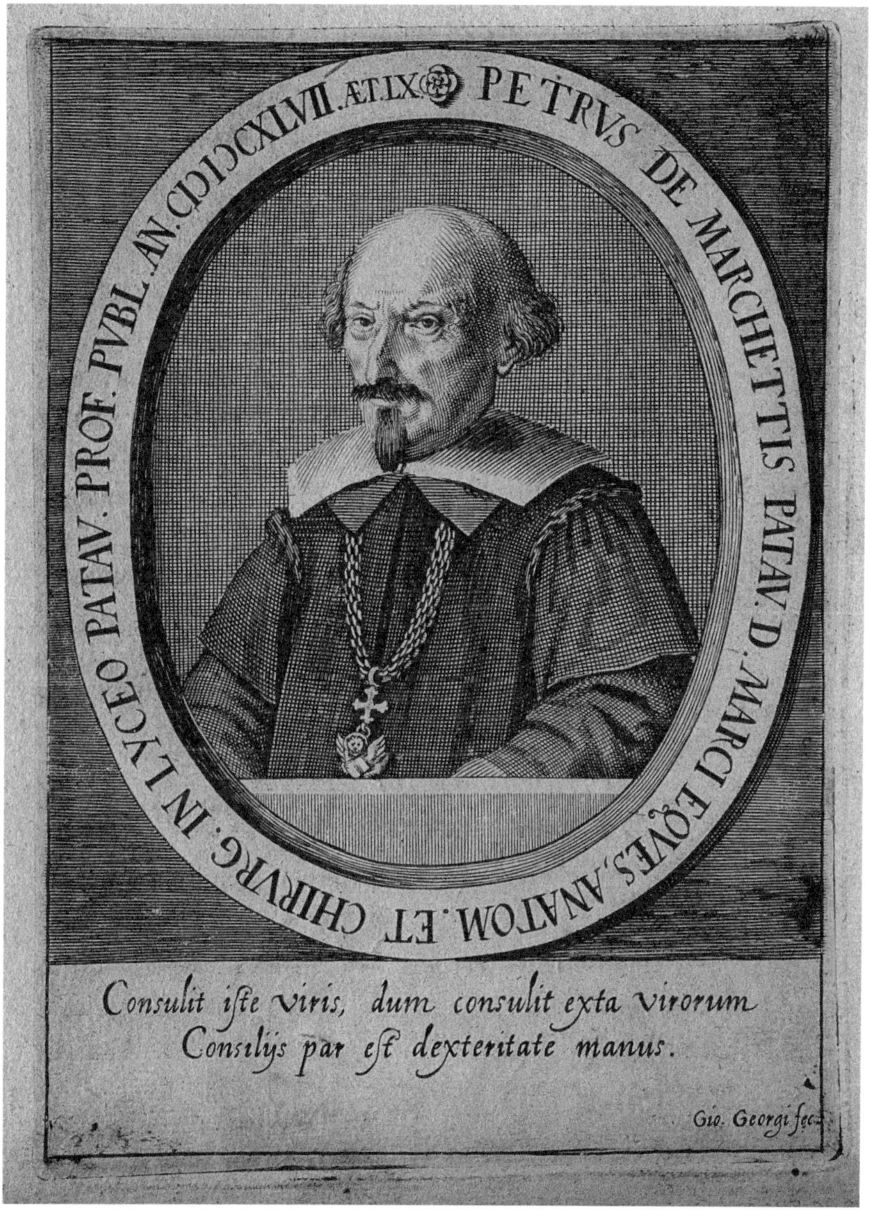

Fig. 1.4 Petrus de Marchettis. Line engraving by G. Giorgi, 1647

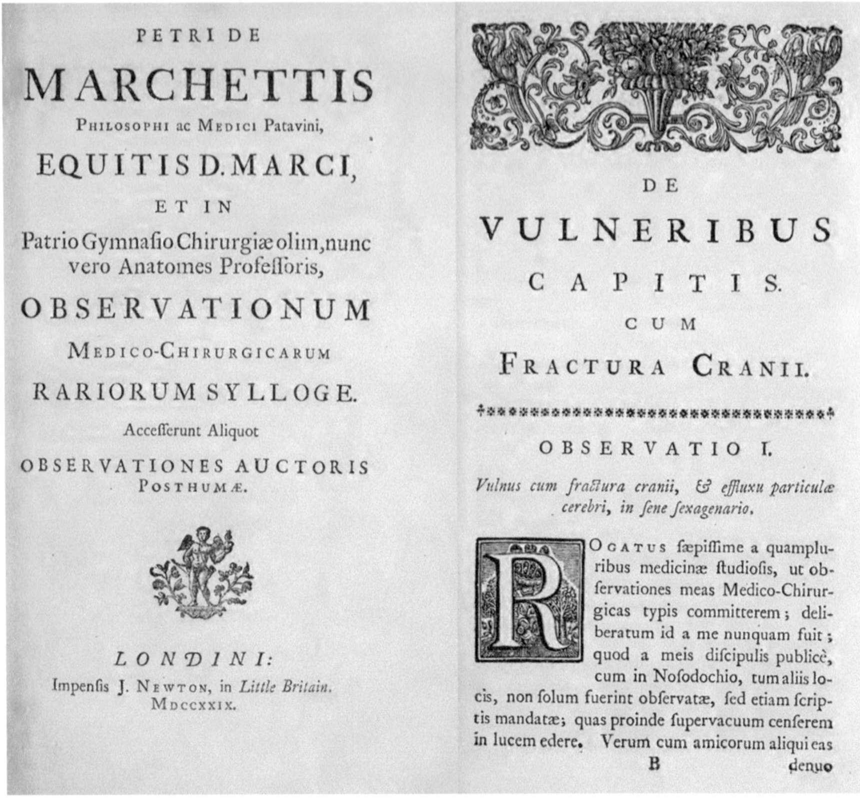

PETRI DE
MARCHETTIS
Philosophi ac Medici Patavini,
EQUITIS D. MARCI,
ET IN
Patrio Gymnaſio Chirurgiæ olim, nunc vero Anatomes Profeſſoris,
OBSERVATIONUM
Medico-Chirurgicarum
RARIORUM SYLLOGE.
Acceſſerunt Aliquot
OBSERVATIONES AUCTORIS
Posthumæ.
LONDINI:
Impenſis J. Newton, in *Little Britain.*
MDCCXXIX.

DE
VULNERIBUS
CAPITIS.
CUM
FRACTURA CRANII.
OBSERVATIO I.
Vulnus cum fractura cranii, & effluxu particulæ cerebri, in ſene ſexagenario.

Rogatus ſæpiſſime a quamplu-ribus medicinæ ſtudioſis, ut ob-ſervationes meas Medico-Chirur-gicas typis committerem; deli-beratum id a me nunquam fuit; quod a meis diſcipulis publicè, cum in Noſodochio, tum aliis lo-cis, non ſolum fuerint obſervatæ, ſed etiam ſcrip-tis mandatæ; quas proinde ſupervacuum cenſerem in lucem edere. Verum cum amicorum aliqui eas
B denuo

Fig. 1.5 “De vulneribus capitis cum fractura cranii,” Pietro Marchetti

Domenico Marchetti’s main work, although he was a skilled surgeon, was a treatise on anatomy, entitled “Anatomia: cui responsiones ad Riolanum, anatomicum Parisiensem, in ipsius animadversionibus contra Veslingium additæ sunt,” published in Padua in 1652 and 1654 and followed by subsequent editions until 1688. It is evident how in the engraving of the frontispiece (Fig. 1.6) and in the complete structuring of the title in his “Anatomy” Domenico Marchetti makes explicit reference to the work of his master Veslingio, to his father Pietro (Fig. 1.7), and to the “diatribes” with his contemporary Jean Riolan “the Younger” (1580–1657) (Fig. 1.8).

It is in Chap. XIII (De partibus Capitis Externis) of his “Anatomy,” on page 167, that Domenico Marchetti describes the ossification of the stylohyoid ligament with the following words (Fig. 1.9):

> Observavi tamen aliquando processum styloideum
> usque ad cornua ossis hyoidei pervenire,
> ipsisque valido nexu devinci.

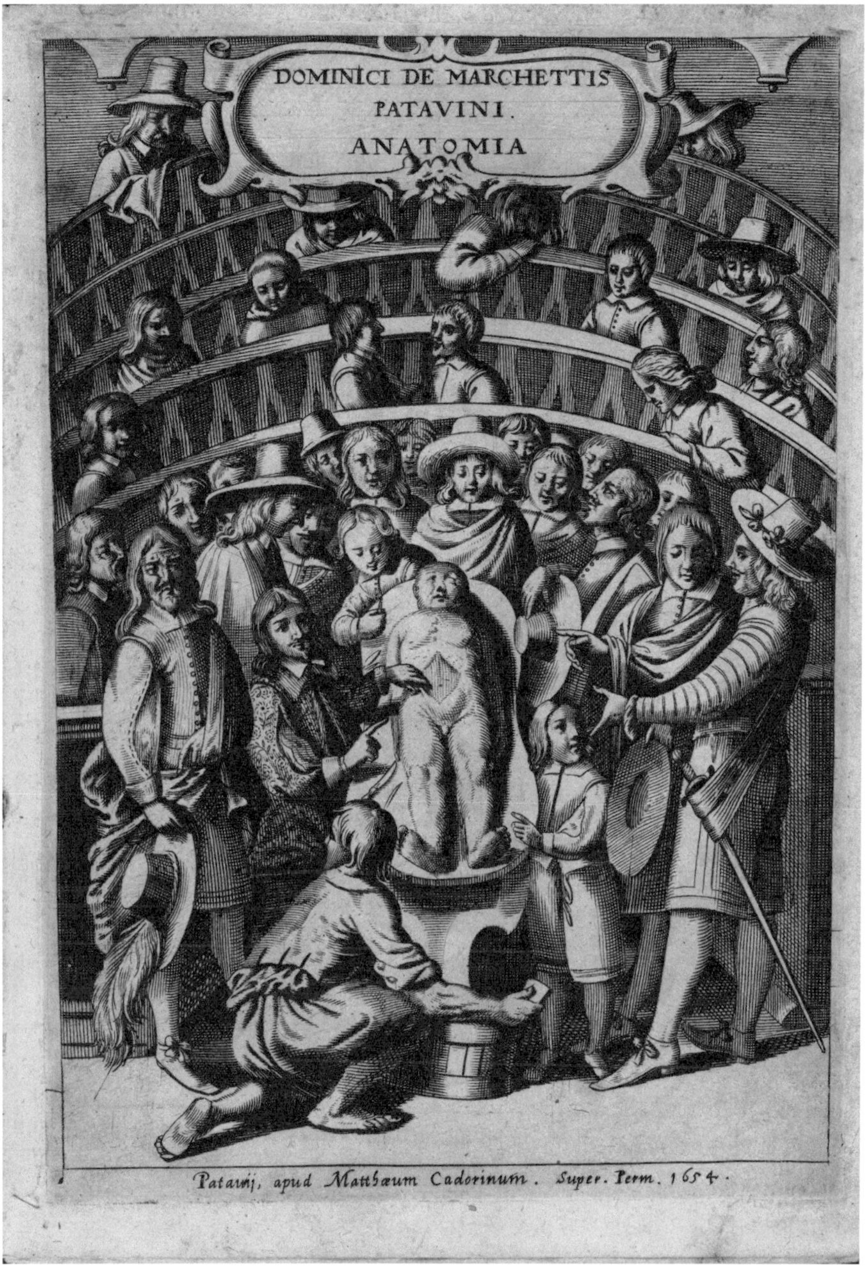

Fig. 1.6 Dominicus de Marchettis "Anatomia." Line engraving by G. Giorgi, 1647

Fig. 1.7 Marchetti's "Anatomia," 1666 edition

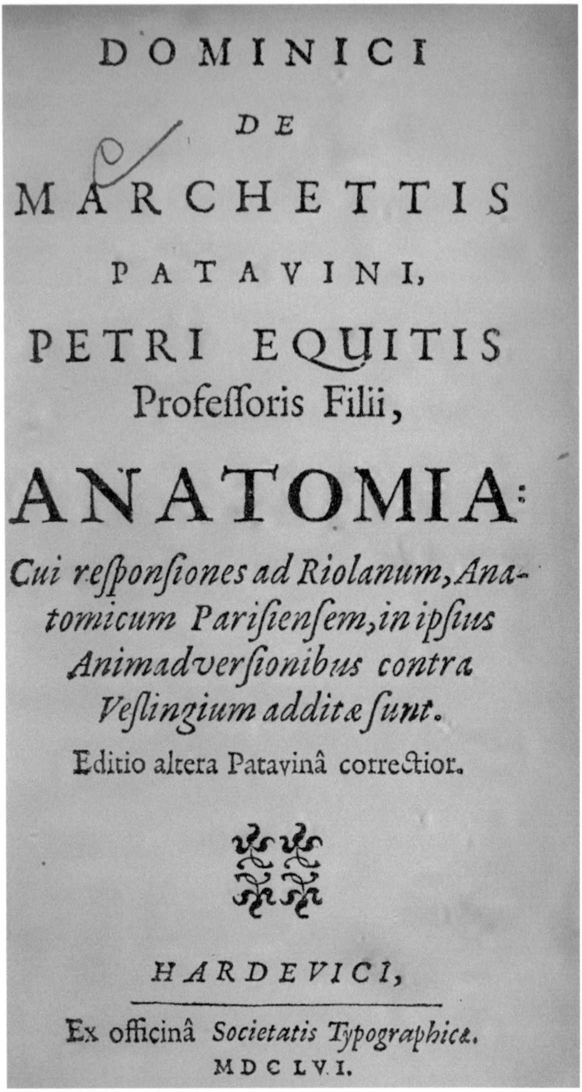

DOMINICI

DE

MARCHETTIS

PATAVINI,

PETRI EQUITIS

Profeſſoris Filii,

ANATOMIA:

Cui reſponſiones ad Riolanum, Ana-
tomicum Pariſienſem, in ipſius
Animadverſionibus contra
Veſlingium additæ ſunt.

Editio altera Patavinâ correctior.

HARDEVICI,

Ex officinâ *Societatis Typographicæ.*

M D C L V I.

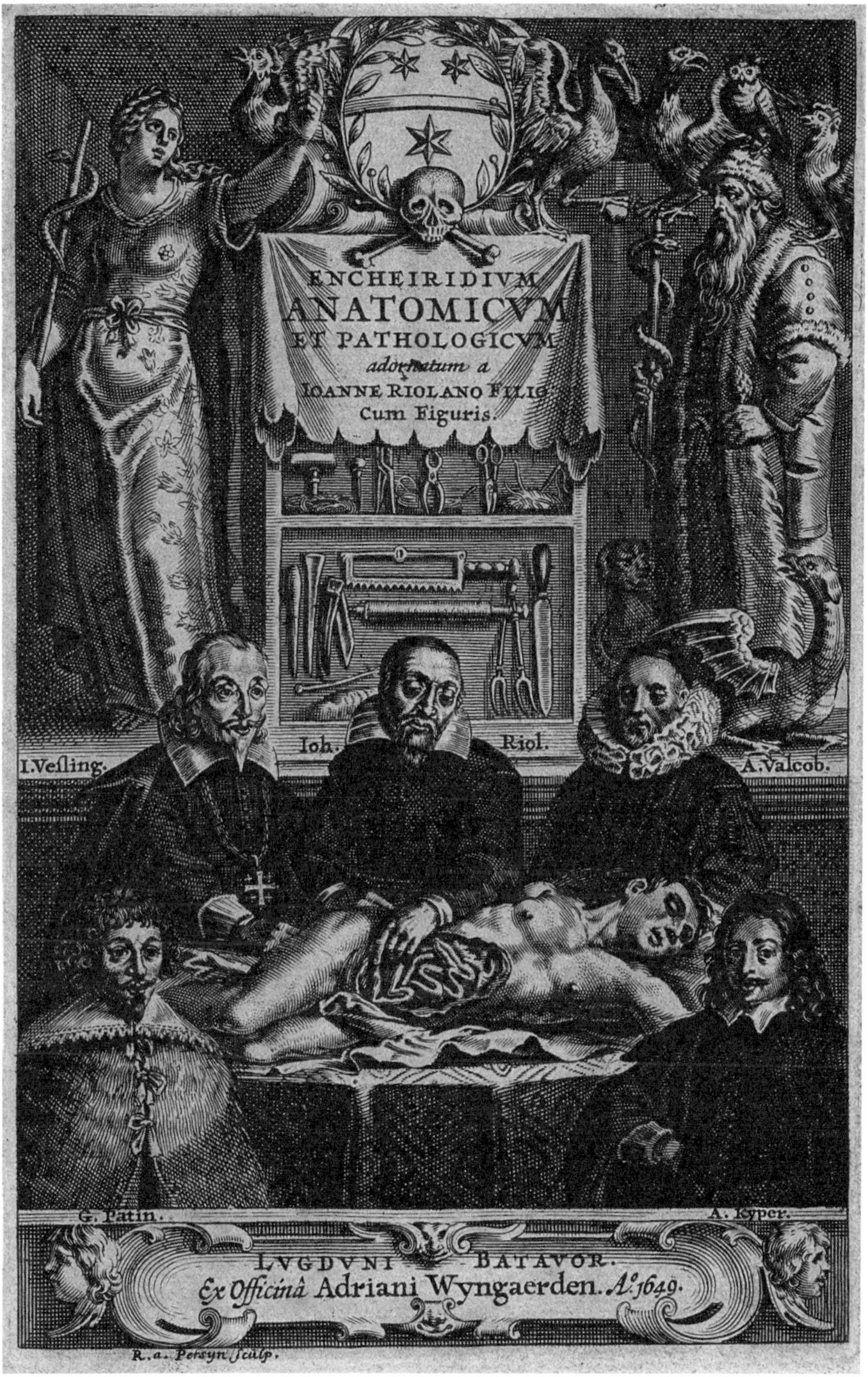

Fig. 1.8 Jean Riolan the Younger (1580–1657). Engraving of 1649 by Reinier van Persyn

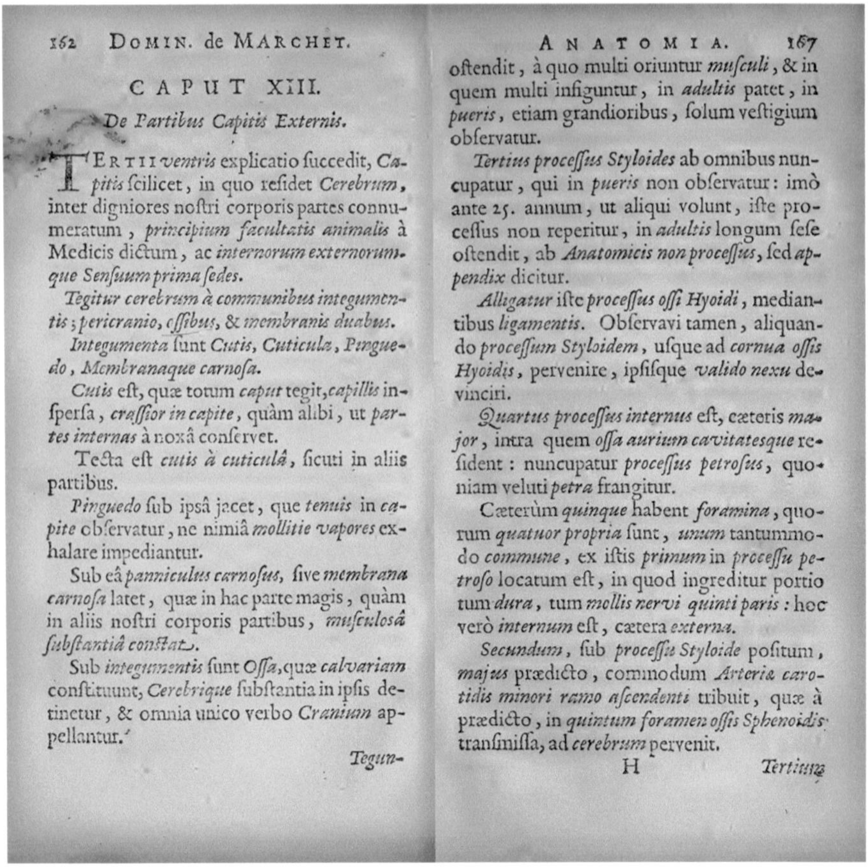

162 DOMIN. de MARCHET.

CAPUT XIII.

De Partibus Capitis Externis.

TERTII *ventris* explicatio ſuccedit, *Capitis* ſcilicet, in quo reſidet *Cerebrum*, inter digniores noſtri corporis partes connumeratum, *principium facultatis animalis* à Medicis dictum, ac *internorum externorumque Senſuum prima ſedes.*

Tegitur cerebrum à communibus integumentis; pericranio, oſſibus, & membranis duabus.

Integumenta ſunt *Cutis, Cuticula, Pinguedo, Membranaque carnoſa.*

Cutis eſt, quæ totum *caput* tegit, *capillis* inſperſa, *craſſior in capite*, quàm alibi, ut *partes internas* à noxâ conſervet.

Tecta eſt *cutis à cuticulâ*, ſicuti in aliis partibus.

Pinguedo ſub ipsâ jacet, que *tenuis* in *capite* obſervatur, ne nimiâ *mollitie vapores* exhalare impediantur.

Sub eâ *panniculus carnoſus*, ſive *membrana carnoſa* latet, quæ in hac parte magis, quàm in aliis noſtri corporis partibus, *muſculosâ ſubſtantiâ conſtat.*

Sub *integumentis* ſunt *Oſſa*, quæ *calvariam* conſtituunt, *Cerebrique* ſubſtantia in ipſis detinetur, & omnia unico verbo *Cranium* appellantur.

Tegun-

ANATOMIA. 167

oſtendit, à quo multi oriuntur *muſculi*, & in quem multi inſiguntur, in *adultis* patet, in *pueris*, etiam grandioribus, ſolum veſtigium obſervatur.

Tertius proceſſus Styloides ab omnibus nuncupatur, qui in *pueris* non obſervatur: imò ante 25. annum, ut aliqui volunt, iſte proceſſus non reperitur, in *adultis* longum ſeſe oſtendit, ab *Anatomicis non proceſſus*, ſed *appendix* dicitur.

Alligatur iſte *proceſſus oſſi Hyoidi*, mediantibus *ligamentis*. Obſervavi tamen, aliquando *proceſſum Styloidem*, uſque ad *cornua oſſis Hyoidis*, pervenire, ipſiſque *valido nexu* devinciri.

Quartus proceſſus internus eſt, cæteris *major*, intra quem *oſſa aurium cavitatesque* reſident: nuncupatur *proceſſus petroſus*, quoniam veluti *petra* frangitur.

Cæterùm *quinque* habent *foramina*, quorum *quatuor propria* ſunt, *unum* tantummodo *commune*, ex iſtis *primum* in *proceſſu petroſo* locatum eſt, in quod ingreditur portio tum *dura*, tum *mollis nervi quinti paris*: hoc verò *internum* eſt, cætera *externa.*

Secundum, ſub *proceſſu Styloide* poſitum, *majus* prædicto, commodum *Arteriæ carotidis minori ramo aſcendenti* tribuit, quæ à prædicto, in *quintum foramen oſſis Sphenoidis* tranſmiſſa, ad *cerebrum* pervenit.

H *Tertium*

Fig. 1.9 Domenico Marchetti, Anatomia, chapter XIII, page 167

1.1.2 The First Clinical Descriptions and Surgical Treatments

From Marchetti's first anatomical report to the first clinical descriptions related to these anatomical-pathological conditions, over three centuries passed. The pain syndrome was, indeed, recognized by Lucke (1870) in Vienna. Weinlecher, in 1872, removed a styloid process to relieve the symptoms. Several other isolated cases have been described: Syme, 1915; Yearsley, 1915; Evans, 1915, Stirling, 1896; and Thigpen, 1932 [4].

A study of great importance, which should be considered a true precursor of Watt Eagle's subsequent anatomical-clinical observations, is that of 1907, published by Thomas Dwight, Professor of Anatomy at Harvard Medical School in Boston [5].

As can be noted (Fig. 1.10), Dwight's study begins by quoting verbatim Marchetti's description of the ossification of the stylohyoid ligament, contained in Chap. XIII of his "Anatomy."

STYLO-HYOID OSSIFICATION.

BY THOMAS DWIGHT, M.D.,

OF BOSTON, MASSACHUSETTS.

Parkman Professor of Anatomy at the Harvard Medical School.

" *Observavi tamen aliquando processum styloideum usque ad cornua ossis hyoidei pervenire, ipsisque valido nexû devinci.*" *de Marchettis.* Anatomia. Patavii, 1652, cap. xiii, p. 205. Probably the earliest reference to this condition.

Although the occasional recurrence of ossification of the second branchial bar, represented by the styloid process, the stylo-hyoid ligament and the lesser horn of the hyoid, has been repeatedly observed in man, yet the number of well described cases is very small. Le Double in his work on the variations of the facial bones finds only some twenty instances of which one or two have never been published and of which others are very inaccessible. This condition has most frequently been recognized in the living by laryngologists, but it may be said that its clinical importance has not been generally appreciated. It appears, moreover, that there is even among anatomists more or less misunderstanding as to what has actually occurred in these cases, and that the nomenclature of the parts involved is very confusing.

This subject has been particularly brought to my attention by the observation of a very perfect case of ossification of practically the whole chain on both sides in a dissecting room subject. Moreover, the peculiarity was discovered before the dissection was very far advanced so that it was possible to have the body X-rayed before the relations which existed in life had been very seriously changed. At almost the same time two extremely long styloid processes, reaching nearly to the hyoid, were observed on another subject which was also X-rayed. So far as I am aware these skiagraphs are the first that have been made of this condition.

In this paper I propose (I) to describe the composition

721

Fig. 1.10 Stylo-Hyoid Ossification, Thomas Dwight, 1907

Dwight's study is extensive and articulated in three sections. The first considers the morphogenesis of the stylohyoid apparatus and its ossification processes, the second reports on osteological morphological findings in various collections of human skulls, and finally the third concerns clinical considerations, related to this anatomical condition, obviously advanced by an anatomist and based on the knowledge of the time.

1.1.2.1 Section 1: Morphogenesis of the "Stylohyoid Chain"

In Section 1, the four classic components of the "stylohyoid chain" are identified, described according to the concepts of classical embryology:

> The second branchial bar or the cartilage of Reichert, extends in early embryonic life downwards and forwards, from the skull to meet its fellow to which it is connected by a cross piece the basi-hyal, which becomes the body of the hyoid. The chain of pieces consists of four elements. (i) The tympano-hyal extending from beside the periotic capsule, which later is enclosed in the petrous portion of the temporal bone, to the lower surface of that bone or a little beyond it. (2) The stylo-hyal, which usually forms the greater part of the styloid process: (3) The cerato-hyal, which is usually represented in the adult by the stylo-hyoid ligament, or by an ossification in the same, and (4) The hypo-hyal which becomes the lesser horn of the hyoid. (Fig. 1.11)

1.1.2.2 Section 2: Anatomical Findings of Ossification of the Stylohyoid Chain

In this second section, some osteological findings of ossification of the stylohyoid chain of particular morphological interest are shown (Fig. 1.12).

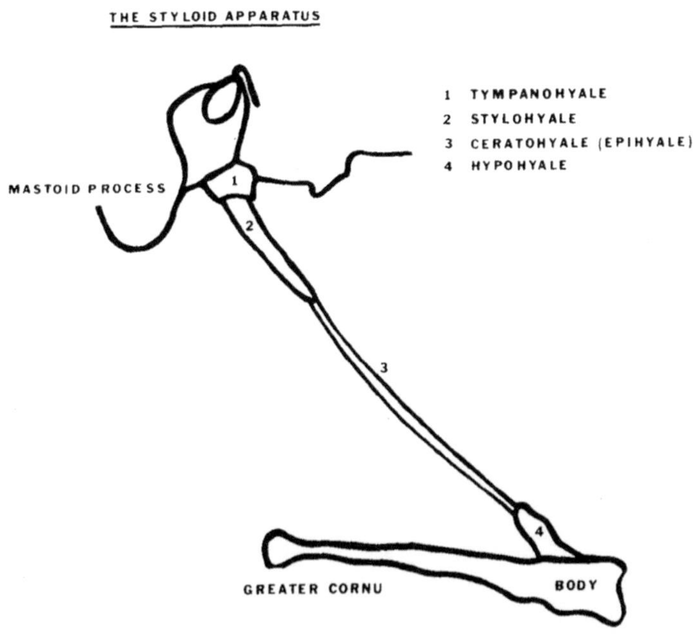

Fig. 1.11 "The styloid apparatus," Dwight, 1907

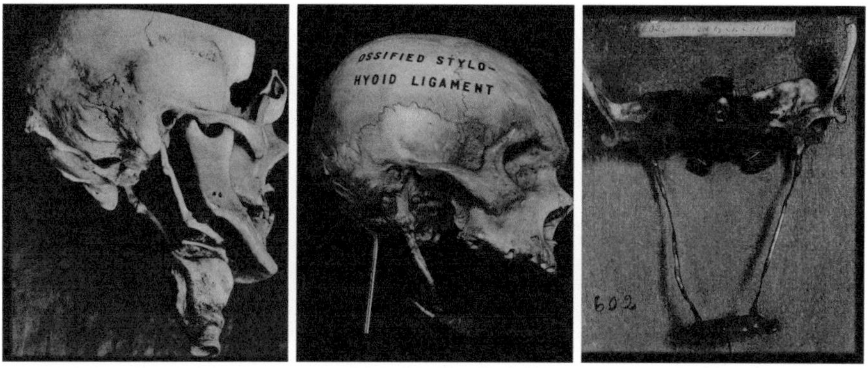

Fig. 1.12 Osteological findings of styloid-hyoid ossification, Dwight, 1907

1.1.2.3 Section 3: Clinical Hypotheses

In the last section, Dwight hypothesizes some clinical disorders correlatable with this anatomical condition: vascular disorders, dysphagia, and unspecified subjective disorders:

> It is not unlikely that the play of one part of the rod on another should give rise to disagreeable subjective symptoms and even to sounds that could be heard by others.

1.1.3 Watt W. Eagle and "Eagle Syndrome"

It is to Watt Eagle, of the Duke University Medical School in Durham, North Carolina, that we owe the nosological systematization of the syndrome (from the Greek Σιν – Δρομε: running together, referring to the set of symptoms related to the pathology), which, to this day, is indicated with the eponym of his surname. The reference publications are five, which appeared in 1937, 1948, 1949, 1958, and 1962. The most important observations of these publications will be considered and reported.

1.1.3.1 Eagle WW. 1937. Elongated Styloid Process. Arch Otolaryngol 25:584–587 (Fig. 1.13)

> Most instances of elongated or otherwise abnormal styloid processes that have been reported were observed by anatomists rather than by clinicians.

With this observation, Watt Eagle's first publication of 1937 begins [6]. They are truly prophetic words, as they point out ab initio the ever-present and unresolved fundamental pathophysiological problem of this syndrome: the discrepancy between the anatomical incidence of the anatomical-pathological picture and the clinical incidence of the symptoms related to it.

In his comprehensive review, Watt Eagle cited the earliest American medical literature reporting cases of elongated styloid processes. Interestingly, one of the

ELONGATED STYLOID PROCESSES

Report of Two Cases

Watt W. Eagle, M.D., Durham, N. C.

Most instances of elongated or otherwise abnormal styloid processes that have been reported were observed by anatomists rather than by clinicians. It is probable that numerous cases of elongated styloid processes have been observed and treated by operation when necessary, but relatively few have been recorded.

From the Department of Otolaryngology, Duke University Medical School and Hospital.

Fig. 1.13 Elongated styloid process. Watt W. Eagle, Arch. Otolaryngol. 1937

first cases, documented by Stirling in 1896, includes a rather anecdotal family history [8]:

> One of the earliest American clinical cases was reported by Stirling, of Atlanta, Ga., in 1896, the patient being his wife.

In his original 1937 publication, Watt Eagle fully describes the first "syndromic" symptom complex and the related diagnostic and therapeutic "pathway": "The symptoms usually arising from elongated styloid processes are localized mainly in the pharynx. A nagging or aching sensation in the throat somewhat similar to chronic pharyngitis is most common. Pains may radiate to the middle ear or the mastoid region. Frequently a sensation of a foreign body having lodged in the pharynx is noticed. There may be difficulty in swallowing. Symptoms similar to those of glossopharyngeal neuralgia have been encountered, and such a condition could easily be possible, owing to the proximity of the glossopharyngeal nerve. Diagnosis is made by digital palpation and roentgenograms. The treatment is accomplished by exposing the styloid process through a pharyngeal approach and biting off with rongeurs the palpable projecting process or the fracture of the process digitally, the fragment being displace laterally."

In this first report, two clinical cases are described, both treated with excision of styloid processes longer than 3 cm, following a pharyngotomy approach. The description of the first clinical case of "Eagle syndrome" treated surgically on September 26, 1935, with immediate resolution of symptoms, is reported in full for its "historical" importance and for being a "faithful mirror of the times": "Case 1.—M. T., a white woman aged 31, for eight years had pain throughout the left side of her throat that radiated into the left middle ear and the tip of the left mastoid. These symptoms occurred immediately after a tonsillectomy performed with the area under local anesthesia. The history was otherwise entirely without significance. The physical examination gave negative results except for a palpable and elongated styloid process in the left tonsillar fossa. The patient had immediate relief from pharyngeal and aural pain on the left side after operation on Sept. 26, 1935. About 2 cm. of the left styloid process was removed. *Unfortunately, roentgenograms were not made in this case.*"

1.1.3.2 Eagle WW. 1948. Elongated Styloid Process, Further Observations and a New Syndrome. Arch Otolaryngol 47:630–640 [7]

This is Eagle's second publication, released 11 years after the first, and should be considered the cornerstone of the nosology of this syndrome (Fig. 1.14).

This study refers to the experience gained from a now considerable clinical caseload, including 254 cases, 43 of which were already published in 1940 by Milo Fritz, also of the Duke University Medical School in Durham [9] (Fig. 1.15).

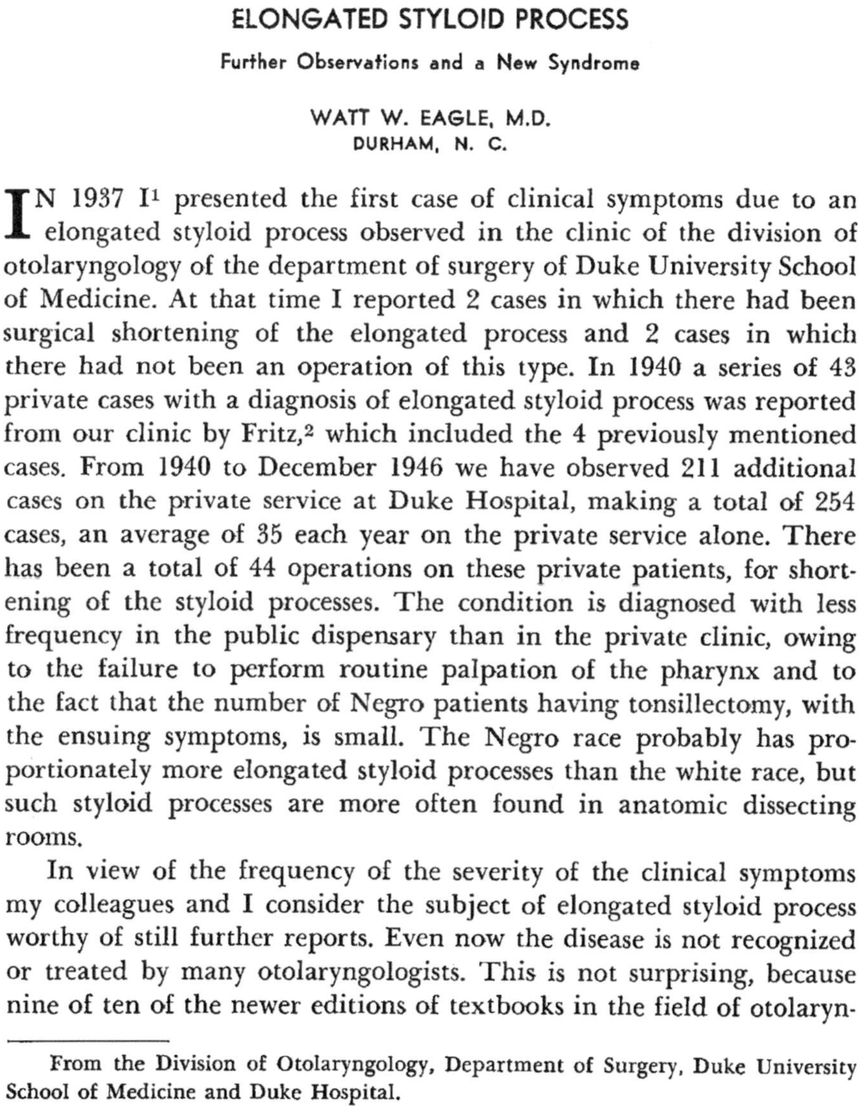

ELONGATED STYLOID PROCESS

Further Observations and a New Syndrome

WATT W. EAGLE, M.D.
DURHAM, N. C.

IN 1937 I[1] presented the first case of clinical symptoms due to an elongated styloid process observed in the clinic of the division of otolaryngology of the department of surgery of Duke University School of Medicine. At that time I reported 2 cases in which there had been surgical shortening of the elongated process and 2 cases in which there had not been an operation of this type. In 1940 a series of 43 private cases with a diagnosis of elongated styloid process was reported from our clinic by Fritz,[2] which included the 4 previously mentioned cases. From 1940 to December 1946 we have observed 211 additional cases on the private service at Duke Hospital, making a total of 254 cases, an average of 35 each year on the private service alone. There has been a total of 44 operations on these private patients, for shortening of the styloid processes. The condition is diagnosed with less frequency in the public dispensary than in the private clinic, owing to the failure to perform routine palpation of the pharynx and to the fact that the number of Negro patients having tonsillectomy, with the ensuing symptoms, is small. The Negro race probably has proportionately more elongated styloid processes than the white race, but such styloid processes are more often found in anatomic dissecting rooms.

In view of the frequency of the severity of the clinical symptoms my colleagues and I consider the subject of elongated styloid process worthy of still further reports. Even now the disease is not recognized or treated by many otolaryngologists. This is not surprising, because nine of ten of the newer editions of textbooks in the field of otolaryn-

From the Division of Otolaryngology, Department of Surgery, Duke University School of Medicine and Duke Hospital.

Fig. 1.14 Eagle WW. 1948. Elongated styloid process, further observations and a new syndrome. Arch Otolaryngol 47:630–640 [7]

ELONGATED STYLOID PROCESS

A CAUSE OF OBSCURE THROAT SYMPTOMS

MILO FRITZ, M.D.
DURHAM, N. C.

The purpose of this communication is to point out that the elongated styloid process is common and that it will often, if sought, be found to be the cause of obscure complaints involving the throat.

Forty-three patients having this condition were found in the private and dispensary services of Duke Hospital, 39 of them between January 1937 and September 1939. Only 11 of the 43 patients came to operation. Four of these patients had been previously reported on.[1]

According to Dwight,[2] the styloid process is derived from the second branchial arch and normally attains the length of 2.5 to 3 cm. (fig. 1). It extends from the under surface of the petrous portion of the temporal bone forward, downward and mesially. The tip is cartilaginous and in the abnormally long styloid process may fuse with the lesser horn of the hyoid bone in the form of a calcified stylohyoid ligament (fig. 2). Such a styloid process is an anatomic curiosity, but it may have clinical significance, as illustrated in case 1, in which a needle was broken off against it during the suturing in a tonsillar fossa (fig. 3). Many styloid processes that are elongated but still are not long enough to reach the hyoid bone are asymptomatic; but if they project abnormally forward and mesially into the tonsillar fossae they not only often give rise to symptoms but may interfere with tonsillectomy.

The symptoms consist of a sensation of fulness in the throat; dysphagia; pain in the throat aggravated by swallowing; dull ache or marked lightning and lancinating pain in the throat radiating to the ear and mastoid tip; a sensation described as neuralgic pain in the throat; pain and soreness in the hard and the soft palate, and a sensation of food having lodged in the throat, necessitating frequent swallowing. Occasionally symptoms are not evident until some days after tonsillectomy. For weeks or years the patient thinks the tonsillar fossa has failed to heal. These symptoms are sometimes indistinguishable from neuralgia of the glossopharyngeal nerve, which lies close to the styloid

From the Department of Otolaryngology, Duke University Medical School and Hospital.

1. Eagle, W. W.: Elongated Styloid Processes: A Report of Two Cases, Arch. Otolaryng. **25**:548 (May) 1937.

2. Dwight, T.: Stylohyoid Ossification, Ann. Surg. **46**:721, 1907.

Fig. 1.15 Fritz, M. (1940). Elongated styloid process: a cause of obscure throat symptoms, Archives of Otolaryngology—Head and Neck Surgery, 31(6), 911–918 [9]

In the 1948 publication, Eagle distinguishes two clinical forms of the syndrome—the typical syndrome and the carotid artery syndrome—of which he provides an accurate clinical description [7]:

Typical Syndrome The characteristic symptoms are: a constant pain or a nagging dull ache in the pharynx, presenting the sensation that the throat did not heal after tonsillectomy; a pain frequently referred to the ear, indicating irritation of the vagus nerve; increased salivation; hesitancy and difficulty in swallowing; gagging; a sensation of a foreign body—even cotton—in the pharynx. These symptoms may be wrongly diagnosed as due to glossopharyngeal neuralgia, but when analyzed they do not fit in with true glossopharyngeal neuralgia, since in that disease one deals with neuralgia of extreme severity, usually lancinating and of momentary duration, but recurrent and frequently stimulated by intake of hot or cold stimuli, such as food or drink, and sometimes stimulated by even the slightest movements of the tongue. The pains due to elongated styloid processes are constantly nagging but rarely severe. The group of cases- presenting the typical syndrome also includes all cases in which there is distortion of nerve function involving the sensory and motor fibers of the fifth, seventh, ninth and tenth cranial nerves. The sensation of taste may be quite distorted. A spasm or contraction of the constrictor muscles of the esophagus and the pharynx may be observed. One patient having spasm of the constrictor muscles was caused much embarrassment each time he attempted to eat. Shortening of his elongated processes allowed him to eat normally.

Carotid Artery Syndrome In August 1946 I had the first data to substantiate an idea which I had entertained for six years that an elongated styloid process might produce pains along the carotid artery distribution. Since 1940 I had encountered patients, probably 12 in all, who had complained of pain beginning in the neck at a point about opposite the tonsillar fossa, which extended upward over the side of the head in a pattern conforming to the distribution of the external or the internal carotid artery. I had made notes that probably a carotid artery was involved in these cases in some way, but I had no definite evidence of this.// I believe that an elongated styloid process which fits so tightly against a carotid artery as to impair its circulation may cause the carotid artery syndrome. I now wonder and even suspect that many patients are treated for migraine, histamine sensitivity, temporal artery and other vascular headache, or atypical headaches and neuralgias, when in reality they may have an elongated styloid process. It is conceivable that even a styloid process of normal length may cause symptoms if there are anatomic malarrangements and variations in the cervical region.

For diagnosis, Eagle considers the clinical history and transoral palpation of an elongated styloid process (>2.5 cm) essential, while the radiographic study is considered as mere confirmation of a diagnosis already made.

> The diagnosis of elongated styloid process should be facilitated by the patient's history. It is confirmed by the palpating finger. When the tonsils have been removed, there is no ques-

tion of the diagnosis if a firm bony resistance is met in the tonsillar fossa, especially at the upper pole of the fossa. If a styloid process is palpable, it is always elongated. The normal length of the styloid process is 1 inch (2.5 cm.), and the normal process can never be palpated, since it lies just that deeply in the parapharyngeal musculature// The elongated process may be palpated through and beneath some tonsils. Roentgenograms are taken merely for confirmation of the diagnosis but are later used as a guide, and are of considerable aid, in the surgical shortening of the process.

Treatment is surgical and is performed via a transoral approach. In Fig. 5 of his publication, Eagle outlines the surgical steps of the procedure (Fig. 1.16).

An incision is made in the tonsillar fossa over the tip of the palpable elongated process. The incision is spread with scissors or a clamp until the tip of the styloid process is palpable through the incision. The muscles attached to the medial surface of the process *are stripped by the finger*. A curved instrument, such as a submucous resection elevator, is used to free the muscles from the lateral and posterior portion of the process. Very little force may be used during the dissection, lest the process be fractured prematurely. After *the muscular stripping*, the styloid process stands out as a white, ivory-appearing rod, usually the caliber of a safety match. The stylohyoid ligament at the tip of the process is easily visualized and palpated during the dissection and is now severed with scissors, unless it is calcified. This maneuver provides easier access *for the finger* and the instruments *to strip any remaining muscular attachments* from the posterior and lateral surface of the process. The length of the portion which is to be removed has been determined prior to operation by study of roentgenograms. The actual fracturing of the portion to be removed is accomplished with

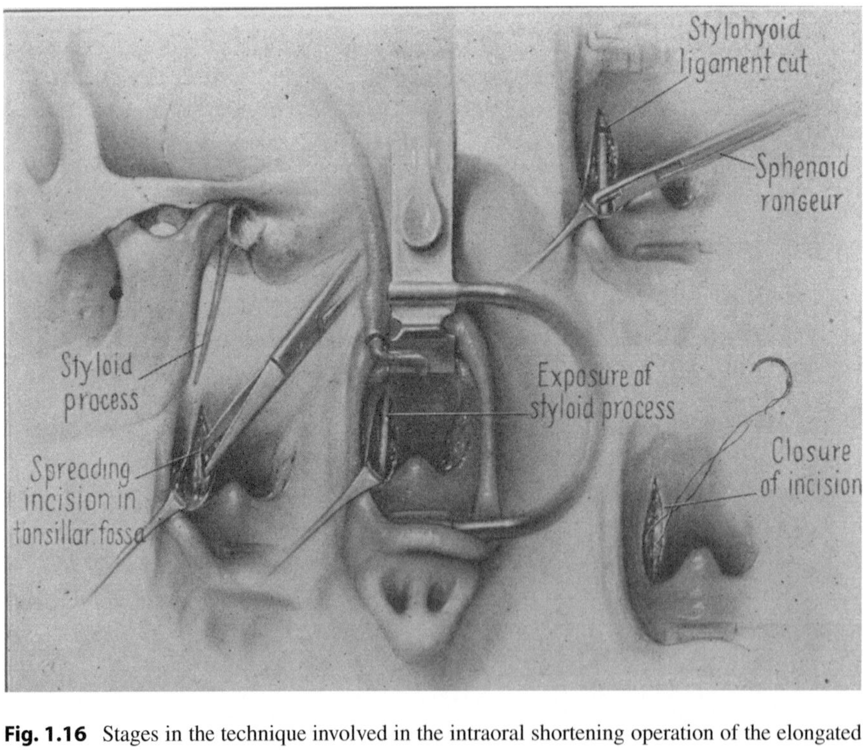

Fig. 1.16 Stages in the technique involved in the intraoral shortening operation of the elongated styloid process [7]

> the Hajek forceps. A curved clamp must have already grasped the distal end of the process to prevent its retraction into the muscles. In removing the fragment by means of this clamp, one must exercise care with regard to the external and internal carotid arteries and the facial nerve, which emerges from the skull posteriorly to the base of the process. The styloid stump is then palpated to determine whether it is too long, and usually it is not.

Eagle reports that, in his experience, this procedure has been free of significant complications, with excellent and long-lasting functional results obtained only with the complete removal of the elongated portion of the styloid process: "When the elongated styloid process is surgically shortened, the results are uniformly excellent and permanent. The elongated portion of the styloid process must be fully shortened, with removal of the fragment, to alleviate all symptoms. There have been 2 cases in which the fragment was pulled back into the musculature by some muscles still attached to the process, and the fragments were never recovered; one of the patients still had mild symptoms one year after the operation."

We will let Eagle's conclusions stand on what is considered the seminal work on Eagle syndrome: "***SUMMARY***: The established syndrome of an elongated styloid process, the syndrome which is typical, is reviewed. An atypical syndrome, referable to involvement of the external or the internal carotid artery, is presented for consideration. The symptoms, the diagnosis and the treatment of both syndromes are discussed. The intraoral surgical technic for shortening the elongated styloid process is described. Complications are reported as minimal, and the intraoral surgical approach is thought to be ideal for excellent and permanent results."

1.1.3.3 Eagle WW. 1949. Symptomatic Elongated Styloid Process: Report of Two Cases of Styloid Process-Carotid Artery Syndrome with Operation. Arch Otolaryngol 49:490–503

In this third publication, Eagle focuses on the carotid artery variant of the syndrome [10] (Fig. 1.17).

Styloid Process-Carotid Artery Syndrome Any styloid process, especially the elongated one, whose tip deviates medially or laterally may cause considerable pressure on the internal or the external carotid artery, not only impairing the function of the vessel by diminishing the caliber, but also causing most pronounced symptoms by irritation of the sympathetic nerve fibers, which form a rich supply to the walls of the carotid artery.

He distinguishes two anatomico-clinical forms—the external carotid artery syndrome and the internal carotid artery syndrome—describing two emblematic clinical cases:

Case 1: External Carotid Artery Syndrome . Mrs. R. S., aged 67, had symptoms suggestive of an elongated styloid process, with impairment of function of the external carotid artery and pain along the distribution of the artery on the left side of the head. The operation for shortening the process was performed in August 1946. The tip of the process was tightly wedged against the left external carotid artery, causing quite

SYMPTOMATIC ELONGATED STYLOID PROCESS

Report of Two Cases of Styloid Process–Carotid Artery Syndrome with Operation

WATT W. EAGLE, M.D.
DURHAM, N. C.

SOME of the obscure, as well as common, pharyngeal pains, painful deglutition and referred otalgia may be traced to an elongated styloid process.[1] It is of interest that these symptoms are usually found only after tonsillectomy. I now hope to establish that the elongated styloid process may also cause facial pain and headache, even when tonsillectomy has not been performed, owing to impingement of the process on a carotid artery. Thus, there exist two distinct syndromes referable to the styloid process; these syndromes present groups of symptoms which differ in their anatomic locations.

The classic, and commoner, syndrome usually relates all symptoms to the pharynx and the ear, but occasionally an atypical group of symptoms may be referred to the hypopharynx and the upper part of the esophagus.[1f] The second syndrome, which I shall designate as the styloid process–carotid artery syndrome, presents symptoms related to the pattern of distribution of either the internal or the external carotid artery.

HISTORICAL REVIEW

The historical background of the elongated styloid process is interesting, but it suffices now merely to recall that the elongated process occurs in approximately 4 per cent of persons, but that only a few of these persons have symptoms. It is of further historical significance that the elongated styloid process had been of anatomic rather than clinical interest until the recent past. The elongated styloid process may be hereditary, as my associates and I have found 3 siblings, the

From the Division of Otolaryngology, Department of Surgery, Duke University Hospital and School of Medicine.

Fig. 1.17 Eagle WW. 1949. Symptomatic elongated styloid process: report of two cases of styloid process-carotid artery syndrome with operation. Arch Otolaryngol 49:490–503

a constriction of the lumen, as well as considerable compression of the sympathetic nerves in the arterial walls. It was resected. The postoperative convalescence was quiet, and the results were excellent with relief of pain immediately after the operation.

Case 2. Internal Carotid Artery Syndrome W. J. P., was a man aged 39. He gave a history of severe pain in the left frontal area and vertex of five years' duration. The pain usually occurred every two to four days and lasted two to four days. All teeth had been extracted and replaced with plates, and there was no suggestion of the temporomandibular joint syndrome. The tonsils and adenoids had been removed, and he had had surgical treatment of the intranasal sinuses many years previously. His hearing and vision had not been impaired, although there was occasional tinnitus in the left ear. The findings on physical examination were normal in every respect except for the bilateral elongated styloid process. Laboratory studies, including serologic tests of the blood revealed no abnormality. The styloid process was definitely elongated bilaterally, the right being a little longer than the left and each being more than 5 cm. in length. Each process showed a medial deviation just above the tip. Since the patient's headache and head pains coincided with the area of distribution of the left internal carotid artery, it was thought that his symptoms were due to impingement of the elongated styloid process on the vessel and the sympathetic nerves in the vessel walls, with disturbance of their function. On Feb. 12, 1948 the patient had bilateral shortening of the elongated styloid process, although only the left process was considered symptomatic. A total of 3.5 cm. was removed on each side. He was seen in a follow-up examination on May 15, 1948 and was found to be completely free of the headaches and head pains.

Even in this circumstance, Eagle's original description, in addition to its value as historical evidence, attests to the ever-present difficulties in the correct diagnostic classification of patients with predominantly "vascular" symptomatology.

Eagle reaffirms the fundamental role of transoral digital palpation of an elongated styloid process, including an extremely effective drawing to define this diagnostic procedure (Fig. 1.18).

Surgical intervention via a transoral approach is indicated:

> There is only one satisfactory and sure method of alleviating the symptoms due to an abnormal styloid process: the surgical shortening of the elongated process or the surgical removal of a tip of a process of normal length that may be impinging on a carotid artery. The intraoral surgical route is preferred and is, indeed, the simpler route of approach.

By performing "radical" surgical procedures, excellent and lasting results are reported:

> The operation for surgical shortening of the styloid process has in our experience always produced excellent results. Other procedures short of the actual shortening of the process, such as fracturing of the process by the palpating finger, have only partially alleviated the symptoms, and the results cannot compare at all with the results of the surgical resection.

The clinical data collected allowed Eagle to draw the following conclusions:

> The symptomatic elongated styloid process produces a characteristic group of symptoms. These symptoms may occur in two distinct groups: (1) the classic syndrome, always occurring after tonsillectomy, with the symptoms involving the pharynx and hypopharynx, with referred pain to the ear, and (2) the styloid process-carotid artery syndrome, in which symptoms are produced along the distribution of an external carotid artery or an internal carotid artery by impingement on the vessel, affecting the circulation in the vessel and producing irritation of the sympathetic nerves in the arterial sheath. A process of normal length may have a deviated tip producing the symptoms, and tonsillectomy does not necessarily precede the onset of symptoms in the styloid process-carotid artery syndrome.

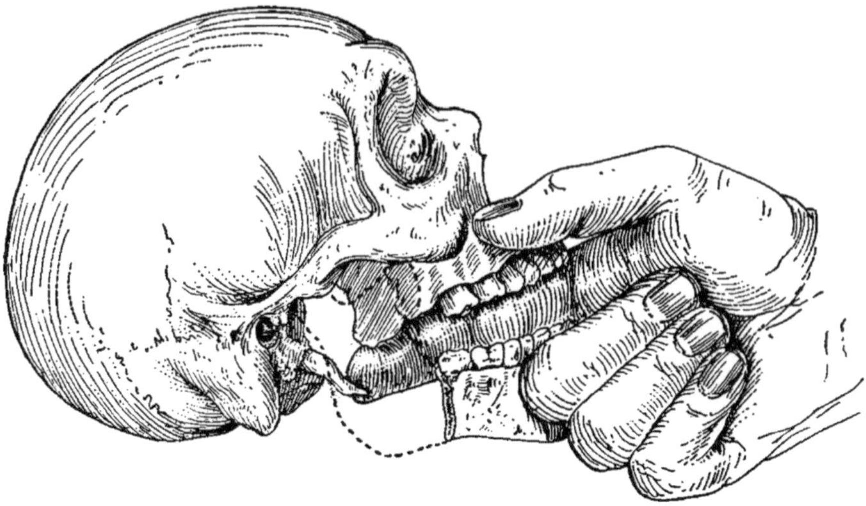

Fig. 1.18 Diagram demonstrating the ease with which the palpating finger locates the elongated styloid process

1.1.3.4 Eagle WW. 1958. Elongated Styloid Process: Symptoms and Treatment. AMA Arch Otolaryngol 67:172–176//Eagle WW. 1962. The Symptoms, Diagnosis and Treatment of the Elongated Styloid Process. Am Surg 28:1–5 [11, 12]

In these last two publications, Eagle (Fig. 1.19 refers to the 1958 article) reiterates the fundamental concepts already expressed in the 1948 and 1949 works [11, 12].

The subdivision of Eagle syndrome into two clinical variants, the importance of intraoral digital palpation as a diagnostic maneuver, and the specific techniques of transoral surgical treatment are confirmed (Fig. 1.20).

Elongated Styloid Process

Symptoms and Treatment

WATT W. EAGLE, M.D., Durham, N. C.

The symptomatic elongation of a styloid process may explain some instances of pharyngeal and ear pains and some headaches, which have defied exhaustive diagnostic studies. I consider that it is a very neglected otolaryngological entity and that it is very deserving of a niche in the diagnostic armentarium of otolaryngologic practice. I venture to state that most of this group, as medical students, learned something about the styloid process from the anatomy books and the cadaver, but never had the opportunity to put this information into clinical application during the latter part of medical school or during residency training. The otolaryngological textbooks—except for a very few—completely omit any reference to the elongated styloid process, and there has been very little in the literature, even the current journals, to place the proper emphasis on this condition. Radiologists in reporting their findings in skull roentgenograms—seeking for the cause of headaches—fail to describe or include the presence of an elongated styloid process when it is very obvious in the film—yet they will describe a questionable platybasia or enostosis frontalis! The alert dentist recognizes the importance of the elongated styloid process, for he, too, occasionally may encounter such an abnormality, which may impede the performance of his planned work, or he may accidentally fracture an elongated styloid process during his routine procedures.

Accepted for publication May 20, 1957.

From the Division of Otolaryngology, Duke University Medical School and Hospital.

Presented at the Sixth International Congress of Otolaryngology, Washington, D. C., May 8, 1957.

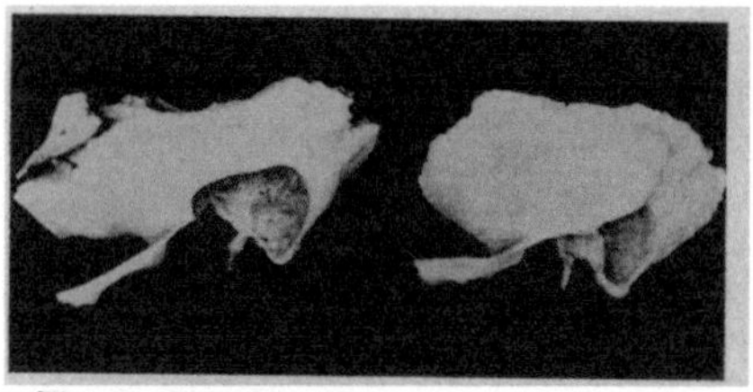

Fig. 1.—Mastoid preparations showing normal length styloid processes.

The normal styloid process is 1 in., or 2.5 cm., in length. The elongated styloid process, which is due to the calcification of the stylohyoid ligament, may be 3 in., or 7.5 cm., or more in length. Three muscles are attached to the styloid process, one extending to the pharynx, one to the tongue, and one to the hyoid bone. There are two ligaments attached to the styloid process, the smaller one to the hyoid bone and the larger one running laterally to the mandible. The distal tip of the normal styloid process lies between the external and the internal carotid arteries. The styloid process originates from the temporal bone on the medial and inferior surface, anterior and medial to the stylomastoid foramen, from which the seventh cranial nerve makes its exit. The process usually points anteriorly and medially, but it may project laterally just inside the mandible; or it rarely may project more posteriorly, being slightly anterior to the cervical spine. The normal-length styloid process is not palpable beneath the tonsillar fossa after tonsillectomy because of the depth of the submucosal tissues. Any process that is palpable beneath the fossa is definitely elongated. Some elongated processes can be palpated through the tonsils. Only about 4% of styloid processes are

Fig. 1.19 Eagle WW. 1958. Elongated styloid process: symptoms and treatment. AMA Arch Otolaryngol 67:172–176

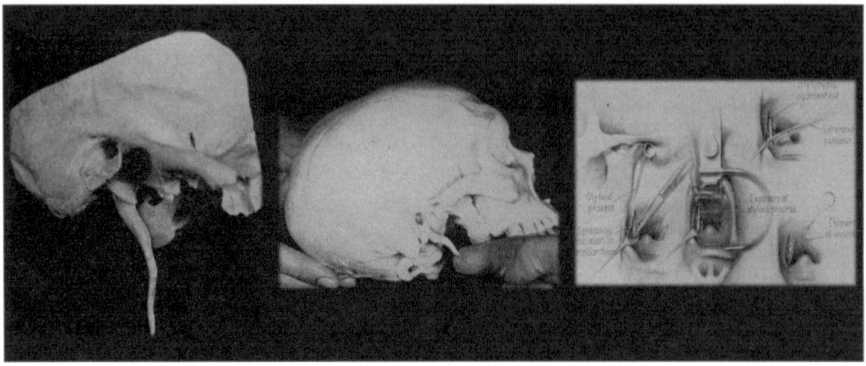

Fig. 1.20 Elongated styloid process, palpation of the tip of styloid process, and technique for shortening of elongated styloid process

1.2 Conclusion

These historical notes on the understanding of "Eagle syndrome," drawing as much as possible on original sources, allow us to delineate a rich doctrinal and clinical path that, from the very beginning, has identified and pinpointed, sometimes expressing a truly far-sighted spirit, the "core" of the peculiarities of this pathology, on an anatomical, physiopathological, and clinical-therapeutic level.

References

1. de Marchetti, Domenico, 1626–1688: Dominici de Marchettis Patavini, Petri Equitis, Professoris Filii, Anatomia: cui responsiones ad Riolanum, anatomicum Parisiensem, in ipsius animadversionibus contra Veslingium additae sunt; Hardevici: Ex officina Societatis typographica; 1656.
2. Vesling, Johann, 1598–1649; "Syntagma anatomicum, publicis dissectionibus, in auditorum usum, diligenter aptatum"; Patavii: Typis Pauli Frambotti bibliopolae; 1647.
3. De Marchetti, Pietro, 1593–1673. Observationum medico-chirurgicarum rariorum sylloge. Londini: J. Newton; edition 1729.
4. Piagkou M, Anagnostopoulou S, Kouladouros K. Giannoulis Piagkos; "Eagle's syndrome: a review of the literature". Clin Anat. 2009;22(5):545–58. https://doi.org/10.1002/ca.20804.
5. Dwight T. Stylo-hyoid ossification. Ann Surg. 1907;46(5):721–35. https://doi.org/10.1097/00000658-190711000-00010.
6. Watt W. Eagle; Elongated styloid process. Arch Otolaryngol. 1937;25:584–7.
7. Eagle WW. Elongated styloid process, further observations and a new syndrome. Arch Otolaryngol. 1948;47:630–40.
8. Stirling A. W.: on bony growths invading the tonsil. J A M A. 1896;27:734.
9. Fritz M. Elongated styloid process: a cause of obscure throat symptoms. Arch Otolaryngol Head Neck Surg. 1940;31(6):911–8. https://doi.org/10.1001/archotol.1940.00660010926002.
10. Eagle WW. Symptomatic elongated styloid process: report of two cases of styloid process-carotid artery syndrome with operation. Arch Otolaryngol. 1949;49:490–503.
11. Eagle WW. Elongated styloid process: symptoms and treatment. AMA Arch Otolaryngol. 1958;67:172–6.
12. Eagle WW. The symptoms, diagnosis and treatment of the elongated styloid process. Am Surg. 1962;28:1–5.

A Patient Prospective

2

Francesca Perfetti

In 2017, I started experiencing a series of symptoms that I will now list:

- A sensation of a lump in my throat, more pronounced on the left side.
- Intermittent pain spreading to the left submandibular area and the left ear. This pain became increasingly severe over time.
- The pain continued to worsen, eventually leading to symptoms of paresthesia and continuous headaches every day, with swollen and enlarged lymph nodes. The enlargement of the lymph nodes led me to undergo surgical interventions, specifically an adenoid biopsy to rule out a possible diagnosis of lymphoma and a tonsillectomy.

Throughout this long journey, I underwent many specialist visits and exams. Without receiving any diagnosis, I continued to wander from one specialist to another, each of them prescribing various tests. I will list a few:

- October 16, 2017 – neurological consultation (cost 82 euros)
- October 17, 2017 – gnathological consultation (cost 122 euros)
- November 29, 2017 – MRI of the facial mass (cost 140 euros)
- December 15, 2017 – angio-MRI (cost 130 euros)
- June 3, 2017 – ENT consultation (cost 86 euros)
- January 18, 2018 – angio-CT scan (cost 370 euros)
- May 18, 2018 – ultrasound of the soft tissues of the neck (cost 110 euros).

Patient affected by Eagle syndrome and treated surgically.
I am Mrs. Francesca Perfetti, an Italian woman, 43 years old. I will now share with you my odyssey, which began in the year 2017.

F. Perfetti (✉)
Department of Control and Computer Engineering, Politecnico di Torino, Turin, Italy

C. Vicini et al. (eds.), *EAGLE Syndrome*,
https://doi.org/10.1007/978-3-031-92829-1_2

- January 7, 2019 – ENT examination (cost 230 euros)
- February 2, 2019 – hematology consultation (cost 300 euros)

All of this was at my own expense, as I was unemployed and unable to work due to the illness I was suffering from.

I wanted to give a voice to all the people who have experienced and are still going through the same ordeal as mine, which had turned into a pilgrimage in search of answers, seeking attention from all the specialists whom I thought cared about the health of the patient.

2019 was my lucky year. During yet another specialist visit, I finally received a much-needed hypothetical diagnosis, obtained solely through a clinical examination (the insertion of a finger into the tonsillar bed). A possible Eagle syndrome was diagnosed, which was later confirmed with a 3D CT scan specifically aimed at diagnosing Eagle syndrome, a rare condition that no one had ever considered.

From the moment I received this diagnosis, I felt a strong desire to do something for those who, like me, suffering from the same condition, could finally have the long-sought answer. This is how I decided to start a group on Facebook called "Eagle Syndrome Italy." The very next day, to my great surprise, I began receiving requests from people seeking help. I am now happy to have been able to guide these people in resolving their problems.

Meanwhile, I continued my search with determination, looking for a professional doctor who, in addition to being familiar with this syndrome, could operate on me.

In 2020, my search had a positive outcome with Professor XX, who immediately conveyed to me a sense of confidence, empathy, and humanity, rare virtues in these times.

On September 14, 2021, I underwent surgery in XX to reduce the size of the styloid process, which was causing most of my problems. Some of them were resolved.

In the group, most people living in Italy have made Professor XX a reference point, as he is considered one of the leading experts in this syndrome and in surgical treatment. Together, united, we will make it!

Best regards.

Eagle Syndrome as a Rare Disease

3

Chiara Bellini, Fabrizio Salvi, and Claudio Vicini

…Nothing is rarer than what is unique…. (Gabriel Girard)

3.1 Introduction

Eagle syndrome (ES) is a rare neck syndrome involving the neurovascular bundle of the neck. An elongated styloid process and/or calcification of the stylohyoid ligament compresses or irritates the neurovascular structure (i.e., carotid artery, jugular vein, and lower cranial nerves). It was described as a syndrome by Watt Weems Eagle in 1937 [1].

Two mayor subtypes of ES have been described: the classic Eagle syndrome (or stylohyoid syndrome, 74% of Eagle disease) with irritation/compression of soft tissue or cranial nerve and vascular Eagle syndrome (stylocarotid syndrome, 23.5%) with symptoms due to the involvement of the common and/or internal carotid artery [2, 3].

Styloid venous syndrome (SVS) or Eagle jugular syndrome is a recently described Eagle syndrome characterized by jugular vein compression between the styloid process and the transverse process of the first cervical vertebral body (bone nutcracker syndrome). The clinical expression of this type of Eagle syndrome may be acute/subacute (thrombosis of the jugular or of the cerebral sinus) or chronic causing intracranial hypertension (headache with papilledema and blurred vision, high opening cerebrospinal pressure, peri-mesencephalic hemorrhage) or chronic

C. Bellini (✉)
Morgagni-Pierantoni Hospital, Forlì, FC, Italy

F. Salvi
Ospedale degli Infermi di Faenza, Faenza, RA, Italy

C. Vicini
University of Ferrara, Cona, FE, Italy
e-mail: claudio@claudiovicini.com

C. Vicini et al. (eds.), *EAGLE Syndrome*,
https://doi.org/10.1007/978-3-031-92829-1_3

cerebrospinal venous insufficiency syndrome (CCSVI). The main clinical features suggesting the presence of a CCSVI are four: headache usually starting on morning awakening with a throbbing character, fatigue, disturbances in working memory, and sleep disorders with a poor quality of the sleep; all of these symptoms have been just described in association with Eagle syndrome [3].

3.2 Eagle Syndrome as a Rare Syndrome?

Rare diseases are by definition diseases with a low prevalence in the general population. In Europe, the diseases with a prevalence of less than 5 over 10,000 citizens are considered rare.

The World Health Organization (WHO) estimates that there are 6000 to 8000 rare diseases that affect in Europe from 27 million to 36 million people.

In Italy, in order to protect persons affected by a rare disease, a special Ministerial Decree, the D.M. number 279/2001, has been identified the diseases and the group of rare diseases, with a specific code, for which the right to exemption from participation in the cost to related health services included in the essential levels of assistance (ELA) has been recognized [4]. According to the D.M. 279/01, the National Network for Rare Diseases, the network is divided into accredited centers for diagnosis and treatment of rare diseases. Every region has its own network, and the centers are individuated on the basis of expertise and numerousness.

National legislation has also provided for the obligation to establish a regional and inter-regional register. The contribution of each register goes to form the national register for rare diseases.

The opportunity to have a regional and national registry for rare diseases allows for timely and uniform epidemiological estimates which ordinary administrative flows would not permit.

The recent Law no. 175/21 aims to protect the right to health of people with rare diseases through:

1. The uniformity of the provision of services and drugs throughout the national territory.
2. The coordination and periodic updating of the ELA and the list of rare diseases.
3. The reorganization of the national network of rare diseases.
4. The creation of transition of paths from childhood to adulthood.
5. The support for scientific research [5].

To make the provisions of the low effective and in particular to extend the ELA and guarantee patients the necessary drugs and aids, the approval of specific implementing Decree will be necessary.

Although epidemiological data indicate that the frequency of an elongated styloid process is present in at least 4% of the general population and that at least 4% of carriers of the elongated styloid process develop Eagle syndrome, the diagnoses of this syndrome remain well below epidemiological estimates and below the prevalence limits of 5 in 10,000 citizens and can therefore be considered a rare disease at the moment [6].

Failure to diagnose a curable disease that can be potentially serious must lead to widespread dissemination of knowledge of the same, including through the channels of rare diseases and scientific societies interested in Eagle syndrome.

The practical impact that the inclusion of Eagle's disease in the National Rare Disease Network would have is primarily concerned with the dissemination of knowledge about the disease.

Eagle syndrome is poorly known and remains in most of the case underrecognized or misdiagnosed.

Eagle syndrome has a wide spectrum of manifestation and its clinical diagnosis is challenging.

Although some symptoms may suggest the diagnosis of Eagle syndrome (i.e., symptoms triggered by head movements, foreign body sensation in the throat, etc.), others instead are nonspecific (Table 3.1) [7–20].

The main specialists that Eagle patients turn to are listed in Table 3.2 [2, 3, 7, 13, 18].

Although epidemiological data suggest a prevalence of at least 16 cases per 10,000 subjects, in reality, the diagnosis of Eagle syndrome is very rare and far below 5 cases per 10,000 [6, 12].

The inclusion of Eagle syndrome in the list of rare diseases would lead to greater knowledge of the disease by specialist and family practice doctors and favor the creation of centers for the diagnosis and treatment of the disease. These centers should have a multidisciplinary approach.

Eagle syndrome manifests itself in most cases with vague symptoms; a better characterization of the symptoms will offer the specialist greater diagnostic possibilities.

Eagle syndrome should be included in the diagnostic workup of patients with stroke, transient ischemic attack, internal carotid artery dissections, and perimesencephalic hemorrhage.

Table 3.1 Symptoms that may suggest ES

Neck pain	During swallowing
	Triggered/worsened by chewing
	Triggered/worsened while turning head to ipsilateral side
	With deep palpation
	Radiated to ear/jaw
Foreign body sensation in the throat	
Unilateral throat pain	
Dysphagia	
Odynophagia	
Otalgia	
Temporomandibular joint pain	
Glossodynia	
Toothache	
Hearing loss	
Ear "popping"	
Dysphonia	
Tinnitus	
Syncope	
Dizziness/fainting	
Seizures	
Headache	
Horner syndrome	
Hemifacial edema	
Peri-mesencephalic hemorrhage	
Convexity subarachnoid hemorrhage	
Internal carotid artery dissection	
Transient ischemic attack	
Stroke	In the territory of internal carotid artery
Jugular thrombosis	
Intracranial hypertension	Due to jugular compression
Papilledema	
Blurred vision	
Facial edema	
Dizziness	
Insomnia	

Table 3.2 Specialists whom ES patients seek for treatment

ENT specialist
Oral and maxillofacial surgeon
Neurologist
Neurosurgeon
Dentist
Pain therapy doctor
Headache center doctor
Palliative care doctor
Psychiatrist
Vascular surgeon
Internal medicine doctor
Stroke unit center doctor
Family practice doctor

References

1. Eagle WW. Elongated styloid processes: Report of two cases. Eagle WW Arch Otolaryngol. 1937;25:584–7.
2. Badhey A, Jategaonkar A, Anglin Kovacs AJ, Kadakia S, De Deyn PP, Ducic Y, Schantz S, Shin E. Eagle syndrome: a comprehensive review. Clin Neurol Neurosurg. 2017;159:34–8. https://doi.org/10.1016/j.clineuro.2017.04.021. Epub 2017 May 6
3. Thielen A, Brizzi V, Majoufre C, Nicot R, Schlund M. Eagle syndrome and vascular complications-a systematic review. Int J Oral Maxillofac Surg. 2024;S0901-5027(24):00377–1. https://doi.org/10.1016/j.ijom.2024.09.011. Online ahead of print
4. Ministero Della Sanita', Gazzetta Ufficiale della Repubblica Italiana, Decreto Legge 18 maggio 2001, n. 279, Allegato n. 1 Elenco Malattie Rare Esentate Dalla Partecipazione AL Costo.
5. Ministero Della Sanita', Gazzetta Ufficiale della Repubblica Italiana DECRETO LEGGE 10 novembre 2021, n. 175, Disposizioni per la cura delle malattie rare e per il sostegno della ricerca e della produzione dei farmaci orfani (21G00189) (GU Serie Generale n.283 del 27-11-2021).
6. Held ME, Farsi S, ERW C, Davis KP, King DL, Suen JY. Eagle syndrome presentation and outcomes in a large surgical case series. Laryngoscope Investig Otolaryngol. 2024;9(4):e1289. https://doi.org/10.1002/lio2.1289. eCollection 2024 Aug. PMID: 39071203
7. Hassani M, Grønlund EW, Albrechtsen SS, Kondziella D. Neurological phenotypes and treatment outcomes in Eagle syndrome: systematic review and meta-analysis. Peer J. 2024;12:e17423. https://doi.org/10.7717/peerj.17423. eCollection 2024
8. Xu Z, Shi P, Zhang P. Eagle syndrome: a rare neuropathic disorder affecting head and neck. Medicine (Baltimore). 2024;103(19):e38128. https://doi.org/10.1097/MD.0000000000038128.
9. Obara K, Furuta T, Yagi C, Nakai N, Suzuki J, Katsuno M, Ito Y. Convexity subarachnoid hemorrhage revealed contralateral internal carotid artery dissection due to eagle syndrome: a case report. BMC Neurol. 2024;24(1):380. https://doi.org/10.1186/s12883-024-03890-y.
10. Calotă RN, Rusu MC, Vrapciu AD. The external carotid artery and the styloid process. Curr Health Sci J. 2024;50(2):232–6. https://doi.org/10.12865/CHSJ.50.02.08. Epub 2024 Jun 30
11. Tadjer J, Béjot Y. Vascular variant of eagle syndrome: a review. Front Neurol. 2024;15:1463275. https://doi.org/10.3389/fneur.2024.1463275. eCollection 2024
12. Campisi R, Caranti A, Meccariello G, Stringa LM, Bianchini C, Ciorba A, Pelucchi S, Vicini C. Transoral robotic styloidectomy for eagle syndrome: a systematic review. Clin Otolaryngol. 2024;49(3):293–8. https://doi.org/10.1111/coa.14145. Epub 2024 Jan 30

13. Liu B, Li Q, Zheng Y, Cai J, Jin H, Lin Y, Wang Y. Ischemic stroke due to stylocarotid artery syndrome: a case report and review. J Int Med Res. 2024;52(5):3000605241253745. https://doi.org/10.1177/03000605241253745.
14. Bargiel J, Gontarz M, Marecik T, Szczurowski P, Gąsiorowski K, Zapała J, Wyszyńska-Pawelec G. Minimally invasive cervical Styloidectomy in stylohyoid syndrome (eagle syndrome). J Clin Med. 2023;12(21):6763. https://doi.org/10.3390/jcm12216763.
15. Xiong L, Heliyon WZ. Intracranial hypertension due to bilateral internal jugular venous occlusion in eagle syndrome: a case report. eCollection. 2023;9(5):e16188. https://doi.org/10.1016/jheliyon2023e16188.
16. Hayashi S, Kumai T, Kishibe K, Takahara M, Katada A, Hayashi T. Internal carotid artery dissection caused by elongated styloid process. Auris Nasus Larynx. 2023;50(6):968–72. https://doi.org/10.1016/j.anl.2023.01.011. Epub 2023 Feb 8
17. Werheim E, Sokol Z, Brown D, Oselkin M. Eagle syndrome causing cerebral sinus hypertension: Case report. Radiol Case Rep. 2023;18(8):2758–62. https://doi.org/10.1016/jradcr202305023. eCollection
18. Zamboni P, Scerrati A, Menegatti E, Galeotti R, Lapparelli M, Traina L, Tessari M, Ciorba A, De Bonis P, Pelucchi S. The eagle jugular syndrome. BMC Neurol. 2019;19(1):333. https://doi.org/10.1186/s12883-019-1572-3.
19. Mantovani G, Zangrossi P, Flacco ME, Di Domenico G, Nastro Siniscalchi E, De Ponte FS, Maugeri R, De Bonis P, Cavallo MA, Zamboni P, Scerrati A. Styloid jugular nutcracker: the possible role of the styloid process spatial orientation-a preliminary morphometric computed study. Diagnostics (Basel). 2023;13(2):298. https://doi.org/10.3390/diagnostics13020298.
20. Zamboni P, Galeotti R, Menegatti E, Malagoni AM, Tacconi G, Dall'Ara S, Bartolomei I, Salvi F. Chronic cerebrospinal venous insufficiency in patients with multiple sclerosis. J Neurol Neurosurg Psychiatry. 2009;80(4):392–9. https://doi.org/10.1136/jnnp.2008.157164. Epub 2008 Dec 5

4 Social (Chats), Websites, and ChatGPT in Eagle Syndrome

Giovanni Cammaroto, Andrea Migliorelli, Stefano Pelucchi, Giuseppe Meccariello, and Andrea De Vito

4.1 Introduction

The application of technology and artificial intelligence (AI) in healthcare has grown exponentially in recent years. This is due to the combination of technological innovations (e.g., Internet connectivity, increased computing power, security of analyzed data, etc.) and the increasing availability of multimodal data (e.g., demographic, clinical, economic, etc.). This development has profoundly changed and improved healthcare models around the world [1].

AI represents an "intelligent machine" that mimics human cognitive functions (learning and problem solving) through algorithms and rules. Therefore, AI aims to enhance and amplify human intelligence and help it perform a very large number of analyses in a shorter amount of time [2].

The strength of AI lies in its ability to learn and recognize relational patterns, thus having the power to deal with problems intelligently and adaptively, and also being dynamic and autonomous systems with the ability to renew themselves as new data become available [3, 4].

AI consists of several subfields, one of the most important being machine learning (ML), which is the study of algorithms that allow programs to improve themselves autonomously [1].

Deep learning (DL) is a system that learns by using a very large number of multilevel interconnected processes and exposing them to a large number of examples.

G. Cammaroto (✉) · G. Meccariello · A. De Vito
ENT Department, Morgagni Pierantoni Hospital, AUSL Romagna, Forlì, Italy

A. Migliorelli · S. Pelucchi
ENT & Audiology Unit, Department of Neurosciences, University Hospital of Ferrara, Ferrara, Italy
e-mail: andrea.migliorelli@ospfe.it; Stefano.pelucchi@unife.it

C. Vicini et al. (eds.), *EAGLE Syndrome*,
https://doi.org/10.1007/978-3-031-92829-1_4

To date, DL is the dominant form of AI, enabling image recognition, for example [5, 6].

The main application of AI in healthcare is in radiological image recognition. Numerous studies have shown that for specific diseases, the performance of AI is comparable to that of experienced radiologists.

Studies have demonstrated its effectiveness in identifying solid tumors and nodules in X-ray, CT, and MRI images. Thus, AI can play an excellent supporting role in imaging [7–9].

The recent development of AI has led to the creation of language models that acquire their capabilities by analyzing articles published on the Internet and thus are able to learn from a vast amount of data [10, 11].

At present, the most widely used of these is ChatGPT, created in 2022, which is now widely used in healthcare and is the subject of numerous scientific publications [12].

In the simplest terms, AI in healthcare can have three different levels of application [1, 13]:

1. Medical assistance: It is a valuable resource that assists the physician from diagnosis to therapeutic choice. With a vast amount of data and knowledge at its disposal, it can assist the physician in managing the patient by suggesting additional examinations, diagnoses, and possible treatment options. While AI should never take the place of a physician, it can provide critical support to healthcare professionals, minimizing the risk of error. In addition, AI can make a fundamental contribution to the management of rare diseases, providing information and assisting the specialist in even the most difficult diagnoses.
2. Education: Having an almost unlimited amount of scientific information available on your computer or smartphone can help students and residents in their education.
3. Patient care: Recent programs, such as ChatGPT, are available to the general population; therefore, they also find their use in answering patients' questions. However, it must be stressed that the information generated by AI is not always correct and thus there is a risk of creating misunderstandings or false concerns for the patient themselves. Therefore, we would like to point out that AI should not replace the healthcare professional yet. However, if used properly, it could certainly guide patients to the right tests or the right specialist for their problem, saving valuable time from symptom onset to diagnosis.

As mentioned earlier, one of the AI's most important roles is in the management of rare diseases. Eagle syndrome is a rare and often unrecognized condition characterized by an elongated styloid process and a nonspecific symptom spectrum [14].

First described by Eagle in 1937, it is divided into a classic form characterized by pharyngeal and laterocervical pain, dysphagia, and hypopharyngeal foreign body sensation and a stylocarotid form in which the elongated styloid process reaches the carotid artery, resulting in parietal and periorbital pain, visual disturbances, and syncope [15–20].

An increased size of the styloid process (more than 30 cm) has been found in 4–7% of the population, a percentage that reaches 22–88% if calcification of the stylohyoid ligament is also considered. However, the incidence of symptomatology is present in only 4–10% of patients with this anatomical anomaly [21–24]. Diagnosis is clinical and radiologic (CT and/or orthopanoramic).

In this rare and often undiagnosed condition, technology and AI can certainly play a key role in the management of these patients by assisting specialists, students, and patients.

4.2 Eagle Syndrome, AI, and Imaging

The styloid process is a bony component located anterior to the stylomastoid foramen. Its length is usually between 20 and 25 mm, but if it exceeds 30 mm, it can cause Eagle syndrome [14, 25].

In order to diagnose this disease, it is essential to perform an imaging study, orthopantography or CT scan, with measurement of the length of the styloid process [14, 25].

Manual interpretation of this value can be subject to variability among healthcare providers, requiring a long time for reporting. This is where AI and DL find their main application. These approaches make it possible to assist the radiologist in the analysis and interpretation of images, improving accuracy and diagnostic efficacy while reducing the workload and time required for reporting.

A recent study investigated the ability of AI to detect an elongated styloid process by analyzing 400 digital orthopantographs and found that the algorithms analyzed had 100% accuracy (no false positives or negatives) in image classification, showing complete agreement with manual radiological assessment [25].

Thus, to date, there is only one study in the literature using AI in the radiologic diagnosis of elongated styloid process [25].

No studies were found that evaluated the role of AI in the detection of elongated styloid process on CT scans.

CT is certainly the most widely used examination in the study of Eagle syndrome, and therefore, the lack of AI in CT evaluation is an important gap in this field that needs to be filled as soon as possible.

However, the role of AI in CT reporting is well established in other osteomuscular diseases, so this bodes well for its role in identifying the elongated styloid process.

Further studies are needed to confirm these hypotheses.

4.3 Website and Chats in Eagle Syndrome

In recent years, the Internet and social media platforms have played an increasingly important role in spreading awareness, facilitating patient communities, and assisting with diagnosis and treatment plans for rare diseases such as Eagle syndrome.

To date, there are many reputable medical websites (such as WebMD, Mayo Clinic, and MedlinePlus) that provide patient-friendly information about Eagle syndrome, covering topics such as symptoms, diagnostic criteria, and treatment options. These sites are often the first port of call for patients seeking to understand the rare disease from which they suffer.

For medical professionals, there are also more specialized websites (e.g., PubMed and UpToDate) that provide in-depth clinical data, research papers, and case studies on Eagle syndrome. These resources are invaluable to physicians who may rarely encounter this condition in their practice.

The abundance of misinformation that can be found on the Internet should always be emphasized, so it is critical that both physicians and patients rely on validated medical sources.

Many hospitals and specialty clinics that treat this condition have websites that provide information on diagnostic procedures, treatment options, and contact information for specialists. They also offer telemedicine consultation options.

Social media also plays an important role in connecting people with the same disorder.

For example, the Facebook group "Eagle Syndrome Group" provides a space for people to share their experiences, symptoms, diagnostic pathways, and treatment outcomes.

Sharing personal stories often helps patients recognize their symptoms and seek a correct diagnosis. The community aspect allows members to ask questions, share their experiences of living with Eagle syndrome, and recommend specialists they have found helpful.

Social media sites such as TikTok, Instagram, and Twitter with hashtags such as #EagleSyndrome or #RareDisease also allow the community to connect with each other.

Many doctors use YouTube to create informative and educational videos about Eagle syndrome, providing visual aids and simple but detailed explanations to help patients understand the disease.

What is missing, however, is an association of Eagle syndrome patients; many other conditions, such as fibromyalgia or Meniere's syndrome, have specific associations that promote awareness of the condition and create a more structured and controlled community than can be created on social media.

The major limitation of the Internet is that the information provided is often not controlled and therefore risks being misleading or even harmful to patients. In addition, participating in social forums or groups with personal profiles puts the patient's own privacy at risk.

The Internet and social media have become valuable tools for raising awareness of Eagle syndrome, providing a platform for patients to share their experiences, and for healthcare providers to access up-to-date medical information. While these tools enhance communication, education, and support, it is important to use them with caution, ensuring that information comes from reliable sources and is used responsibly to complement professional medical advice.

4.4 Eagle Syndrome and ChatGPT

ChatGPT is an advanced language model that is part of the generative pre-trained transformer (GPT) family developed by OpenAI. It uses DL techniques to produce appropriate and contextually relevant human-like responses [12, 26].

AI, particularly natural language processing tools such as ChatGPT, is increasingly becoming a valuable resource in medical practice. ChatGPT has the potential to aid research, support clinical decision-making, and improve communication and patient education for rare diseases such as Eagle syndrome [27].

ChatGPT can quickly retrieve and summarize a wealth of medical information about Eagle syndrome, helping healthcare professionals learn about the pathophysiology, symptoms, and treatment options for the condition. Medical professionals can use ChatGPT to access current research, guidelines, and clinical cases that are not readily available in traditional textbooks and can be time-consuming.

For example, a young physician encountering Eagle syndrome for the first time can use ChatGPT to quickly review the etiology of the condition, understand its clinic, and evaluate recommended imaging techniques for diagnosis.

In addition, ChatGPT can provide patients with easy-to-understand explanations of their condition, including the causes, symptoms, and treatment options for Eagle syndrome. In this way, healthcare professionals can use artificial intelligence as a tool to help patients understand their condition.

Furthermore, ChatGPT can be used by healthcare providers to generate a differential diagnosis based on a patient's symptoms. However, to date, by listing the typical symptoms of classic Eagle syndrome to ChatGPT, it is not mentioned among the diseases that are included in the differential diagnosis.

This is a limitation of this model, probably dictated by the fact that more common and probable pathologies are mentioned. On the other hand, if the patient has imaging that shows an elongated styloid process, ChatGPT immediately raises the question of Eagle syndrome [27].

When the patient then asks ChatGPT what Eagle syndrome is, the answer is as follows:

Eagle Syndrome is a rare condition characterized by pain and discomfort in the head, neck, or face due to an elongated or misshapen **styloid process** (a small pointed bone just below the ear) or **calcification** of the **stylohyoid ligament**. This syndrome can lead to various symptoms when these structures impinge on surrounding tissues, such as blood vessels or nerves.

Causes of Eagle Syndrome

- **Elongated Styloid Process**: In most people, the styloid process is about 2.5 cm long. In those with Eagle syndrome, it can be significantly longer.
- **Calcification of the Stylohyoid Ligament**: This ligament, which connects the styloid process to the hyoid bone, may become hardened or calcified.

Symptoms

- **Throat and Facial Pain**: A sharp, shooting pain in the throat, jaw, or face, often worse when swallowing, yawning, or turning the head.
- **Ear Pain**: Often experienced without any apparent ear infection.
- **Dysphagia (Difficulty Swallowing)**: Due to pressure on the throat or related nerves.
- **Tinnitus**: A ringing or buzzing in the ear.
- **Headaches**: Sometimes localized to one side of the head or face.

In some cases, the syndrome can also compress the **internal carotid artery**, leading to vascular symptoms like dizziness, vision changes, or even **transient ischemic attacks (TIAs)**, though these cases are rare.

Diagnosis

- **Physical Examination**: The doctor may feel the elongated styloid process through the throat.
- **Imaging**: X-rays, CT scans, or 3D reconstructions can confirm the diagnosis by showing the abnormal styloid process or ligament calcification.

Treatment

- **Conservative Approaches**: Anti-inflammatory medications, pain relievers, or corticosteroid injections can be used to manage symptoms.
- **Surgical Intervention**: In severe cases, surgery (styloidectomy) is performed to shorten or remove the elongated styloid process.

While Eagle syndrome can be debilitating, it's treatable, especially when properly diagnosed.

The advantage of ChatGPT is that one can continue to inquire about Eagle syndrome in all its aspects, from diagnosis to treatment, providing an important amount of useful and understandable information for both the user and the healthcare provider.

In addition, ChatGPT can summarize the latest evidence-based treatment approaches for Eagle syndrome, from conservative therapies such as anti-inflammatory drugs, pain management techniques, and steroid injections to more invasive surgical options.

Finally, ChatGPT can help create personalized care plans for follow-up care of patients recovering from surgery. This can include advice on postoperative pain management, dietary recommendations, and when to seek medical attention in case of complications.

The massive and increasing use of AI and ChatGPT has led the literature to ask some ethical questions about it (27).

It must first be emphasized that although ChatGPT can provide useful information, it is essential to always verify the accuracy of its answers. Healthcare providers should use ChatGPT as a supplementary tool rather than the sole source of decision-making.

In addition, when using AI tools in clinical settings, care must be taken to protect patient confidentiality. Clinicians should avoid entering sensitive patient information into AI systems that are not explicitly designed to handle protected health information.

Finally, it should be remembered that the responses of ChatGPT and analogs are based on the data they were trained on, so if they are incorrect, the tool could provide biased and erroneous information.

In conclusion, ChatGPT represents an important advance in the medical field, offering physicians and patients new ways to deal with rare diseases such as Eagle syndrome. However, its use must always be complemented by clinical expertise, evidence of efficacy, and careful ethical considerations. Moreover, in the context of Eagle syndrome, it still has some gaps in the field of differential diagnosis, so further developments and updates are needed to expand and improve its use.

4.5 Future Perspectives

AI has recently been introduced and applied in healthcare. We are still at the beginning of its application, but we can already feel its limitless potential. For rare diseases, it would be important to create global databases by analyzing them with ML methods to predict their trends and facilitate their knowledge and diagnosis by healthcare professionals.

For Eagle syndrome, we believe that AI can play a key role in the near future. The groundwork we have is already solid; it just needs some adjustments and refinements (Fig. 4.1).

We believe that the patient with Eagle syndrome symptoms can first contact the AI, such as ChatGPT, and describe their symptoms. The AI should ask the patient further questions to narrow down the differential diagnosis. Once the basis of the differential diagnosis is established, the patient should go to his or her primary care physician who, if clinically suspicious for Eagle syndrome, can prescribe the appropriate radiologic investigations.

It should be emphasized that even the general practitioner or other specialist, if unaware of Eagle syndrome or unwilling to consider it, could use AI to do so and be guided in prescribing imaging.

The imaging could then be analyzed by DL methods to confirm or not confirm Eagle syndrome.

At this point, the patient and physician should use AI and the website to analyze possible treatment options and evaluate the presence of a possible specialist who treats this condition in the area of residence.

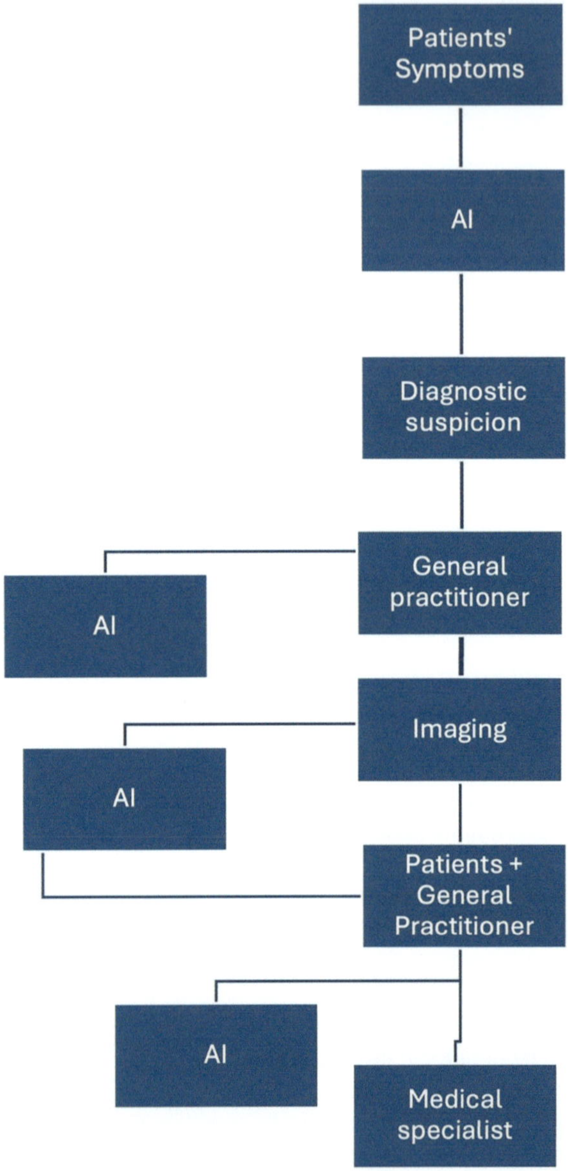

Fig. 4.1 Our proposal for the use of AI in the management of Eagle syndrome

4.6 Conclusion

The exponential development of technology since the beginning of the twentieth century has also led to the implementation of AI and websites and their use in healthcare. This is of fundamental importance in assisting the doctor and guiding the patient. The main implications of AI are the role it can play in rare diseases and in the analysis of radiological images.

This chapter has described the important role of AI and the Internet in a rare disease such as Eagle syndrome. However, much can be improved in terms of accuracy and control of information, association/forum, and privacy.

We believe that these small changes can be made in a relatively short period of time and would bring enormous benefits to the disclosure of a rare disease such as Eagle syndrome.

References

1. Bajwa J, Munir U, Nori A, Williams B. Artificial intelligence in healthcare: transforming the practice of medicine. Future Healthc J. 2021. 34286183;8(2):e188–94. https://doi.org/10.7861/fhj.2021-0095.
2. McCarthy J. What is artificial intelligence? John McCarthy; 1998.
3. Shukla SS, Jaiswal V. Applicability of artificial intelligence in different fields of life. IJSR. 2013;e 1:28–35.
4. Binns R, Gallo V. Trade-offs. Information Commissioner's Office. 2019. https://ico.org.uk/about-the-ico/news-and-events/ai-blog-trade-offs.
5. The Royal Society. Machine learning: the power and promise of computers that learn by example. The Royal Society; 2017.
6. LeCun Y, Bengio Y, Hinton G. Deep learning. Nature 2015 e 436–44., 521.
7. Sahoo PK, Mishra S, Panigrahi R, Bhoi AK, Barsocchi P. An improvised deep-learning-based mask R-CNN model for laryngeal cancer detection using CT images. Sensors (Basel). 2022;e 22:8834.
8. Jing X, Wielema M, Cornelissen LJ, van Gent M, Iwema WM, Zheng S, Sijens PE, Oudkerk M, Dorrius MD, van Ooijen PMA. Using deep learning to safely exclude lesions with only ultrafast breast MRI to shorten acquisition and reading time. Eur Radiol. 2022;e32:8706.
9. Khan E, Rehman MZU, Ahmed F, Alfouzan FA, Alzahrani NM, Ahmad J. Chest X-ray classification for the detection of COVID-19 using deep learning techniques. Sensors (Basel). 2022;e 22:1211.
10. Vaswani A, Shazeer NM, Parmar N, Uszkoreit J, Jones L, Gomez AN, Kaiser L, Polosukhin I. Attention is all you need. NIPS. https://proceedings.neurips.cc/paper_files/paper/2017/file/3f5ee243547dee91fbd053c1c4a845aa-Paper.pdf. Accessed 1 June 2023.
11. Radford A, Narasimhan K, Salimans T, Sutskever I. Improving language understanding by generative pre-Training. https://s3-us-west-2.amazonaws.com/openai-assets/research-covers/language-unsupervised/language_understanding_paper.pdf. Accessed 1 June 2023.
12. OpenAI, ChatGPT: Optimizing language models for dialogue. https://openai.com/blog/chatgpt/. Accessed 1 June 2023).
13. Karako K, Song P, Chen Y, Tang W. New possibilities for medical support systems utilizing artificial intelligence (AI) and data platforms. Biosci Trends. 2023;17(3):186–9. https://doi.org/10.5582/bst.2023.01138.
14. Badhey A, Jategaonkar A, Anglin Kovacs AJ, et al. Eagle syndrome: a comprehensive review. Clin Neurol Neurosurg. 2017;159:34–8. https://doi.org/10.1016/j.clineuro.2017.04.021.
15. Eagle WW. Elongated styloid processes: report of two cases. Arch Otolaryngol Head Neck Surg. 1937;25(5):584–7. https://doi.org/10.1001/archotol.1937.00650010656008.
16. Eagle WW. Sphenopalatine ganglion neuralgia. Arch Otolaryngol Head Neck Surg. 1942;35(1):66–84. https://doi.org/10.1001/archotol.1942.00670010067004.
17. Eagle WW. Elongated styloid process e further observations and a new syndrome. Arch Otolaryngol. 1948;47(5):630–40.
18. Eagle WW. Symptomatic elongated styloid process e report of two cases of styloid process-carotid artery syndrome with operation. Arch Otolaryngol. 1949;49(5):490–503.

19. Eagle WW. Elongated styloid process e symptoms and treatment. AMA Arch Otolaryngol. 1958;67(2):172–6.
20. Eagle WW. The symptoms, diagnosis and treatment of the elongated styloid process. Am Surg. 1962;28:1–5.
21. Kaufman SM, Elzay RP, Irish EF. Styloid process variation: radiologic and clinical study. Arch Otolaryngol. 1970;91(5):460–3.
22. Carroll MKO. Calcification in the stylohyoid ligament. Oral Surg Oral Med Oral Pathol. 1984;58(5):617–21. https://doi.org/10.1016/0030-4220(84)90089-6.
23. Miller D. Eagle's syndrome and the trauma patient. Significance of an elongated styloid process and/or ossified stylohyoid ligament. Funct Orthod. 1997;14(2):30–5.
24. Murtagh RD, Caracciolo JT, Fernandez G. CT findings associated with eagle syndrome. Am J Neuroradiol. 2001;22(7):1401–2.
25. Jeevitha SJ, Kumar SL, Yadalam PK. Artificial intelligence: a reliable tool to detect the elongation of the styloid process. Cureus. 2023;15(11):e49541. https://doi.org/10.7759/cureus.49541. Published 2023 Nov 28.
26. Radford, A., Narasimhan, K., Salimans, T., and Sutskever, I. (2018). Improving language understanding by generative pre-training.
27. Dave T, Athaluri SA, Singh S. ChatGPT in medicine: an overview of its applications, advantages, limitations, future prospects, and ethical considerations. Front Artif Intell. 2023;6:1169595. https://doi.org/10.3389/frai.2023.1169595. Published 2023 May 4

Glossary, Definitions, and Related Terms

5

Alberto Caranti and Claudio Vicini

Come, let us go down and there confuse their language, so that they may not understand one another's speech. (Genesis 11:7)

5.1 Eagle Syndrome (ES)

It is the eponymic name coming from the first ENT surgeon who first described the clinical entity in 1937 [1]. In the original description is depicted only the so-called typical Eagle (see below).

5.2 Typical Eagle Syndrome

It is the first variant of ES based on glossopharyngeal pain and mechanical pharyngeal symptoms. It is the only entity described in the first Eagle paper.

5.3 Classic Styloid Syndrome

It is the same as typical styloid syndrome.

A. Caranti
University of Ferrara, Cona, FE, Italy

Otorinolaringoiatria, S. Pier Damiano di Faenza - GVM care & research, Faenza, Italia

C. Vicini (✉)
University of Ferrara, Cona, FE, Italy
e-mail: claudio@claudiovicini.com

C. Vicini et al. (eds.), *EAGLE Syndrome*,
https://doi.org/10.1007/978-3-031-92829-1_5

5.4 Stylalgia

The term, literally "pain from styloid," emphasizes the main symptom (pain) related to styloid process [2, 3].

5.5 Styloid Syndrome

The term emphasizes the multiple clinical symptoms related to a pathological styloid process [4].

5.6 Classic Stylalgia

It may be considered as equivalent to classic styloid syndrome [5].

5.7 Styloid Process Neuralgia

This term emphasizes the concept of a secondary neuralgia produced by the interaction of a sensory nerve with a pathological styloid process [6].

5.8 Carotid Artery Syndrome

This variant was described by Dr. Eagle on 1948 in his second paper [7]. In the original Eagle's paper, carotid artery syndrome is produced by the compression of the carotid artery instead of the glossopharyngeal nerve as in classic variant. The compression produces pain mainly irradiated to the temporal area (carotid plexus stimulation), but major arterial complications (TIA, stroke, carotid dissections) are possible. It is assumed but not included into the definition the responsibility of the styloid process [8].

5.9 Styloid Jugular Nutcracker (SJN)

It refers to the special mechanism of jugular vein compression like a nut between an elongated styloid and a prominent C1 lateral mass (the nutcracker) [9].

5.10 Eagle Jugular Syndrome (EJS)

It is a more recent syndrome centered on the jugular vein instead of the glossopharyngeal nerve [10].

5.11 Venous Vascular Variant of Eagle Syndrome

It is the same as Eagle jugular syndrome, emphasizing the concept of venous vs arterial [9].

5.12 Styloidogenic-Cervical Spondylotic Internal Jugular Venous Compression

It is a comprehensive term describing the combined responsibility of cervical spine C1 and styloid in the extrinsic compression of internal jugular vein [11].

5.13 Styloid-Induced Internal Jugular Vein Stenosis

It refers to the responsibility of the elongated styloid process in narrowing the internal jugular vein lumen [12].

5.14 Stylo-Carotid Artery Syndrome

It is the same as carotid artery syndrome [13].

5.15 Elongated Styloid Process

The term emphasizes the main pathological finding: the excessive length of the styloid process. It is a truly anatomical description, without any detail about the induced clinical picture [14, 15].

5.16 Syndrome of Elongated Styloid Process

It is simply a wide box including all the symptoms produced by an elongated styloid process [16].

5.17 Calcification of the Stylohyoid Ligament

It is a frequently used term. It refers to an elongation of the stylohyoid ligament produced by a calcified fibrous tissue, without a real bone metaplasia [17, 18].

5.18 Ossification of the Stylohyoid Ligament

It is probably the most common situation in which the fibrous connection of the stylohyoid ligament to the tip of the styloid underwent a progressive bone metaplasia [19]. It produces a slow elongation of the styloid process by means of a very dense and strong growing bone tissue with a sharp tip [20].

5.19 Stylohyoid Pain Syndrome

It simply stresses the main symptom of the classic form with the responsibility of a pathological stylohyoid complex [21].

5.20 First-Bite Syndrome

First-bite syndrome (FBS) is characterized by pain in the parotid and retromandibular region when taking the first bite in a meal and occurs more or less invariably and may accompany untreated ES [22]. First-bite syndrome (FBS) may occur after operations on parapharyngeal space, including resection of the styloid process. It is usually self-resolving [23].

5.21 Insertion Tendonitis

Insertion tendonitis in a broader way is a disorder caused by repetitive tendon strain and subsequent tendon inflammation. "Insertion tendonitis can resemble Eagle syndrome. However, it usually causes tenderness over the greater horn of the hyoid bone. An elongated styloid process can be palpated by intraoral palpation, placing the index finger in the tonsillar fossa, and applying gentle pressure" [4].

5.22 Trigeminal Neuralgia Post-styloidectomy in Eagle Syndrome

In the literature, Blackett JW reported an anecdotal case in 2012 [24]. "In this report we present a case of Eagle syndrome exhibiting the typical findings of glossopharyngeal nerve involvement, as well as unusual involvement of the trigeminal nerve. Notably, this patient developed a classical trigeminal neuralgia post-styloidectomy."

References

1. Eagle WW, Durham NC. Elongated styloid processes. Report of two cases. Arch Otolaryngol Head Neck Surg. 1937;25:584–7.
2. Härmä R. Stylalgia: clinical experiences of 52 cases. Acta Otolaryngol. 1966;63(224):149–55. https://doi.org/10.3109/00016486709123570.
3. Lambor DV, Shetgaunkar RR, De Sa C. Stylalgia: our experience of 101 cases treated by intraoral Styloidectomy. Indian J Otolaryngol Head Neck Surg. 2022;74(S2):2198–204. https://doi.org/10.1007/s12070-020-02074-7.
4. Bokhari MR, Graham C, Mohseni M. Eagle syndrome. In: StatPearls [Internet]. Treasure Island (FL): StatPearls Publishing; 2023. 2024 Jan–.
5. Bargiel J, Gontarz M, Marecik T, Szczurowski P, Gąsiorowski K, Zapała J, Wyszyńska-Pawelec G. Minimally invasive cervical Styloidectomy in stylohyoid syndrome (Eagle syndrome). J Clin Med. 2023;12(21):6763. https://doi.org/10.3390/jcm12216763.
6. Papadiochos I, Papadiochou S, Sarivalasis ES, Goutzanis L, Petsinis V. Treatment of Eagle syndrome with transcervical approach secondary to a failed intraoral attempt: surgical technique and literature review. J Stomatol Oral Maxillofac Surg. 2017;118(6):353–8. https://doi.org/10.1016/j.jormas.2017.06.017.
7. Eagle WW. Elongated styloid process; further observations and a new syndrome. Arch Otolaryngol. 1925). 1948;47(5):630–40. https://doi.org/10.1001/archotol.1948.00690030654006.
8. Sultan S, Acharya Y, Soliman O, Hynes N. Stylohyoid Eagle syndrome and EXTracranial INternal carotid arTery pseudoaneurysms (EXTINCT) with internal jugular vein nutcracker syndrome: a challenging clinical scenario. BMJ Case Rep. 2022;15(4):e249558. https://doi.org/10.1136/bcr-2022-249558.
9. Mantovani G, Zangrossi P, Flacco ME, Di Domenico G, Nastro Siniscalchi E, De Ponte FS, Maugeri R, De Bonis P, Cavallo MA, Zamboni P, Scerrati A. Styloid jugular nutcracker: the possible role of the styloid process spatial orientation-a preliminary morphometric computed study. Diagnostics (Basel). 2023;13(2):298. https://doi.org/10.3390/diagnostics13020298.
10. Zamboni P, Scerrati A, Menegatti E, Galeotti R, Lapparelli M, Traina L, Tessari M, Ciorba A, De Bonis P, Pelucchi S. The eagle jugular syndrome. BMC Neurol. 2019;19(1):333. https://doi.org/10.1186/s12883-019-1572-3.
11. Scerrati A, Norri N, Mongardi L, Dones F, Ricciardi L, Trevisi G, Menegatti E, Zamboni P, Cavallo MA, De Bonis P. Styloidogenic-cervical spondylotic internal jugular venous compression, a vascular disease related to several clinical neurological manifestations: diagnosis and treatment-a comprehensive literature review. Ann Transl Med. 2021;9(8):718. https://doi.org/10.21037/atm-20-7698.
12. Li M, Gao X, Rajah GB, Liang J, Chen J, Yan F, Bao Y, Jiao L, Zhang H, Ding Y, Ji X, Meng R. Styloidectomy and venous stenting for treatment of styloid-induced internal jugular vein stenosis: a case report and literature review. World Neurosurg. 2019;130:129–32. https://doi.org/10.1016/j.wneu.2019.06.100.
13. Kesav P, Hussain SI, Dogar MA, John S. Stylo-carotid syndrome causing bilateral cervical carotid artery dissection requiring endovascular intervention. Clin Neurol Neurosurg. 2020;195:105943. https://doi.org/10.1016/j.clineuro.2020.105943.
14. Bakshi SS. Elongated styloid process. J Oral Maxillofac Surg. 2017;75(12):2484. https://doi.org/10.1016/j.joms.2017.07.165.
15. Nogueira-Reis F, de Oliveira RL, Fontenele RC, Freitas DQ, Tabchoury CPM. Prevalence and features of elongated styloid process on imaging studies: a systematic review and meta-analysis. Clin Oral Investig. 2022;26(2):1199–215. https://doi.org/10.1007/s00784-021-04285-w.
16. Czako L, Simko K, Thurzo A, Galis B, Varga I. The syndrome of elongated styloid process, the Eagle's syndrome-from anatomical, evolutionary and embryological backgrounds to 3D printing and personalized surgery planning. Report of Five Cases Medicina (Kaunas). 2020;56(9):458. https://doi.org/10.3390/medicina56090458.

17. Monteagudo PT, Rossinol VL, do Nascimento Verreschi IT, Dias-da-Silva MR. Stylohyoid ligament calcification: a greater-than-expected cause of otalgia in turner syndrome. J Endocr Soc. 2019;3(7):1403–8. https://doi.org/10.1210/js.2019-00009.
18. Searle E, Searle A. An overview of Eagle's syndrome. Br J Pain. 2021;15(4):388–92. https://doi.org/10.1177/2049463720969741.
19. Piagkou M, Anagnostopoulou S, Kouladouros K, Piagkos G. Eagle's syndrome: a review of the literature. Clin Anat. 2009;22(5):545–58. https://doi.org/10.1002/ca.20804.
20. Saccomanno S, Quinzi V, D'Andrea N, Albani A, Coceani Paskay L, Marzo G. Traumatic events and Eagle syndrome: is there any correlation? A systematic review. Healthcare (Basel). 2021;9(7):825. https://doi.org/10.3390/healthcare9070825.
21. Waters CM, Ho S, Luginbuhl A, Curry JM, Cognetti DM. Surgical Management of Stylohyoid Pain (Eagle's) syndrome: a 5-year experience. Ann Otol Rhinol Laryngol. 2019;128(3):220–6. https://doi.org/10.1177/0003489418816999.
22. Gauthier B, Ségolène G, Bruno C. First-bite syndrome and Eagle syndrome. J Oral Med Oral. 2018;24(1):36–9. https://doi.org/10.1051/mbcb/2017025.
23. Cernea CR, Hojaij FC, De Carlucci D, Plopper C Jr, Vanderley F, Guerreiro CA, Viana MS. First-bite syndrome after resection of the styloid process. Laryngoscope. 2007;117(1):181–2. https://doi.org/10.1097/01.mlg.0000245059.40028.ed.
24. Blackett JW, Ferraro DJ, Stephens JJ, Dowling JL, Jaboin JJ. Trigeminal neuralgia post-styloidectomy in Eagle syndrome: a case report. J Med Case Rep. 2012;6:333. https://doi.org/10.1186/1752-1947-6-333.

Stylohyoid Complex Embryology

6

Elio Maria Cunsolo, Alberto Caranti, Ruggero Campisi, Stefano Pelucchi, and Claudio Vicini

6.1 Introduction

The embryology of the stylohyoid complex and its ossification process has been investigated since the first anatomical and clinical reports of the complex syndrome [1], which, according to Watt Eagle, was given the eponym of Eagle syndrome [2]. However, the embryologic history of the styloid process, stylohyoid ligament, and hyoid bone remains a subject of debate. Schematically, three historical periods related to the knowledge of this topic can be distinguished:

(a) The phase of morphological description, based on the classical conception of the embryology of the branchial apparatus.
(b) The phase of serial histological studies, conducted on human embryos at different gestational ages.
(c) The current phase of "molecular" embryology.

Alongside studies on human embryology, investigations on the morphology and morphogenesis of these structures in non-human mammals have been carried out [3], with the aim of clarifying the role of this anatomical complex in the morphological evolution of the upper airways, in relation to the acquisition of articulated

E. M. Cunsolo (✉)
Policlinico di Modena, Modena, MO, Italy

A. Caranti · R. Campisi · C. Vicini
University of Ferrara, Cona, FE, Italy
e-mail: claudio@claudiovicini.com

S. Pelucchi
ENT & Audiology Unit, Department of Neurosciences, University Hospital of Ferrara, Cona, FE, Italy
e-mail: stefano.pelucchi@unife.it

C. Vicini et al. (eds.), *EAGLE Syndrome*,
https://doi.org/10.1007/978-3-031-92829-1_6

language [4]. Indeed, it is a fact that the hyoid apparatus in mammals provides the skeletal scaffolding supporting the tongue, upper vocal tract, and larynx and thus forms the core of the vocal production system [5].

In this paper, we will focus on the morphogenesis of the stylohyoid complex in humans.

6.2 Classical Morphological Conception

According to the classical morphological conception, the stylohyoid complex derives from Reichert's cartilage (RC) of the second branchial arch (pharyngeal arch). According to Revilla and Stuyt [6], the styloid process, stylohyoid ligament, and lesser horn of the hyoid bone derive from the endochondral ossification of RC. At the third month of fetal life, RC gives rise to four distinct components, defined in a cranio-caudal sense: tympanohyal, stylohyal, ceratohyal, and hypohyal. The fifth segment, basihyal, does not strictly belong to the stylohyoid complex (Fig. 6.1 and Table 6.1).

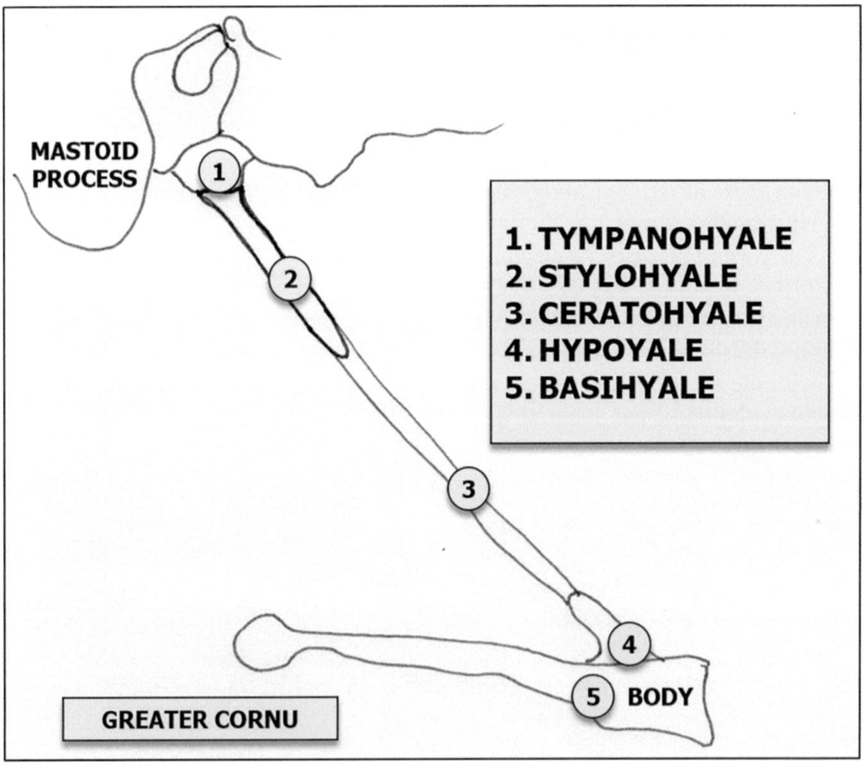

Fig. 6.1 The stylohyoid chain

Table 6.1 Development of the hyoid apparatus in humans

Divisions of the embryonal Reichert's cartilage, from cranial to caudal side	Derivatives in adulthood
Tympanohyal	Styloid process (proximal part)
Stylohyal	Styloid process (distal part)
Ceratohyal	Stylohyoid ligament (partially possible participation in styloid process formation)
Hypohyal	Small horn of the hyoid bone
Basihyal	Upper body of the hyoid bone

The tympanohyal, which will subsequently be incorporated into the bony portion of the temporal bone, extends downward and anteriorly from the periotic capsule to reach the underlying stylohyal. This gives rise to the styloid process, which, in turn, extends toward the ceratohyal. In the adult, this component gives rise to the stylohyoid ligament or an ossification thereof. The ceratohyal continues into the hypohyal, from which the lesser horn of the hyoid bone will form. The basihyal gives rise to the superior portion of the body of the hyoid bone, which, as previously mentioned, does not strictly belong to the stylohyoid complex.

According to this classical conception, the morphogenesis of the styloid process can be schematized as follows: both the tympanohyal and stylohyal undergo ossification to produce normal-sized styloid processes. When only the tympanohyal ossifies, a short styloid process forms. In cases of extremely long styloid processes or the complete ossification of the hyoid apparatus, the ceratohyal does not degenerate but undergoes ossification and completes the bony stylohyoid chain.

6.3 Contemporary Histological Understanding

The revision of the "classical" conception of the styloid complex morphogenesis is based on in-depth studies of serial sections conducted on human embryos. The reference studies are those of Rodriguez-Vázquez and collaborators, published in 2006, 2011, and 2015 [7–9], and Bakker et al. in 2017 [10]. Rodriguez-Vázquez and collaborators distinguish the morphogenesis of the stylohyoid complex that occurs during the embryonic period from that which occurs during the fetal period.

6.3.1 Embryonic Period

During the embryonic period (O'Rahilly stages 20, 21, 22, and 23), RC, belonging to the second pharyngeal arch, is composed of two distinct segments. The cranial segment is the longer one. The cranial end of this cartilaginous structure is curved into a hook shape, joining the side of the otic capsule and appearing as a prolongation from it.

The smaller, inferior segment is angled and located in proximity to the oropharynx. This segment is in contact with the body and the greater horn of the hyoid bone.

Between each segment of Reichert's cartilage, there is no cartilaginous connection (Fig. 6.2).

There is a mesenchymal condensation that joins the cranial segment with the caudal segment. Between these two segments, there is no cartilaginous connection, but rather a dense mesenchyme (Fig. 6.3).

At the end of the embryonic period, the cartilage of the second pharyngeal arch adopts the following arrangement:

- Cranial or styloid segment, longer and larger: This cartilaginous segment has two ends—the superior end, joined to the otic capsule, and the inferior end, which is angulated. This clear angulation occurs where the cartilage is in close proximity to the external carotid artery.
- Caudal or hyoid segment: This short cartilaginous segment terminates caudally in the hyoid cartilaginous structure between the body and the greater horn.

The studies of Rodriguez-Vázquez and collaborators highlight a morphologic finding of great importance for a pathogenetic interpretation of Eagle syndrome.

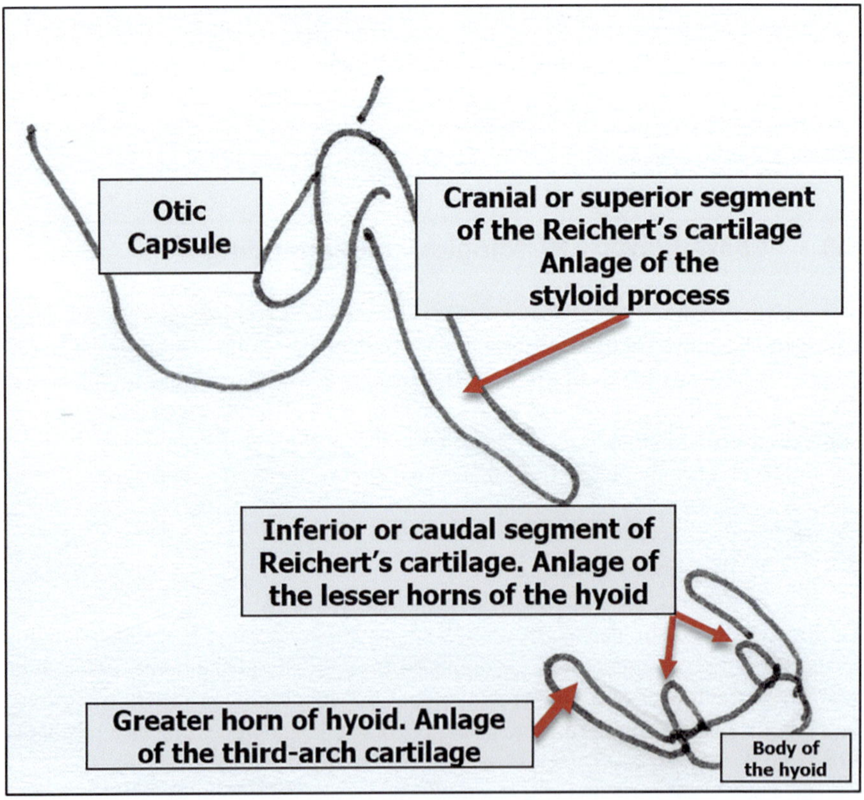

Fig. 6.2 Formation of bone and cartilage within mandibular and hyoid arches

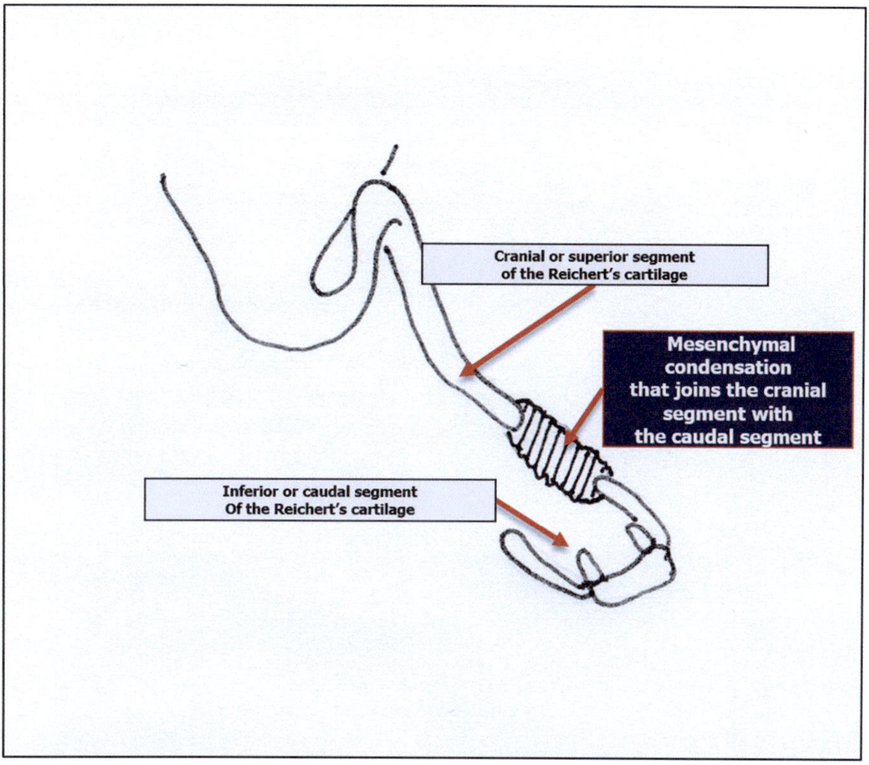

Fig. 6.3 The mesenchymal condensation extends from Reichert's cartilage to the hyoid cartilaginous structure, finishing at the area where the body joins the greater horn

This anatomical finding is the documented angulation between the most cranial and the most distal segment of the superior portion, or "styloid segment," of RC (Fig. 6.4).

6.3.2 Fetal Period

During the fetal period, the superior end of the hook-shaped cranial or styloid segment of RC remains continuous with the inferior extension of the otic capsule. Both structures contribute to the formation of the vertical portion of the facial nerve canal.

The angled segment between the cranial and caudal portions of the styloid segment of RC cartilage also establishes an anatomical relationship with the glossopharyngeal nerve. After crossing the inferior surface of the stylopharyngeal muscle, this nerve lies medial to the angled end of RC, running between this structure and the pharyngeal wall.

At a post-conception age of 13 weeks, the angulation of the inferior end of the cranial or styloid segment may vary, resulting in different degrees of angulation and

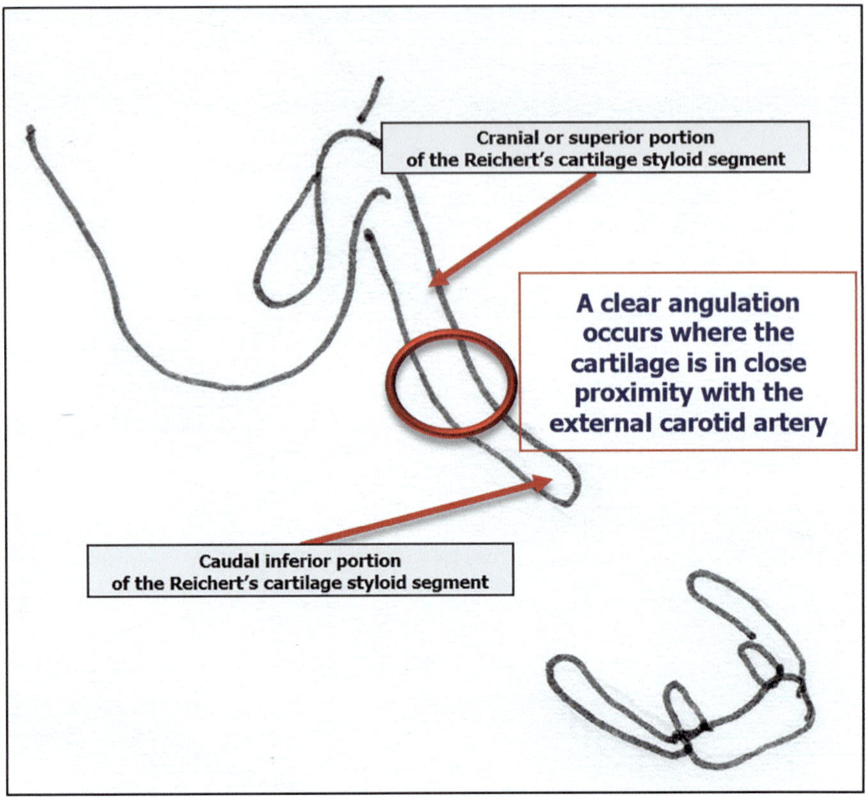

Fig. 6.4 Morphogenesis of the stylohyoid complex during the embryonic period

lengths of this segment. The caudal segments of RC are in contact with the hyoid bone, forming the lesser horns. The mesenchymal condensation, which was present during the embryonic period, is observed at the start of the fetal period but then disappears, leaving no trace during the rest of the fetal period.

During the fetal morphogenesis phase, the three main anatomical relationships established by the stylohyoid complex can be summarized as follows:

- Anatomical relationships with the pharynx: When the angulation of the inferior end of the cranial or styloid segment persists, the end of the cartilage may be very close to the pharyngeal wall, depending on the degree of angulation.
- Anatomical relationships with the glossopharyngeal nerve: This nerve crosses medial to the inferior end of the cranial segment. The more angulated this segment, the closer the nerve crosses to its end.
- Anatomical relationships with the external carotid artery: The artery, surrounded by the external carotid nerves, passes through the hiatus or space defined by RC and the stylohyoid muscle. This occurs where RC changes direction and begins to angulate.

The most recent studies by Rodriguez-Vázquez and colleagues have documented the "fate" of the mesenchymal formation (MF) found between the two segments of RC. The disappearance of the MF begins at the eighth week of development and progresses until the tenth week, at which point it is no longer detectable. This results in a substantial disconnection between the cranial and caudal segments of RC and the absence of structures resembling the "stylohyoid ligament" or "ceratohyal" in the classical four-segment description of RC, as observed in the histological sections of Rodriguez-Vázquez's studies. Consequently, according to these authors, the perichondrium of RC does not act as a "guide" for the formation of the stylohyoid ligament, which has a fascial origin, arising from the "tensor-vascular-styloid fascia." This fetal "disconnection" between the proximal and distal segments of RC, according to this interpretation, represents a fundamental factor for the postnatal ontogenetic descent of the hyoid, necessary for the development of the human vocal tract and, therefore, the ability to produce articulate speech. In studies of serial histological sections conducted on human embryos, the Rodriguez-Vázquez group has documented morphogenetic abnormalities in the development of RC, responsible for anatomical variations of the stylohyoid complex, which could have an impact on the pathogenesis of established cases of Eagle syndrome. These morphogenetic variations of the stylohyoid complex can be divided into four groups:

1. *Variations on the angulation of the cranial segment of RC* (Fig. 6.5)
2. *Continuous RC variation* (Fig. 6.6): Continuous RC variation run, unilaterally or bilaterally between the otic capsule and the hyoid. The cartilage exhibits a double incurvation caudally and next to the oropharynx. Overall, the cartilage presents a bayonet-like morphology. The angulation is arranged close to the pharyngeal wall. The cartilage extends caudally and makes contact with the cartilaginous formation of the hyoid.
3. *Isolated cartilaginous formation* (Fig. 6.7)
4. Elongated cranial segment of the RC (Fig. 6.8)

If these altered morphologies are maintained in the adult, they are likely to explain a major symptom associated with the classic and carotid types of Eagle syndrome.

More recently (2017), a group of Dutch researchers [10] proposed a "revisit" of the development of the hyoid-laryngeal complex. By applying three-dimensional (3D) study techniques to histological sections of human embryos, they developed a simplified theory compared to the classical one, regarding the morphogenesis of the branchial system. They replaced the conventional scheme, which envisages a five-arch system (Fig. 6.9), with a simplified three-arch scheme.

Only the first three pharyngeal arch cartilages develop as pharyngeal arch cartilages. The thyroid and cricoid cartilages develop separately from each other from mesenchymal condensations.

The body of the hyoid bone develops from one growth center (anlage), without the contribution of the second and third pharyngeal arch cartilages (Fig. 6.10).

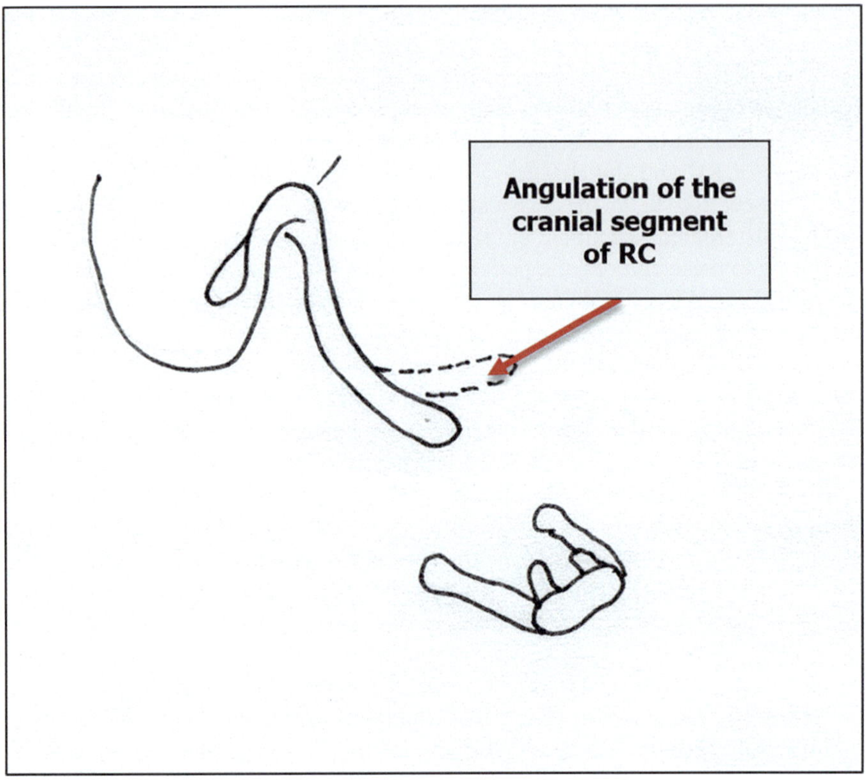

Fig. 6.5 In these cases, the tip of the caudal end had a close contact with the glossopharyngeal nerve as well as the pharyngeal wall

The authors "observed a less complicated development of the hyoid-larynx complex from only the second and third pharyngeal arch cartilages, in combination with a single hyoid body anlage. The fourth and sixth pharyngeal arch cartilages, which were expected to give rise to the thyroid and cricoid cartilages, were not observed as cartilaginous bars. Instead, the thyroid and cricoid were immediately discernible as mesenchymal condensations in the neck region, without being preceded in their development by a cartilaginous bar."

Based on these findings, they proposed a true "3D flow chart" summarizing the stages of embryonic development of the hyoid-laryngeal complex (Fig. 6.11).

The rapid morphogenesis of the hyoid-laryngeal complex can be summarized as follows: the hyoid body anlage develops in stage 18 (44–48 days), the greater horns (third pharyngeal arch cartilages) and thyroid cartilages develop in stage 19 (48–51 days), and the cricoid cartilage first arises in stage 20 (51–53 days). It takes approximately 55 days for the tracheal rings to develop.

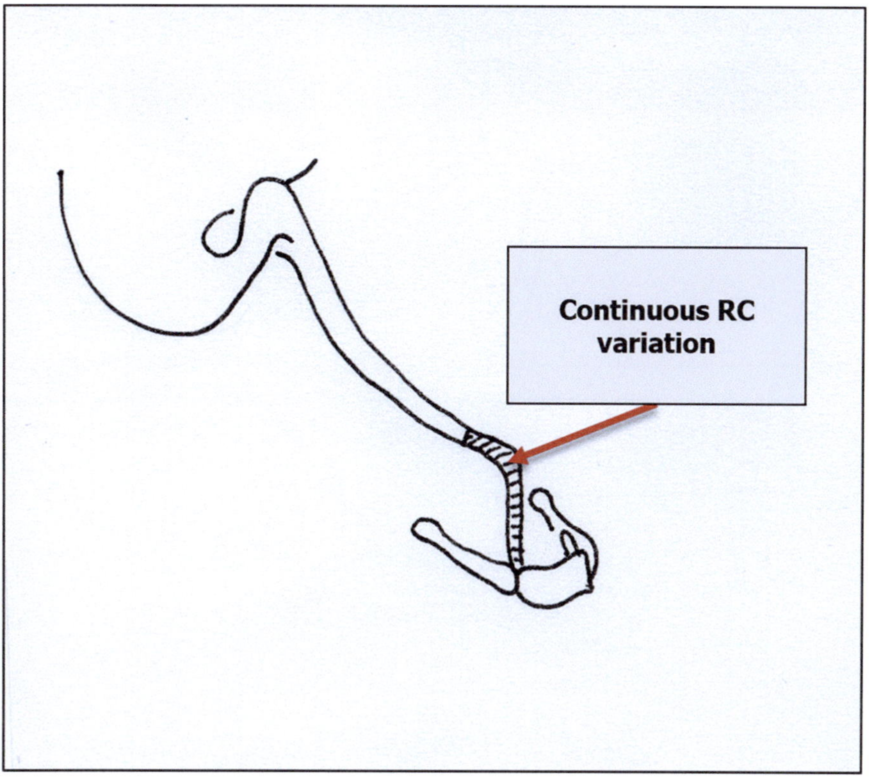

Fig. 6.6 Continuous RC variation

6.3.3 Current Knowledge in Molecular Embryology

These studies represent the state of the art in scientific and doctrinal knowledge of embryology. Specifically, models of craniofacial development in mice and zebrafish are studied to investigate the gene regulatory networks directing the patterning and osteochondrogenesis of the mandibular and hyoid arches, which are actually conserved among all gnathostomes [11]. The cited review is divided into three parts: the first part describes the anatomy and development of mandibular and hyoid arches in both species. The second part analyzes cell signaling and transcription factors that ensure the specificity of individual structures along the anatomical axes. The third part discusses the genes and molecules that control the formation of bone and cartilage within mandibular and hyoid arches and how dysregulation of molecular signaling influences the development of skeletal components of the viscerocranium (Fig. 6.12).

Despite the advancements, these contemporary studies continue to build upon the foundation of classical embryological morphology, drawing on its concepts and terminology (Table 6.2).

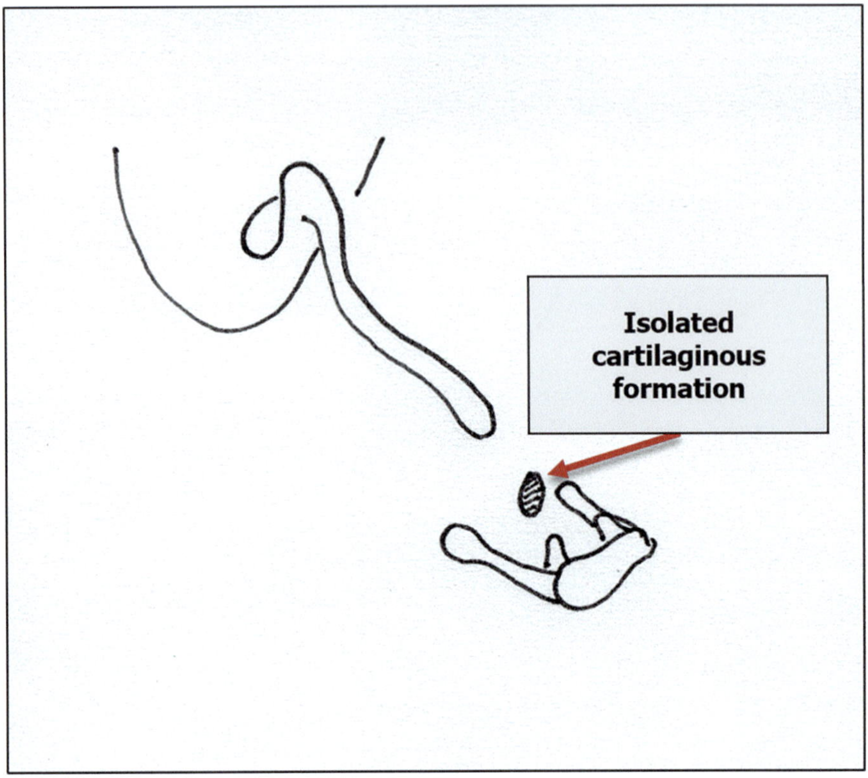

Fig. 6.7 Isolated cartilaginous formation

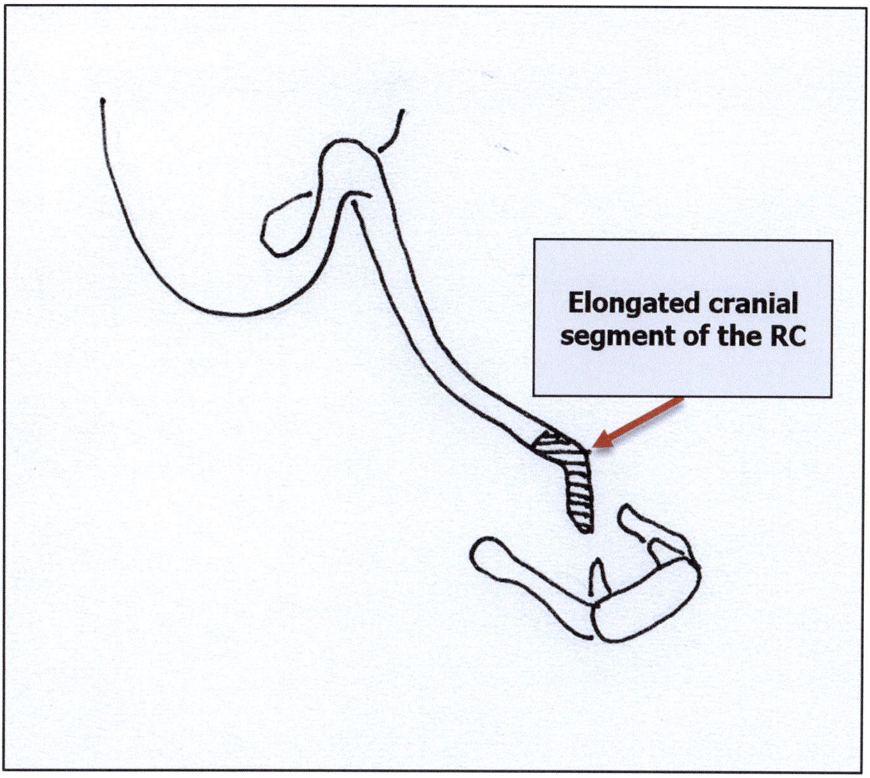

Fig. 6.8 The cranial segment of the RC is elongated, stretching almost to the cartilaginous hyoid. The lesser horns may be absent

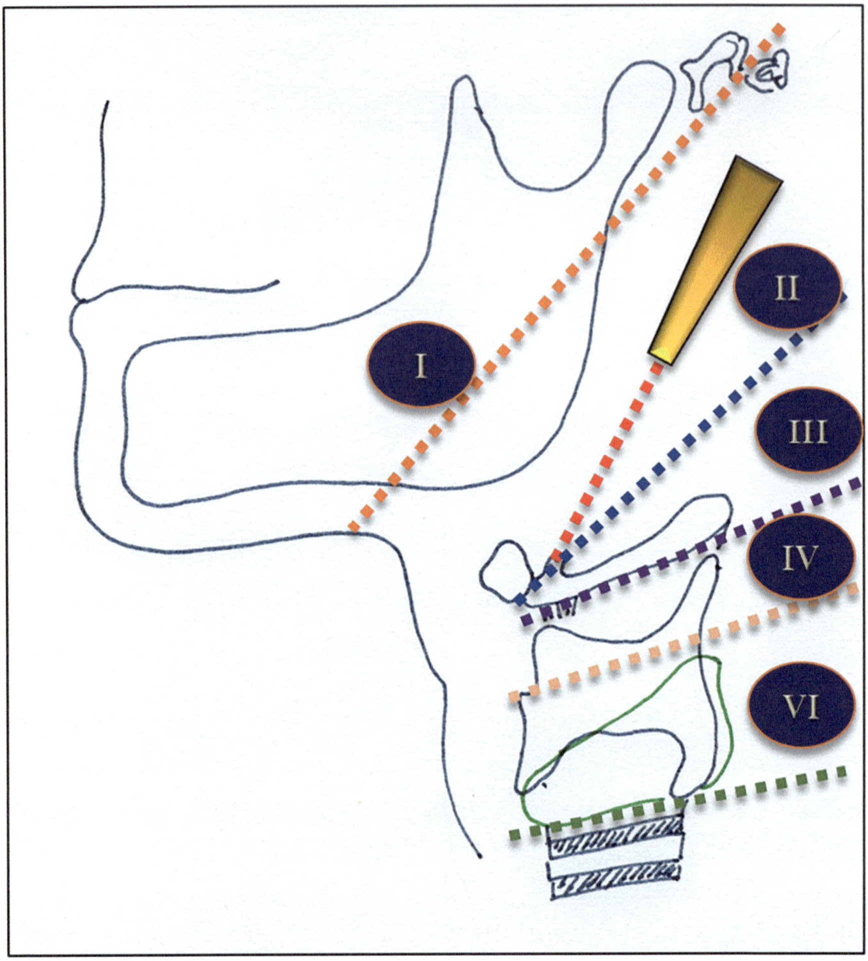

Fig. 6.9 Embryonic development of the hyoid-larynx complex. The current opinion of the division of the neck region in five pharyngeal arch zones, depicting the origin of each component of the hyoid-larynx complex

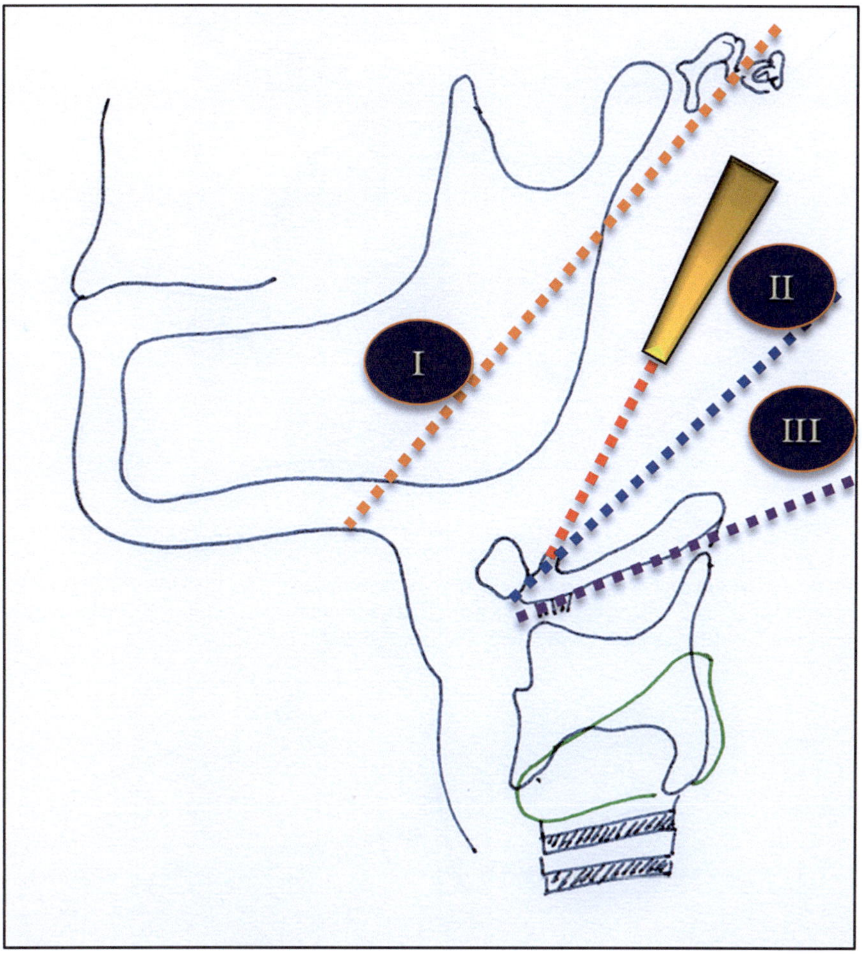

Fig. 6.10 Development of the hyoid-larynx complex from only the second and third pharyngeal arch cartilage, in combination with a single hyoid body anlage

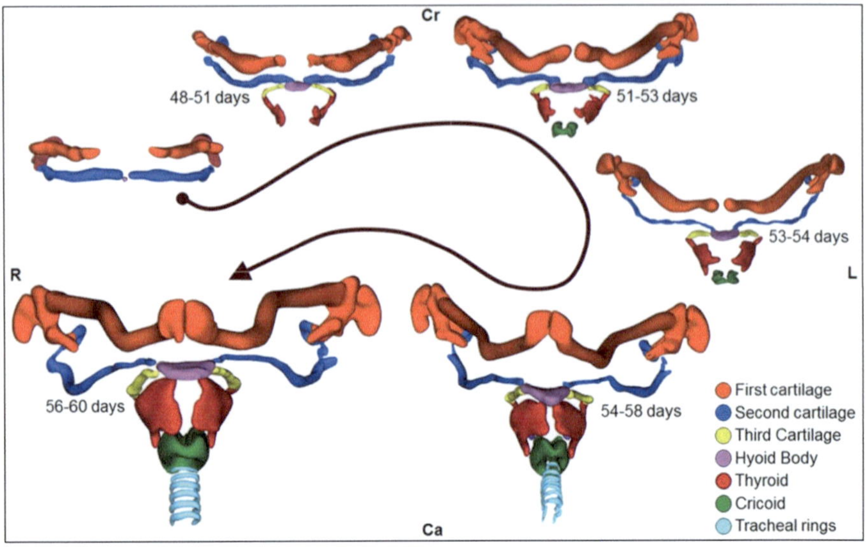

Fig. 6.11 The fundamental stages of the embryonic development of the hyoid-laryngeal complex are remarkably rapid, completing within a mere 10 days (from Bakker e coll. The development of the human hyoid-larynx complex revisited; The Laryngoscope, 2017 [10])

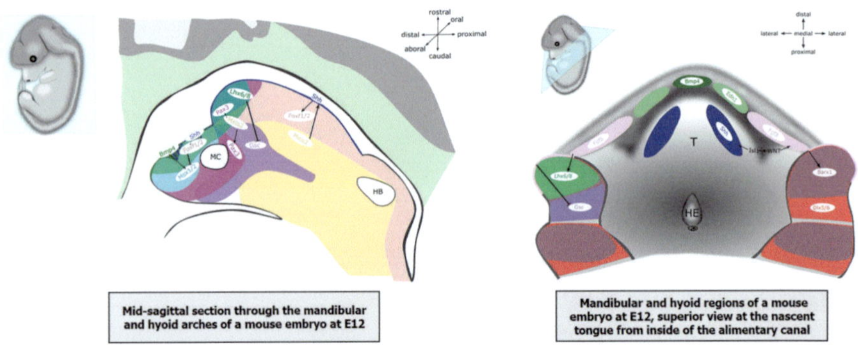

Fig. 6.12 Formation of bone and cartilage within mandibular and hyoid arches (modifications by Jaroslav Fabik, Viktorie Psutkova, and Ondrej Machon. The Mandibular and Hyoid Arches—From Molecular Patterning to Shaping Bone and Cartilage; Int J Mol Sci. 2021 Jul 14;22(14):7529)

Table 6.2 Skeletal derivatives of pharyngeal arches in the mouse and zebrafish

Viscerocranium	Mouse		Zebrafish	
	Cartilaginous	Membranous	Cartilaginous	Membranous
First pharyngeal arch (the mandibular)	Palatoquadrate cartilage: Alisphenoid Incus	Premaxilla Maxilla Zygomatic bone Temporal squama	Palatoquadrate Cartilage: Quadrate Metapterygoids Palatines	Premaxilla Maxilla Ectopterygoid Entopterygoid
	Meckel's cartilage: Mandibular symphysis Lingula of the mandible Sphenomandibular ligament Spine of sphenoid Anterior ligament of malleus Malleus	Dentary bone	Meckel's cartilage: Retroarticular	Dentary Anguloarticular Coronomeckelian
Second pharyngeal arch (the hyoid)	Stapes Styloid process of the temporal bone Stylohyoid ligament Lesser horns of the hyoid bone		Basihyal Ceratohyal Epihyal Hypohyal Hyomandibula Interhyal Symplectic	Urohyals Branchiostegal rays Interopercle Opercles Preopercles Subopercles
Third pharyngeal arch	Greater horns of the hyoid bone		Basibranchials Ceratobranchials Epibranchials Hypobranchials Pharyngobranchials	

6.4 Conclusion

The embryology of the stylohyoid complex is a complex topic that continues to be investigated. Classical embryological principles remain essential for understanding this region and form the basis for modern research, bridging the gap between basic science and clinical practice.

References

1. Dwight T. Stylo-hyoid ossification. Ann Surg. 1907;46(5):721–35. https://doi.org/10.1097/00000658-190711000-00010.
2. Watt W. Eagle; Elongated styloid process. Arch Otolaryngol. 1937;25:584–7.
3. Weissengruber GE, Forstenpointner G, Peters G, Kubber-Heiss A, Fitch WT. Hyoid apparatus and pharynx in the lion (Panthera leo), jaguar (Panthera onca), tiger (Panthera tigris), cheetah (Acinonyxjubatus) and domestic cat (Felis silvestris f. catus). J Anat. 2002;201:195–209.

4. Nishimura T. Comparative morphology of the hyo-laryngeal complex in anthropoids: two steps in the evolution of the descent of the larynx. Primates. 2003;44:41–9.
5. Czako L, Simko K, Thurzo A, Galis B, Varga I. The syndrome of elongated styloid process, the eagle's syndrome-from anatomical, evolutionary and embryological backgrounds to 3D printing and personalized surgery planning. Report of five cases; Medicina (Kaunas). 2020;56(9):458. https://doi.org/10.3390/medicina56090458.
6. Revilla Borjas C, Stuyt MT. El sindrome estiloideo: a proposito de 3 casos. In: Annales de Otorrinolaringologia Iberoamericana; 1989. p. 659–66.
7. Rodríguez-Vázquez JF, Mérida-Velasco JR, Verdugo-López S, Sánchez-Montesinos I, Mérida-Velasco JA. Morphogenesis of the second pharyngeal arch cartilage (Reichert's cartilage) in human embryos. J Anat. 2006;208:179–89.
8. Rodríguez-Vázquez JF, Kim JH, Verdugo-Lopez S, Murakami G, Cho KH, Asakawa S, Abe S-i. Human fetal hyoid body origin revisited. J Anat. 2011;219:143–9.
9. Rodriguez-Vazquez JF, Verdugo-Lopez S, Abe H, Murakami G. The origin of the variations of the hyoid apparatus in human. Anat Rec. 2015;298:1395–407.
10. de Bakker BS, de Bakker HM, Soerdjbalie-Maikoe V, Dikkers FG. The development of the human hyoid-larynx complex revisited. Laryngoscope. 2018;128(8):1829–34. https://doi.org/10.1002/lary.26987. Epub 2017 Dec8
11. Fabik J, Psutkova V, Machon O. The mandibular and hyoid arches-from molecular patterning to shaping bone and cartilage. Int J Mol Sci. 2021;22(14):7529. https://doi.org/10.3390/ijms22147529.

"Normal" Clinical Anatomy of the Styloid Complex and Anatomical Variants of the Stylohyoid-Laryngeal Complex

7

Elio Maria Cunsolo, Alberto Caranti, Ruggero Campisi, Stefano Pelucchi, Chiara Bianchini, and Claudio Vicini

7.1 Introduction

The clinical anatomy relevant to understanding Eagle syndrome is quite complex due to the "irregular" morphology of the lateral base of the skull, to which it belongs, and to the important visceral, vascular, and neural relationships that derive from it. These basic problems are exacerbated by the great morphological and dimensional variability of the stylohyoid complex, a variability linked to the articulated embryology of this anatomical-functional unit. Therefore, the basic and topographic anatomy of the stylohyoid complex and the systematization of its morphological variants will be considered, with particular attention to those that represent the anatomical substrate of Eagle syndrome.

E. M. Cunsolo (✉)
Policlinico di Modena, Modena, MO, Italy

A. Caranti · R. Campisi · C. Vicini
University of Ferrara, Cona, FE, Italy
e-mail: claudio@claudiovicini.com

S. Pelucchi
ENT & Audiology Unit, Department of Neurosciences, University Hospital of Ferrara, Ferrara, Italy
e-mail: stefano.pelucchi@unife.it

C. Bianchini
ENT & Audiology Unit, University Hospital of Ferrara, Cona, FE, Italy
e-mail: chiara.bianchini@unife.it

C. Vicini et al. (eds.), *EAGLE Syndrome*,
https://doi.org/10.1007/978-3-031-92829-1_7

7.2 "Normal" Human Anatomy of the Styloid Complex

The styloid process is a long, thin prominence emerging from the inferior surface of the skull base. Although typically straight, it is occasionally curved. Its attachment is anterior and medial to the mastoid process, lateral to the jugular foramen, posterior and lateral to the carotid canal orifice, and immediately anterior and slightly medial to the stylomastoid foramen [1, 2] (Fig. 7.1).

The relationship of the styloid process to the jugular foramen and carotid canal orifice is crucial to the ultimate pathophysiology of Eagle syndrome (Fig. 7.2).

Two ligaments attach to the styloid process: the stylohyoid and stylomandibular ligaments. The stylohyoid ligament is attached to the tip of the styloid process and extends to the lesser cornu of the hyoid bone. Stylohyoid and stylomandibular ligaments help to regulate the movements of the mandible, the hyoid bone, the tongue, and the pharynx. Many important anatomic structures are closely located to the styloid process and the stylohyoid ligament. Lateral to the styloid process, one finds the facial and hypoglossal nerves, the occipital artery, and the posterior belly of the digastric muscle. The facial nerve emerges from the stylomastoid foramen posteriorly and passes laterally through the parotid gland. Medial to the styloid process (from posterior to anterior), the internal jugular vein (with the accessory, hypoglossal, vagus, and glossopharyngeal nerves) and the internal carotid artery are seen. The superior constrictor muscle and the pharyngobasilar fascia are situated medially to the tip of the styloid process and adjacent to the tonsillar fossa. The styloid process begins to ossify at the end of pregnancy and continues to undergo calcification over the first 8 years of life. The ossification time and degree of ossification vary greatly. The length and direction of the styloid process and styloid chain (styloid process, styloid ligaments, styloid musculature) are highly variable. This

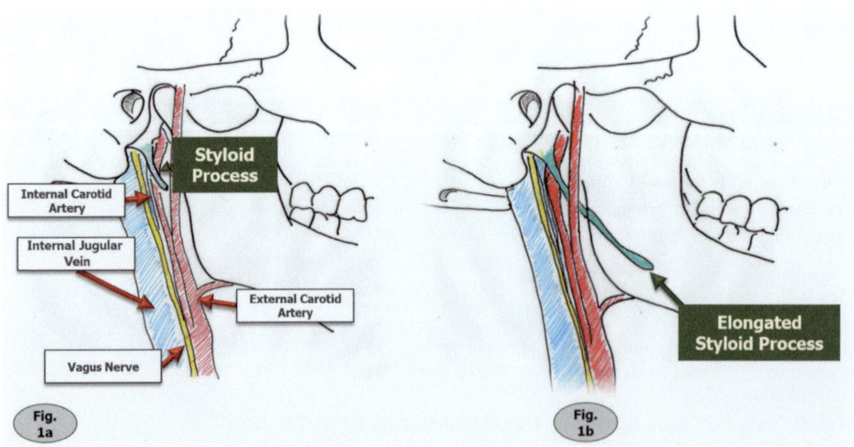

Fig. 7.1 Normal anatomy of the styloid process (Fig. **1a**). Elongated styloid process as found in patients with Eagle syndrome (Fig. **1b**)

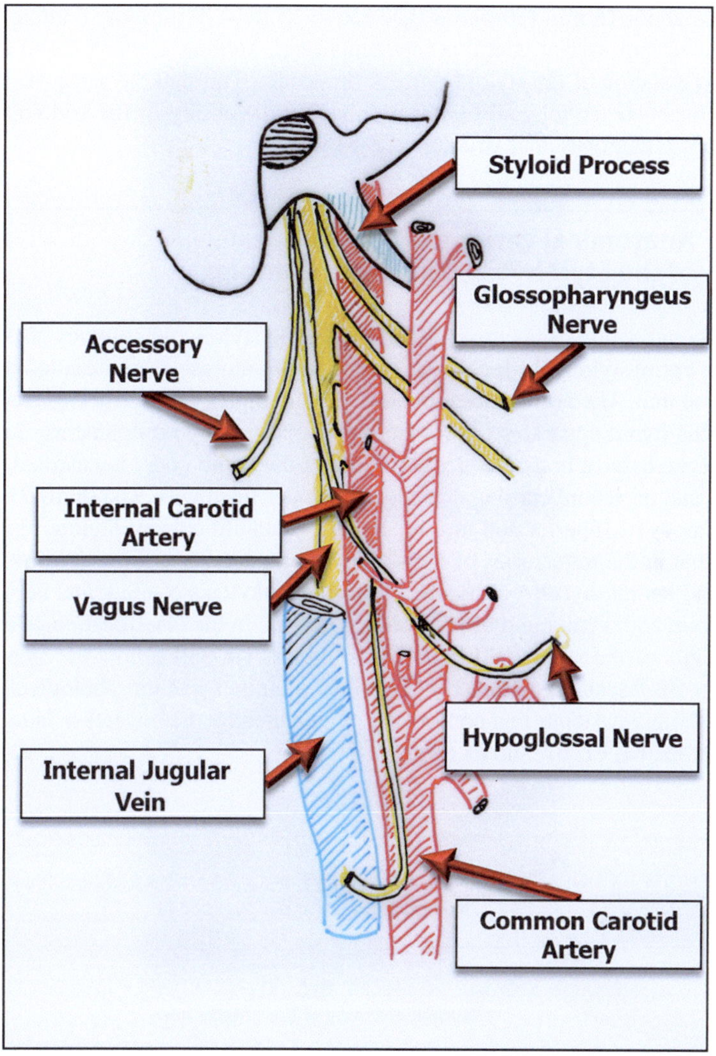

Fig. 7.2 Styloid process anatomy. From posterior to anterior are located the internal jugular vein (with the accessory, hypoglossal, vagus, and glossopharyngeal nerves) and the internal carotid artery

variability leads to a wide range of relationships between the chain and the aforementioned neurovascular elements of the neck [1–3]. The mean length of the styloid process ranges from 21 mm to 29.5 mm. By consensus, a styloid process longer than 30 mm confers an increased risk of Eagle syndrome. A longer styloid process confers greater translational capacity at its distal end, increasing the risk of adjacent neurovascular compromise. Consider the simple example of mild neck extension, during which about 30 degrees of angular motion is generated in the tip of the styloid process. If the length of the styloid process is 30 mm, then the tip movement measures about 15 mm (30 mm × 0.52 rad ≈ 15 mm). With more complex movements involving medial-lateral components (e.g., holding a telephone to the ear), further translation of the styloid process tip occurs. Through the same mechanism, elongation of the stylohyoid ligament enhances the ability of the styloid chain to compromise neurovascular structures [1–3].

7.3 Anatomical Variants of the Stylohyoid-Laryngeal Complex

The systematization of anatomical variants of the stylohyoid complex should consider the entire stylohyoid-laryngeal system, which represents a true anatomical and functional unit. The normal adult hyoid-larynx complex is described as a combination of the hyoid apparatus (i.e., styloid process, stylohyoid ligaments, and lesser horns of the hyoid); body and greater horns of the hyoid bone; uncalcified thyroid, cricoid, and arytenoid cartilages; and their proper ligaments. The thyroid cartilage encompasses its superior and inferior horns. No additional cartilaginous structures are present in the trajectories of the stylohyoid ligaments, median thyrohyoid ligament, and lateral thyrohyoid ligaments, and no ankylosis of the joints between the hyoid body and greater and/or lesser horns occurs. In the classification of anatomical variants of the stylohyoid-laryngeal complex, we will follow the system proposed by BS Backer et al. in 2019 [4], which identifies five morphological classes, starting from a basic normal conformation indicated by the lowercase letters of the alphabet: a1, b1, c1, d1, and e1 (Fig. 7.3).

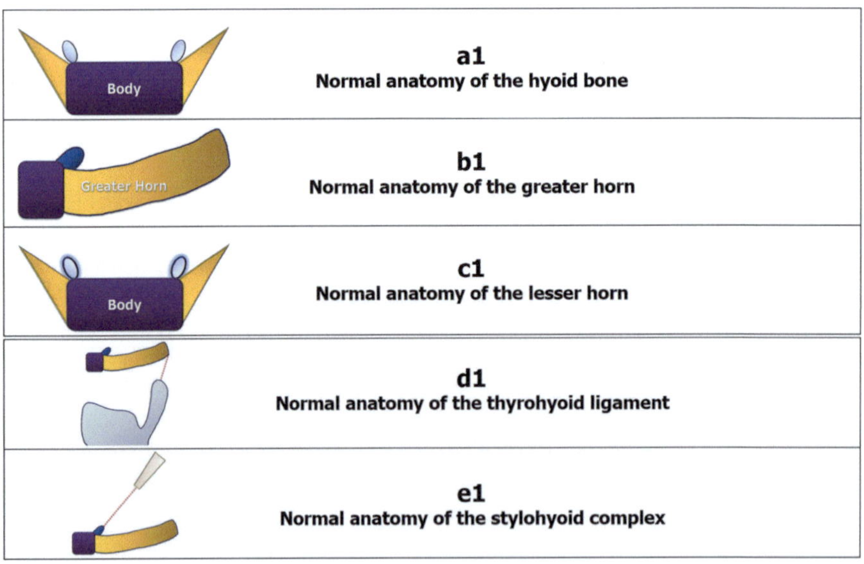

Fig. 7.3 Normal anatomy of the stylohyoid-laryngeal complex [4]

It is evident that, for the purpose of systematizing the morphological picture of Eagle syndrome, the anatomical class of interest is e1.

In the following figures, the main morphological variations of the stylohyoid-laryngeal complex will be schematized (Fig. 7.4), reserving a detailed description for the variations of class e1 (Figs. 7.5 and 7.6).

The anomalies of "class e" are those strictly involved in the determination of Eagle syndrome. The adopted classification [4] refers to the concepts and terminology of classical embryology [5, 6], which are recalled here (Fig. 7.6).

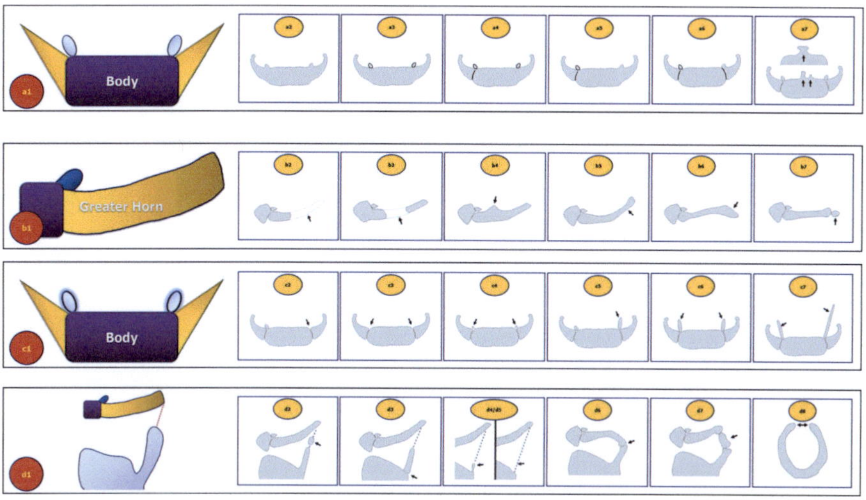

Fig. 7.4 Anatomical variants of classes a, b, c, and d, indicated for each subsite with increasing numerical values

Fig. 7.5 Classical embryological concept and terminology of the stylohyoid complex

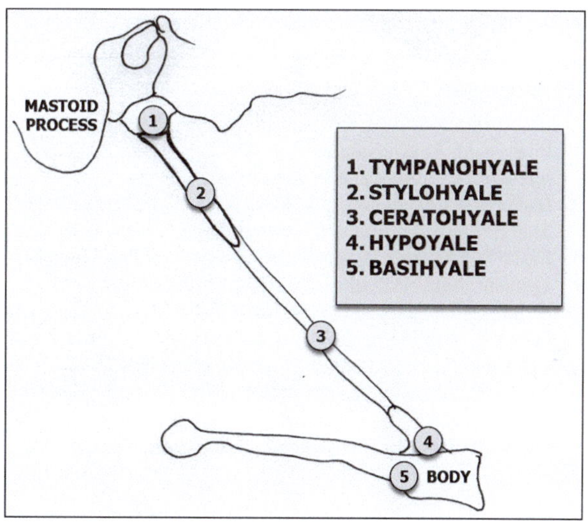

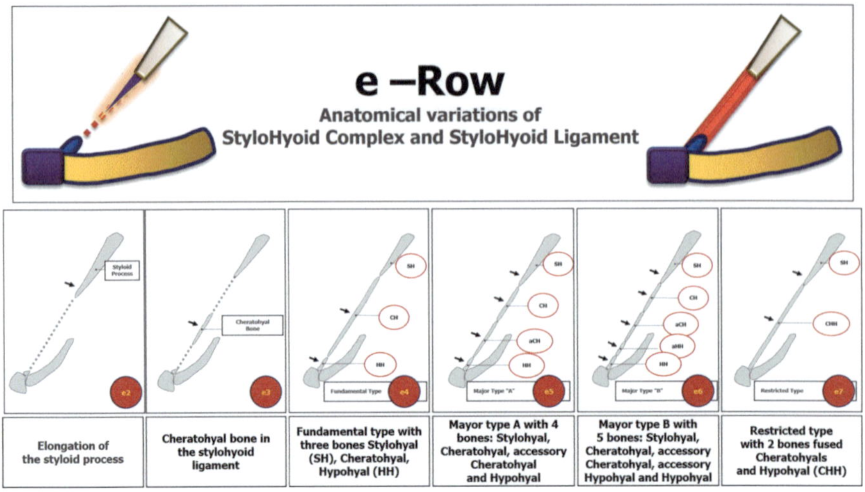

Fig. 7.6 Lateral view on variations of stylohyoid complex and stylohyoid ligament

In Fig. 7.6, the main anatomical variations of the stylohyoid complex are schematized.

7.4 Conclusions

These notes confirm the complex anatomy of the stylohyoid complex and, even more so, the resulting pathogenetic problems. The proposed classification system is based on concepts and terminology derived from "classical" embryology, which may be obsolete when compared to current hyper-specialized doctrinal knowledge, but which maintain an undoubted utility in clinical practice.

References

1. Piagkou M, Anagnostopoulou S, Kouladouros K, Piagkos G. Eagle's syndrome: a review of the literature. Clin Anat. 2009;22:545–58.
2. Badheya A, Jategaonkara A, Kovacsb AJA, Kadakiaa S, De Deync PP, Ducicd Y, Schantza S, Shin E. Eagle syndrome: a comprehensive review. Clin Neurol Neurosurg. 2017;159:34–8.
3. Fusco DJ, Asteraki S, Spetzler RF. Eagle's syndrome: embryology, anatomy, and clinical management. Acta Neurochir. 2012;154:1119–26.
4. de Bakker BS, de Bakker HM, Soerdjbalie-Maikoe V, Dikkers FG. Variants of the hyoid-larynx complex, with implications for forensic science and consequence for the diagnosis of eagle's syndrome. Sci Rep. 2019;9(1):15950. https://doi.org/10.1038/s41598-019-52476-z.
5. Olivier E. Lappareil Hyoıdien. Son ossification comple'te chez l'homme. Paris: Libraire Louis Arnette; 1923.
6. Dwight T. Stylo-hyoid ossification. Ann Surg. 1907;46:721–35.

Surgical Anatomy Pearls

8

Claudio Vicini, Pierfrancesco Bettini, Alberto Caranti, Ruggero Campisi, and Chiara Bellini

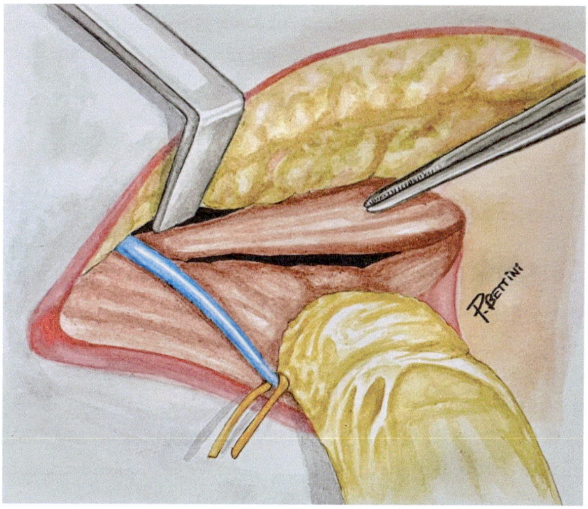

The foundations of the anatomical knowledge are laid at the beginning of the medical study. Anatomy remains an important part of the knowledge of operations throughout training as a specialist. ***Even after that, surgeons will need anatomical knowledge time and time again if they wish to adopt a new procedure or a variant of an existing procedure.*** *Prof Dr Theo Wiggers Jan 18, 2021*

C. Vicini (✉) · P. Bettini · A. Caranti · R. Campisi
University of Ferrara, Cona, FE, Italy
e-mail: claudio@claudiovicini.com; pierfrancesco.bettini@unife.it

C. Bellini
Morgagni-Pierantoni Hospital, Forlì, FC, Italy

C. Vicini et al. (eds.), *EAGLE Syndrome*,
https://doi.org/10.1007/978-3-031-92829-1_8

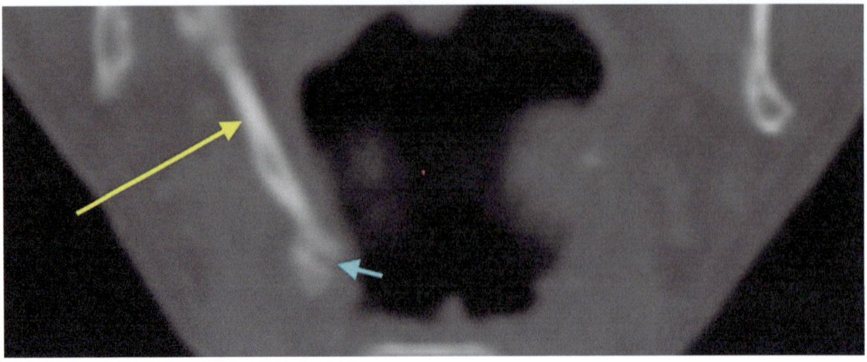

Fig. 8.1 Monolateral pathological elongation of the styloid process. The yellow arrow depicts the long distance of the superior half of the styloid bone from the neck skin. The light blue arrow points out the small distance between styloid process tip and pharyngeal wall

The study of the structure and morphological features of the tissues and organs of the body that are related to surgery is defined as surgical anatomy. In the special case of ES surgery, surgical anatomy must be considered as the description and discussion of the different anatomical structures that are encountered inside the surgical field during the progression of the surgical dissection from the mucosal or skin surface to the depth targeting the elongated styloid as the final goal of any procedure. Some anatomical structures are landmarks to be followed for keeping the best and most safe way. Some other must be recognized to be spared in order to avoid possible complications. Last but not least, some crucial structures (jugular vein, carotid artery, etc.) must be kept in mind even if immediately around the surgical pathway and not strictly in sight inside the dissection field for their importance in case of unaware damage. In the next pages, we will focus into the styloidectomy surgical procedures for classic Eagle syndrome. Two different surgical anatomies will be discussed in comparison: the anatomy of the external route and the anatomy of the internal route. Anatomical pearls will be described and summarized as "take-home messages" (THM) in order to simplify the reader for keeping that in mind.

In Fig. 8.1 is shown a TC slice of a monolateral ES. Some of the main differential anatomical features of the open route vs the transoral route is evident at a glance. The longer pointing up arrow depicts the long distance of the superior half of the styloid bone from the neck skin. The smaller arrow offers an immediate perception of the reduced distance between the pharyngeal wall and the inferior tip of the styloid bone in the transoral approach.

8.1 THM No. 1

Transoral approach allows a less extensive tissue dissection than open approach [1, 2].

8.2 THM No. 2

Due to its medial inclination, the styloid is encountered at its lower aspect in transoral approach and in its superior aspect in external route. In Fig. 8.2 is schematically reproduced the anatomical relations between the styloid complex (styloid bone, stylohyoid ligament, and styloid muscle bundle), posterior belly of the digastric muscle, and neck jugular-carotid axis [3, 4]. The main issue is that the plane of the elongated styloid is lateral to the major vascular axis [5]. Point number 2: the stylohyoid bundle intersects jugular vein superficially in a somehow oblique way [6]. The external carotid artery is more anteriorly located than the internal one and may intersect the styloid bundle on its external surface or sometimes inside the bundle [7]. A couple of medium-sized arteries (occipital and posterior auricular, average diameter of 4.0 mm, range 3.8–4.2 mm and 0.7–1.2 mm, respectively) run in a parallel way along the digastric and styloid bundle complex in strict relation to them branching posteriorly from the external carotid artery [8]. Occipital artery travels in a supero-posterior direction, deep (and parallel) to the posterior belly of the digastric muscle. The posterior auricular artery arises from the external carotid artery at the level of the styloid process tip. It travels in a superior direction, passing between the parotid gland (anterior) and the styloid process (posterior).

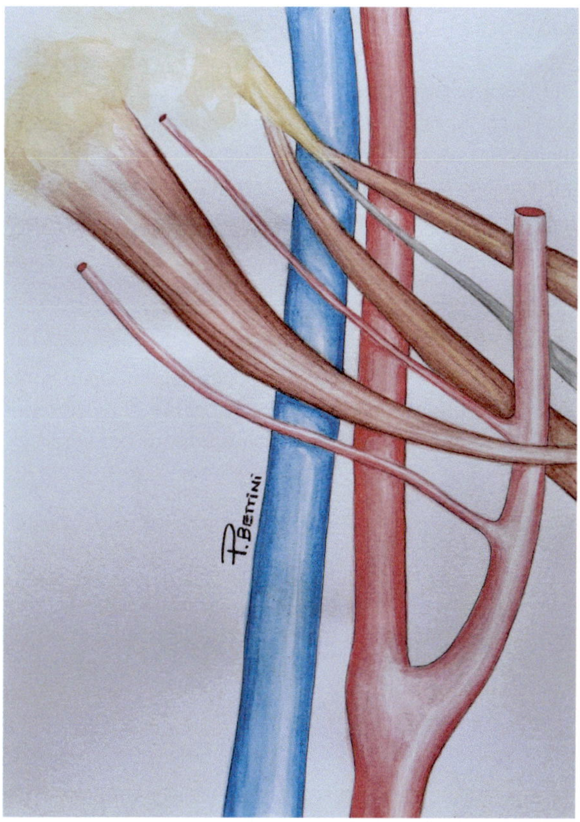

Fig. 8.2 Schematic representation of the styloid process and its anatomical relations with surrounding muscles, nerves, and vessels

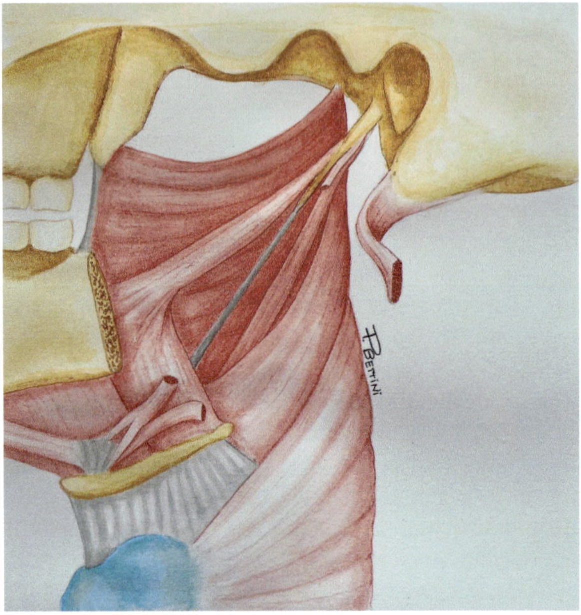

Fig. 8.3 An external view of superior pharyngeal constrictor and its direct relationships with the stylohyoid complex

8.3 THM No. 3

In the same way of the homo-hyoid muscle in the lower neck, in our surgical area, the posterior belly of the digastric muscle overlies the jugular-carotid axis and warns the surgeon about the course of the major vessels below the upper third of the digastric muscle. On the other hand, in the internal approach, the transoral route finds the major vessels first and styloid in the depth (Fig. 8.3).

8.4 THM No. 4

The external carotid artery is encountered in open surgery more inferiorly along the posterior belly of the digastric muscle but in more superficial plane where it must be identified and spared. It is not an issue for transoral approach.

8.5 THM No. 5

The occipital artery is identified at the inferior or posterior surface of the digastric muscle and retracted superiorly in the cervical approach.

8.6 THM No. 6

The posterior auricular artery is usually found in strict relations with the styloid muscle and if necessary ligated and cut.

Fig. 8.4 The facial nerve crosses the lateral aspect of the styloid process in its superior portion close to the skull base

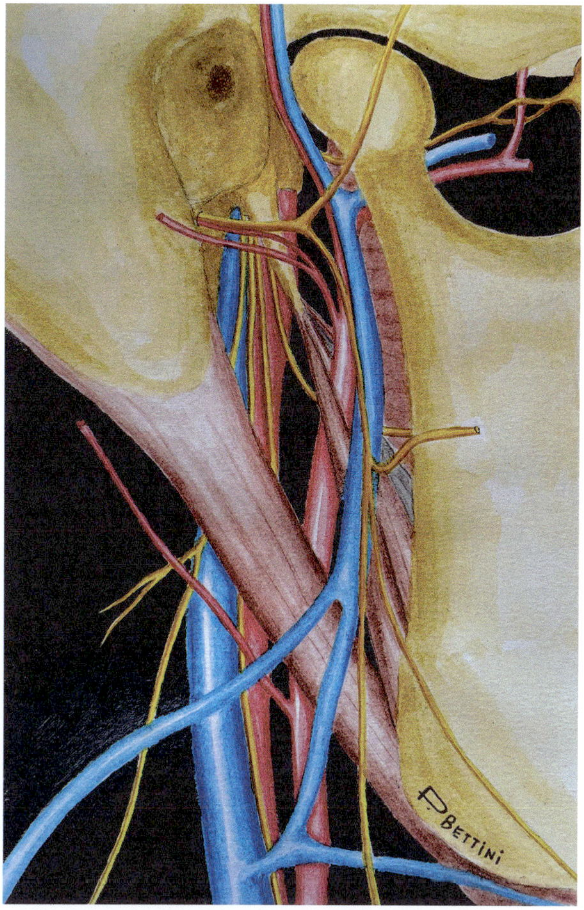

8.7 THM No. 7

The facial nerve crosses lateral to the styloid process and medial to the posterior belly of the digastric muscle. The crossing point is close to the origin of the styloid process (Fig. 8.4).

In case of total resection of the styloid process, keep in mind the position of the facial nerve trunk on the lateral aspect of the styloid.

References

1. Fitzpatrick TH 4th, Lovin BD, Magister MJ, Waltonen JD, Browne JD, Sullivan CA. Surgical management of eagle syndrome: a 17-year experience with open and transoral robotic styloidectomy. Am J Otolaryngol. 2020;41(2):102324. https://doi.org/10.1016/j.amjoto.2019.102324.
2. Wang J, Liu Y, Wang ZB, Yan KS. Intraoral and extraoral approach for surgical treatment of eagle's syndrome: a retrospective study. Eur Arch Otorrinolaringol. 2022;279(3):1481–7. https://doi.org/10.1007/s00405-021-06914-2.

3. Mantovani G, Zangrossi P, Flacco ME, Di Domenico G, Nastro Siniscalchi E, De Ponte FS, Maugeri R, De Bonis P, Cavallo MA, Zamboni P, Scerrati A. Styloid jugular nutcracker: the possible role of the styloid process spatial orientation-a preliminary morphometric computed study. Diagnostics (Basel). 2023;13(2):298. https://doi.org/10.3390/diagnostics13020298.
4. Buono U, Mangone GM, Michelotti A, Longo F, Califano L. Surgical approach to the stylohyoid process in eagle's syndrome. J Oral Maxillofac Surg. 2005;63(5):714–6. https://doi.org/10.1016/j.joms.2004.10.013.
5. Müderris T, Bercin S, Sevil E, Beton S, Kırıs M. Surgical management of elongated styloid process: intraoral or transcervical? Eur Arch Otorrinolaringol. 2014;271(6):1709–13. https://doi.org/10.1007/s00405-013-2664-0.
6. Jayaraman MV, Boxerman JL, Davis LM, Haas RA, Rogg JM. Incidence of extrinsic compression of the internal jugular vein in unselected patients undergoing CT angiography. AJNR Am J Neuroradiol. 2012;33(7):1247–50. https://doi.org/10.3174/ajnr.A2953.
7. de Barros JF, Rodrigues MV, Barroso LA, Amado IC. Eagle syndrome: an underdiagnosed cause of orofacial pain. BMJ Case Rep. 2021;14(1):e238161. https://doi.org/10.1136/bcr-2020-238161.
8. Breda D, Ferreira S, Colino M, Cerqueira É, Amado I. Recurrent syncope related to carotid compression in eagle syndrome: a case report. Cureus. 2023;15(9):e45134. https://doi.org/10.7759/cureus.45134.

Stylohyoid Complex Imaging

9

Giorgio Mantovani, Paolo Zamboni, and Alba Scerrati

Imaging of the stylohyoid complex (SHC) is all about untangling the relationship between the bony components (the styloid process (SP) and the hyoid bone) and their surrounding structures such as muscles, ligaments, arteries, veins, and nerves. Given the mostly unknown nature of the precise boundary between physiological variations and pathology, imaging must always be integrated with a careful clinical evaluation. Classically, by consensus, a bony SP longer than 30 mm could be considered pathological, but, for example, a recent review found that an elongated SP can be found in up to 30.2% of the general asymptomatic population, without correlation with sex, age, or geography [1]. Increasing evidences in the last years prove that SP length is not the only important element in SHC pathologies. Also, it must be kept in mind that SHC is located in one of the most mobile segments of the human body, and head position greatly influences the relations of its different components. In a physiological range of movement, during a neck extension, the tip of the styloid process shows around 30 degrees of angular motion, and considering a styloid process length of 30 mm, then the tip movement measures about 15 mm [2, 3]. From this consideration comes the importance of functional and dynamic imaging (such as ultrasonography, angiography, and venogram) alongside with static and purely anatomical ones.

G. Mantovani · A. Scerrati (✉)
Neurosurgery Department, University of Ferrara, Cona, FE, Italy
e-mail: giorgi01.mantovani@edu.unife.it; alba.scerrati@unife.it

P. Zamboni
Vascular Diseases Center, University of Ferrara, Cona, FE, Italy
e-mail: zambo@unife.it

C. Vicini et al. (eds.), *EAGLE Syndrome*,
https://doi.org/10.1007/978-3-031-92829-1_9

9.1 X-Ray

A panoramic radiography (PR) often constitutes the first level of imaging for Eagle syndrome (ES), thus prompting further exams. Other monoplanar projections to determine the dimensions of SP include the lateral cephalograms, lateral views of the neck, and posterior-anterior views of the skull that are nowadays mostly abandoned in favor of multiplanar techniques.

Comparative studies recently showed that SHC measurements on PR have a high correlation with CT ones, assessing then the reliability of this method [4]. Even though, in PR, the structures located medially have higher magnification and distortion. For this reason there is an increased risk for measurement errors, especially when morphological variations are present.

Population-based studies using radiography give precious epidemiological information on prevalence and association of SHC ossification [5–8].

Most studies found that more than one-third of patients of the general population could present an elongated SP on PR and around 10% harbor SHC calcifications. Associations with increasing age and female sex are inconstant and sometimes contradictory between studies. Curiously, in the Spanish population is reported a prevalence of 72.75% of elongated SP (>30 mm), far higher than other similar studies [7].

Artificial intelligence (AI) algorithms have been developed to improve the accuracy and fasten the identification of elongated SP with high level of precision analyzing a standard PR [9].

It is to note that, in differential diagnosis of ES, a negative PR has no negative predictive value, since neurovascular impingement can come from muscular and tendinous structures such as non-ossified stylohyoid ligament and digastric muscle. In other words, a negative PR in a patient with suggestive symptoms doesn't exclude ES.

9.2 CT Scan

Computed tomography (CT) scan is considered the gold standard technique for SHC assessment giving precise information on SP length, calcification, angulation, and presence of anatomical variations. The main advantages of CT are that it overcomes the intrinsic limits of two-dimensional imaging, such as distortion, magnification, and superimposition of images while giving quantitative information on distance and relationship between the involved structures. 3D reconstruction for a better evaluation of structure relationship is possible.

In oral and maxillofacial surgery, classic CT scan is frequently replaced by cone-beam computed tomography (CBCT) that offers clinicians three-dimensional and multiplanar views for a more accurate diagnosis and treatment without the financial burden and radiation exposure of conventional CT.

The most common anatomical variations of SP reported in the literature are:

- Double (or triple) proximal origin.
- Segmentation (interruption of the cortical calcified profile).
- Bending of the lower end.
- Unilateral or bilateral absence (complete or partial) [10–13].

SP shape is usually scalariform with a large base and a thinner tip; other presentations are:

- Linear (constant thickness on the entire length).
- Moniliform (thin base and large tip).
- Pseudoduplicated.

Usual patterns of calcification include calcified outline and nodular complex; complete calcification is less frequent. The mean thickness of the SP is reported to be around 5 mm, with positive correlation with length [10].

Calcification of the stylohyoid ligament is found in around 13–15% of individuals, with occasional pseudo-articulation between the different segments up to rare cases of complete ossification of the SHC from the temporal bone to the hyoid.

In a comparative study, it has been found that the short distance of the SP tip from the tonsillar fossa (mean 12.7 mm in ES patients) was more strongly associated with ES than the SP length itself, thus suggesting that the distance to the tonsillar fossa may be a more appropriate diagnostic criterion for ES than SP length. This evidence is coherent with the hypothetical neural stretching pathogenesis of classic ES [14].

Spatial direction of the SP is another important factor in the genesis of SHC pathologies. Normally, the SP directs antero-inferiorly and medially from the base to the tip, thus forming one angle on the sagittal plane and one on the transverse (coronal) plane, respectively.

Quantification of these angles is a matter of debate in the literature, as different definition of the reference points from which take the measure led to different results, particularly for the sagittal angle:

- The angle between the long axis of the SP and the skull base line connecting the nasion and the opisthion (Chamberlain's line). Mean sagittal angle of 93.5° [13].
- The angle between the long axis of the SP and the skull base line connecting the anterior and posterior margins of the foramen magnum (basion to opisthion, McRae's line). Mean sagittal angle of 63.6° [10].
- The angle between the long axis of the SP and the skull base. Mean angle of 53.98° [15].
- The angle between the skull base and the long axis of the SHC. Mean angle 72.24° [16].

Generally, there is a consensus between studies that a narrow sagittal angle is more probably associated with pathogenic features, as several structures (such as the internal jugular vein, the internal carotid artery, and cranial nerves IX–XII) can be compressed between the SP and the cervical spine.

Also, the lateral-medial angle data in the literature are variable between 66.74° and 72.7° [13, 15]. The common reference line adopted is the one connecting the two temporal base of the SP. As for sagittal angle, it is intuitive that a narrow lateral-medial angulation could be implied in pathological constriction of neurovascular structure.

Recently, a semi-automatic software that processes CT images has been developed, giving quantitative information about distance and direction of the SP in a three-dimensional space [17]. Healthy controls were compared to patients suffering from styloid jugular nutcracker syndrome, and it has been found that the sagittal angle is more strongly associated with the disease than the SP length itself, confirming that the spatial direction of the SP is an essential feature in pathological conditions.

9.3 Advanced Imaging for Neurovascular Compression

To fully detail the functional relationship of the SHC different components with the surrounding structures, second- and third-level diagnostics are frequently required. Furthermore, dynamic imaging such as multi-position CT scan and ultrasonography are emerging techniques to investigate movement-related disorders.

9.3.1 Angio-CT Scan

A contrast-enhanced CT scan with arterial and venous acquisition shows vascular compression with the internal carotid artery (ICA) and the internal jugular vein (IJV), and it is nowadays considered essential in the diagnostic workup of the SHC pathologies.

The stylo-carotid syndrome is due to mechanical irritation of the sympathetic plexus around the ICA wall by an elongated or dysmorphic SP. The mean distance from the SP tip to the ICA has been measured at around 8.2 mm [18]. It is to note that the pressure on ICA can be due not only by the tip of SP but also from its medial deviation.

It is well known that SP elongation is a risk factor for spontaneous ICA dissection, a common cause of stroke in young adults and a non-negligible cause of mortality, probably underdiagnosed. A recent case-control study found that SP-ICA intercentric distance and SP-ICA marginal distance are positively correlated to ICA dissection [19]. Also, a comparative study found that the SP lateral-medial angle of patients suffering from ICA dissection tends to be more acute, with a shorter distance between the SP and the anterior arch of C1 [20].

Angio-CT scan is an essential tool also for venous pathology related to SHC.

Styloid jugular nutcracker (SJN) (aka styloidogenic-cervical spondylotic internal jugular venous compression, styloid-induced internal jugular vein stenosis, or

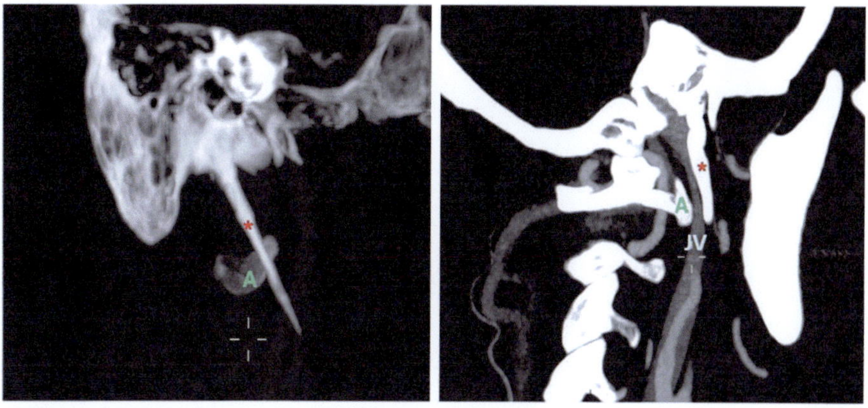

Fig. 9.1 CT and angio-CT scan showing the elongated styloid process (*) and its relationship with the arch of C1 (A) and the jugular vein (JV)

Eagle jugular syndrome) is caused by the compression of the IJV between the SP and the anterior arc of C1 [21] (Fig. 9.1).

It has been consistently linked to headache, tinnitus, and insomnia. Also, the IJV has been recognized to be a risk factor for idiopathic non-aneurismal subarachnoid hemorrhage (aka sine materia SAH) [22]. To evaluate the presence of SAH, a standard CT scan is performed, showing bleeding in the subarachnoid space. In the sine materia SAH, no vascular malformation is found at angio-CT scan. This same exam with venous phase acquisition is also required to properly assess the severity of IJV compression and it is recommended, together with Doppler ultrasound of the neck.

It has been reported that arterial and venous compression can be present at the same time, caused by a dysmorphic SHC. Sultan et al. report a case of a patient with SJN and an Eagle carotid variant syndrome with traumatic pseudoaneurysm of the ICA [23]. Patient complains of neck pain, dizziness, intermittent diplopia, right-sided headache, tinnitus, and eye bloating resolved after styloidectomy and ICA end-to-end anastomosis. 3D reconstruction can be useful for better understanding the spatial relationship between bony and vascular structures (Fig. 9.2).

Recently, a semi-automatic software that processes angio-CT images, giving quantitative information about the distance and direction of the styloid process in a three-dimensional space, was developed and applied in eight cases of Eagle jugular syndrome with good results [17].

9.3.2 Ultrasonography

Ultrasound examination of the neck is the most powerful tool to investigate the hemodynamic effect of SHC impingement on the arterial and venous vessels. A linear array probe with Doppler module is usually sufficient, with a vascular preset. Progressive adjustment of gain, depth, and focus is required to obtain good-quality images. All patients should be in a good hydration state, supine, and breathing

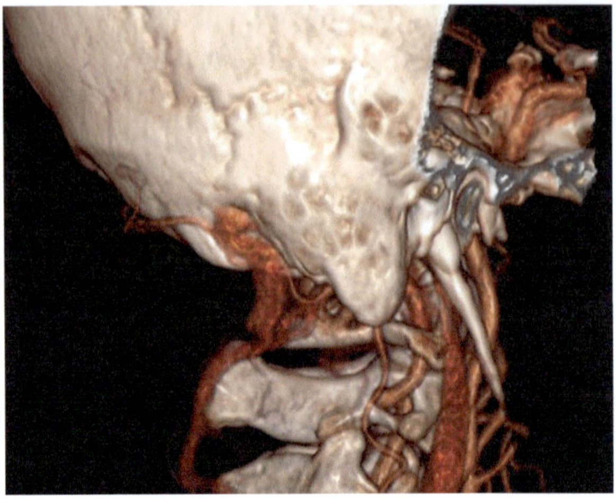

Fig. 9.2 3D reconstruction of angio-CT showing the relationship between the bony and vascular structures

normally through the nose. Valsalva maneuver can be useful to identify collapsed vein and differentiate between hypoplasia/agenesia and hypovolemia or stenosis.

Ideally, a complete examination should include three components:

1. Anatomical identification of landmark structures on B mode.

   Standard transverse and longitudinal sections of the infra-hyoid region are used to assess the ICA and the IJV (the two most caudal sections J2 and J3) in their carotid space together with the vagus nerve, infra-hyoid muscles (sternohyoid, omohyoid, sternothyroid, and thyrohyoid), sternocleidomastoid muscle, esophagus, trachea, and thyroid gland.

   Oblique coronal and oblique transverse sections are used to assess the contents of the supra-hyoid region, using the submandibular gland and the parotid gland (in the gap between the mastoid and the mandible ramus) and acoustic windows. In this crowdy space, it is possible to identify the SP with the attached muscles, the superior portion of ICA and IJV (J1), and the parapharyngeal space delimited by the air in the nasopharynx, the tonsils, and the mylohyoid, digastric, hyoglossus, genioglossus, and geniohyoid muscles. It has been proven that ultrasonography is a reliable method to assess the shape of the SP and its distance to the main structures involved in the SHC pathologies, namely, the ICA and the pharyngeal tonsils, compared to the CT scan [24].
2. Vascular flow assessment on Doppler mode.

   Color Doppler and spectral Doppler give, respectively, qualitative and quantitative information on the direction, velocity, and turbulence of the vascular flow into the ICA and IJV. To ensure a reliable measurement, a large amount of ultrasonic gel should be used to reach a complete coupling between the transducer and the patient's skin. Also, the insonation angle should be maintained between 45° and 60°. Pulsatility index (PI), peak systolic velocity (PSV), spectral broadening, and trickle flow are parameters that demonstrate the presence of a general stenosis in the vessel with augmented or turbulent flow. They are fundamental in

SHC pathologies to explore the external compression site and severity on ICA and IJV.

3. Dynamic imaging.

   Perhaps the most important aspect of ultrasound examination in SHC pathologies is the possibility to replicate the insonation with the head in different position. Generally, five positions are recommended: rest position, maximum extension, maximum flexion of the head, maximum right rotation, and maximum left rotation. However, the exam can be performed differently if the patient has a clear provoking position.

   This kind of procedure should be performed each time there is the possibility of a positional syndrome in the differential diagnosis, as it can reveal a hidden vascular variant of ES [25, 26]. Of course, a high index of suspicion is necessary a priori.

9.3.3 Magnetic Resonance Imaging

Magnetic resonance imaging (MRI) provides the anatomic details on soft tissue of the neck that usually lack in a CT scan. It is also a valuable method to assess the intracranial effects of a vascular variant of ES: diffusion sequences (DWI) can show even little areas of ischemia, and susceptibility-weighted imaging (SWI) is highly sensitive for micro-hemorrhages due to venous retrograde hypertension.

MRI angiography is the noninvasive gold standard to assess arterial vessel compression as it does not require contrast enhancement. On the other hand, phase-contrast techniques (e.g., 2D TOF MRV) give the possibility of a semi-quantitative venography, with or without contrast enhancement.

MRI is usually performed with the head in rest position. This can hide positional compression or impingement caused by the SHC components. It is possible to perform MRI in different head positions, as for ultrasonography, but its clinical application is challenging due to the long acquisition time needed.

9.3.4 Digital Subtraction Angiography and Venography

Direct arterial and venous visualization through invasive puncture remain the gold standard method to study neck vessel flow (Fig. 9.3).

On the other side, angiography does not give information on surrounding structures causing compression, and so it needs complementary diagnostic examinations.

Diversely from other diagnostic techniques, angiography also offers therapeutic possibility through the positioning of arterial and venous stenting, alone or as adjunctive treatment after surgery. However, the literature about stenting effectiveness is scarce and prospective studies are needed.

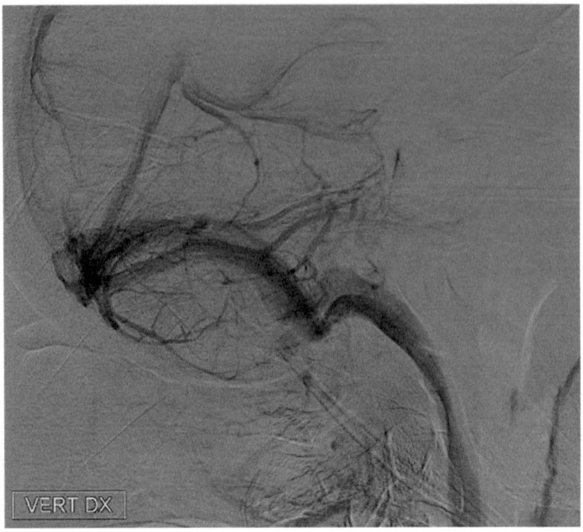

Fig. 9.3 DSA showing a reduction of left internal jugular vein flow in a patient suffering from Eagle jugular syndrome

References

1. Nogueira-Reis F, de Oliveira RL, Fontenele RC, Freitas DQ, Tabchoury CPM. Prevalence and features of elongated styloid process on imaging studies: a systematic review and meta-analysis. Clin Oral Investig. 2022;26(2):1199–215. https://doi.org/10.1007/s00784-021-04285-w.
2. Werne S. Studies in spontaneous atlas dislocation. Acta Orthop Scand Suppl. 1957;23:1–150.
3. H S. Anatomical and mechanical considerations of the atlantoaxial articulations. J Bone Joint Surg Am. 1968;50:1481–2.
4. Dudde F, Bergmann W, Schuck O, Schunk J, Barbarewicz F. Accuracy in the diagnostics of styloid process – panoramic radiograph vs. computed tomography: a comparative study. In Vivo. 2024;38(3):1390–6. https://doi.org/10.21873/invivo.13580.
5. Acikgoz A, Akkemik O. Prevalence and radiographic features of head and neck soft tissue calcifications on digital panoramic radiographs: a retrospective study. Cureus. 2023;15(9):e46025. https://doi.org/10.7759/cureus.46025.
6. Bruno G, De Stefani A, Balasso P, Mazzoleni S, Gracco A. Elongated styloid process: an epidemiological study on digital panoramic radiographs. J Clin Exp Dent. 2017;9(12):e1446–52. https://doi.org/10.4317/jced.54370.
7. Assiri Ahmed H, Estrugo-Devesa A, Roselló Llabrés X, Egido-Moreno S, López-López J. The prevalence of elongated styloid process in the population of Barcelona: a cross-sectional study & review of literature. BMC Oral Health. 2023;23(1):674. https://doi.org/10.1186/s12903-023-03405-0.
8. Vieira EMM, Guedes OA, Morais SD, Musis CRD, Albuquerque PAAD, Borges ÁH. Prevalence of elongated styloid process in a central Brazilian population. J Clin Diagn Res. 2015;9(9):ZC90–2. https://doi.org/10.7860/JCDR/2015/14599.6567.
9. Jeevitha SJ, Kumar SL, Yadalam PK. Artificial intelligence: a reliable tool to detect the elongation of the styloid process. Cureus. 2023;15(11):e49541. https://doi.org/10.7759/cureus.49541.
10. Ramadan SU, Gokharman D, Tunçbilek I, Kacar M, Koşar P, Kosar U. Assessment of the stylohoid chain by 3D-CT. Surg Radiol Anat. 2007;29(7):583–8. https://doi.org/10.1007/s00276-007-0239-8.
11. Ekici F, Tekbas G, Hamidi C, et al. The distribution of stylohyoid chain anatomic variations by age groups and gender: an analysis using MDCT. Eur Arch Otorrinolaringol. 2013;270(5):1715–20. https://doi.org/10.1007/s00405-012-2202-5.

12. Ayyildiz VA, Senel FA, Dursun A, Ozturk K. Morphometric examination of the styloid process by 3D-CT in patients with eagle syndrome. Eur Arch Otorrinolaringol. 2019;276(12):3453–9. https://doi.org/10.1007/s00405-019-05602-6.
13. Onbas O, Kantarci M, Murat Karasen R, et al. Angulation, length, and morphology of the styloid process of the temporal bone analyzed by multidetector computed tomography. Acta Radiol. 2005;46(8):881–6. https://doi.org/10.1080/02841850500335085.
14. Kent DT, Rath TJ, Snyderman C. Conventional and 3-dimensional computerized tomography in eagle's syndrome, glossopharyngeal neuralgia, and asymptomatic controls. Otolaryngol Head Neck Surg. 2015;153(1):41–7. https://doi.org/10.1177/0194599815583047.
15. Andrei F, Motoc AGM, Didilescu AC, Rusu MC. A 3D cone beam computed tomography study of the styloid process of the temporal bone. Folia Morphol (Warsz). 2013;72(1):29–35. https://doi.org/10.5603/fm.2013.0005.
16. Buyuk C, Gunduz K, Avsever H. Morphological assessment of the stylohyoid complex variations with cone beam computed tomography in a Turkish population. Folia Morphol (Warsz). 2018;77(1):79–89. https://doi.org/10.5603/FM.a2017.0061.
17. Mantovani G, Zangrossi P, Flacco ME, et al. Styloid jugular nutcracker: the possible role of the styloid process spatial orientation—a preliminary morphometric computed study. Diagnostics (Basel). 2023;13(2):298. https://doi.org/10.3390/diagnostics13020298.
18. Eraslan C, Ozer MA, Govsa F, Alagoz AK, Calli C. Relationship of stylohyoid chain and cervical internal carotid artery detected by 3D angiography. Surg Radiol Anat. 2017;39(8):897–904. https://doi.org/10.1007/s00276-017-1812-4.
19. Venturini G, Vuolo L, Pracucci G, et al. The proximity between styloid process and internal carotid artery as a possible risk factor for dissection: a case–control study. Neuroradiology. 2023;65(5):915–22. https://doi.org/10.1007/s00234-023-03121-0.
20. Tardivo V, Castaldi A, Baldino G, et al. Internal carotid artery dissection related to abnormalities of styloid process: is it only a matter of length? Neurol Sci. 2022;43(1):459–65. https://doi.org/10.1007/s10072-021-05350-8.
21. Zamboni P, Scerrati A, Menegatti E, et al. The eagle jugular syndrome. BMC Neurol. 2019;19(1):333. https://doi.org/10.1186/s12883-019-1572-3.
22. Scerrati A, De Bonis P, Zamboni P, et al. A new insight in nonaneurysmal subarachnoid hemorrhage: the potential role of the internal jugular veins. J Neurol Surg A Cent Eur Neurosurg. Published online October 22. 2021:s-0041-1733895. https://doi.org/10.1055/s-0041-1733895.
23. Sultan S, Acharya Y, Soliman O, Hynes N. Stylohyoid eagle syndrome and EXTracranial INternal carotid arTery pseudoaneurysms (EXTINCT) with internal jugular vein nutcracker syndrome: a challenging clinical scenario. BMJ Case Rep. 2022;15(4):e249558. https://doi.org/10.1136/bcr-2022-249558.
24. Zang Y, Chen S, Zang G, et al. The anatomic basis for ultrasound in the diagnosis and treatment of styloid process-related diseases. Ann Transl Med. 2020;8(24):1666. https://doi.org/10.21037/atm-20-7781.
25. Siniscalchi EN. Dynamic imaging in suspected eagle syndrome. Eur Arch Otorrinolaringol. 2020;277(1):307. https://doi.org/10.1007/s00405-019-05678-0.
26. Tanaka Y, Anami H, Kurihara H, et al. Eagle syndrome with hidden stylocarotid syndrome examined using dynamic ultrasonography: illustrative case. J Neurosur: Case Lessons. 2021;1(26):CASE21286. https://doi.org/10.3171/CASE21286.

10 Eagle Imaging 2

Ruggero Campisi, Claudio Vicini, Alberto Caranti, Filippo De Carli, Priscilla Visani, and Giuseppe Monetti

10.1 X-Ray

For historical and technological reasons, it is not surprising that the first radiological method to accompany clinical evaluation in Eagle syndrome (ES) was X-ray radiography. Eagle WW himself, in his 1937 work in which he introduced ES, published two lateral X-rays (referred to as roentgenograms in the original text) of a patient with an elongated styloid process [1].

It is therefore not surprising that, for a long time, radiographic studies remained the reference method for investigating patients with clinical presentations suggestive of ES and that numerous reports of elongated styloid processes or calcifications of the styloid process were described in the dental literature as anatomical curiosities [2].

It is emblematic that Hardin FM reported that many patients were referred for ENT evaluation for suspected ES by dental colleagues, due to mandibular or cervical pain not related to dental issues, rather than for the finding of an elongated styloid process on panorex film [3].

Of interest in this regard is the study by Keur JJ and colleagues in 1986, in which they conducted a retrospective analysis of 1135 edentulous patients undergoing panoramic tomograms to investigate the prevalence of styloid process anomalies. They based this on the premise that the increasing use of panoramic tomograms at the time was leading to more frequent findings. Indeed, the authors found anomalies of the styloid complex in 32.9% of the women examined (out of a total of 739

R. Campisi (✉) · C. Vicini · A. Caranti
University of Ferrara, Cona, FE, Italy
e-mail: claudio@claudiovicini.com

F. De Carli · P. Visani · G. Monetti
Primus Medical Center, Forlì, FC, Italy
e-mail: fdecarli@gvmnet.it; pvisani@gvmnet.it; info@muskultrasound.it

C. Vicini et al. (eds.), *EAGLE Syndrome*,
https://doi.org/10.1007/978-3-031-92829-1_10

women with a mean age of 66 years) and in 28.5% (out of a total of 396 men with a mean age of 68 years). However, of the patients with one or two elongated styloid processes, 47% of the women and 60% of the men did not have any clinical symptoms. This observation led the authors to state that the radiological finding of an elongated styloid process or a calcified stylohyoid ligament is a relatively frequent radiological finding, especially in older patients, but is meaningless unless correlated with clinical symptoms suggestive of ES [4].

However, as already noted, the panoramic tomogram is not the only imaging technique capable of detecting a styloid process anomaly. In fact, such anomalies can be identified using various methods, which include panoramic radiography, posteroanterior skull view, lateral cephalogram, lateral oblique mandible view, Towne's view, and open-mouth odontoid view [5].

Alongside the use of different imaging techniques, over the years, the literature has also seen a succession of various classifications, which we will quickly review.

10.1.1 Gossman and Tarsitano's Classification

In a study conducted on 4200 patients in 1977, the 2 authors classified the styloid process into 4 different categories:

1. Slightly elongated.
2. Crooked.
3. Segmented.
4. Very elongated [5].

In the following years, this classification was criticized for not taking into account variants such as joint-like or pseudo-articulated variants, as reported by other authors [6, 7].

10.1.2 Langlais' Classification

In this study conducted in 1986, the authors proposed a more detailed classification, identifying three types of radiological appearances (Fig. 10.1) and four patterns of calcification or mineralization of the process (Fig. 10.2) [6].

A subsequent addition to this classification was introduced in 2001 by MacDonald and Jankowski, who added a fourth category to the radiological aspects, including under letter D a calcification of the styloid process not in continuity with the cranial base [8].

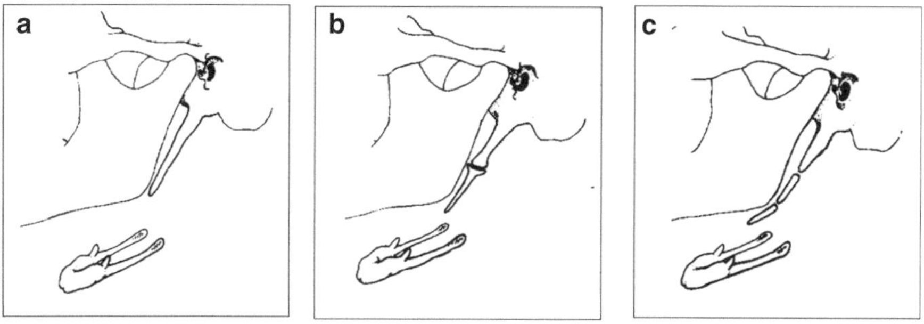

Fig. 10.1 The classification of the radiographic appearance devised by Langlais et al. (**a**) Elongated variant (where the authors used a reference value of >25 mm to define an elongated process). (**b**) Pseudo-articulated variant (the styloid process is apparently joined to the mineralized stylomandibular or stylohyoid ligament by a single pseudo-articulation). (**c**) Segmented variant (short or long noncontinuous portions of the styloid process or interrupted segments of mineralized ligament)

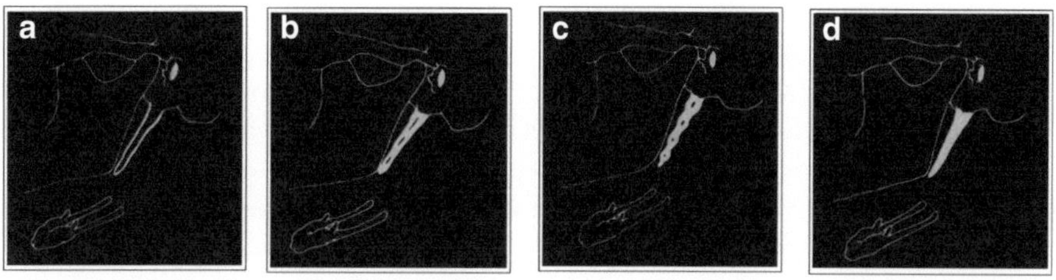

Fig. 10.2 The classification of calcification patterns. (**a**) Calcified outline (radiopaque border with a central radiolucency). (**b**) Partially calcified (thicker radiopaque outline and almost complete opacification, but with small, sometimes discontinuous radiolucent cores). (**c**) Nodular complex (knobby or scalloped outline; it may be partially or completely calcified with varying degrees of central radiolucency). (**d**) Completely calcified process (totally radiopaque with no evidence of a radiolucent interior)

10.1.3 O'Carroll and Jackson Classification

In 1984, O'Carroll MK proposed a very simple classification of styloid process elongation, based on its relationship with the mandibular foramen (Fig. 10.3) [9].

This classification was revisited by several authors, including Öztas B and Orhan K, who evaluated a cohort of 2000 patients treated at the Faculty of Dentistry at Ankara University, using the O'Carroll and Jackson classification to standardize their results [10].

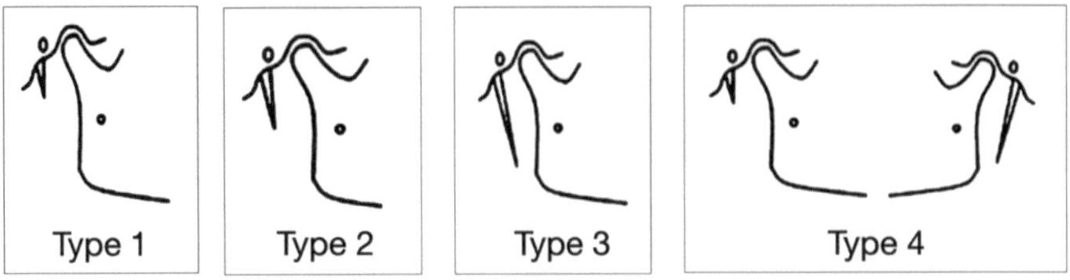

Fig. 10.3 O'Carroll's classification based on the relationship between the styloid process and the mandibular foramen: Type 1—the tip of the styloid process is higher than the mandibular foramen. Type 2—the tip of the styloid process is at the same level as the mandibular foramen. Type 3—the tip of the styloid process extends beyond (lower than) the mandibular foramen. Type 4—the styloid process has different lengths on the two sides

Imaging methods based on X-rays certainly contributed to the knowledge acquired over decades regarding the prevalence, age, sex, and racial distribution, as well as the patterns of elongation and calcification of the styloid process. However, it is also important to acknowledge the limitations pointed out by some authors, such as those reported in the work of Ferrario et al. in 1990 [11]. In this study, the authors noted that traditional radiographic techniques can distort the dimensions of the styloid process, with the magnification of the X-ray image varying depending on the angle of the process itself. Furthermore, the length can sometimes be difficult to estimate because the emergence of the process may be obscured due to the overlap with the mastoid process. More generally, Sokler K and Sandev S also emphasize that the true length of the styloid process could be obscured by the overlap of other anatomical structures, including the contralateral styloid process [12]. For these reasons, compared to other imaging methods listed earlier, the orthopantomogram, with its panoramic view, has established itself as the reference radiological method, allowing the simultaneous visualization of both styloid processes. However, even this method is not without potential errors, still due to the interposition of other structures and an enlargement of the styloid process estimated by Keur JJ et al. to be around 11% or an average error margin of 2.5 mm [2, 4].

10.2 CT Scan

Today, the gold standard for imaging diagnostics in suspected cases of ES is the CT scan [13]. This role has been established due to the CT scan overcoming all the limitations of traditional radiology, particularly the enlargement of the styloid process and, therefore, the overestimation of its length, as well as the overlap of other structures. Specifically, the advent of CT has allowed for much more precise information to be obtained regarding substantial details necessary to determine the pathogenesis of ES and its vascular variants, such as the length of the styloid process, its angle/inclination, its proximity to the pharyngeal wall, and its relationship with adjacent structures, particularly vascular and neural [14–17]. These capabilities have been further refined and enhanced by the advent of 3D reconstruction. Multi-slice CT with 3D reconstruction has allowed for a precise understanding of the three-dimensional structure of the styloid process, which is useful not only for diagnostic purposes but also for planning potential surgical interventions [17].

10.2.1 Length of the Styloid Process

For decades, the literature has discussed the maximum length beyond which the styloid process should be considered pathological. It is now widely accepted that the average length of the styloid process is between 20 and 30 mm and that a styloid process exceeding 30 mm should be considered elongated [18]. This finding is supported by recent studies conducted using CT scans, for example, by Onbas et al., who reported the average length of the SP to be 26.8 mm (in a study conducted on 283 patients), and by Ceylan et al., who reported an average SP length of 28.3 mm (in a study conducted on 61 patients) [19, 20].

Thanks to cadaver studies and radiological studies based on CT scans, we have been able to obtain important information about the distribution of SP length among asymptomatic patients and those affected by ES.

Specifically, in a study conducted by Balcioglu HA et al., it was found that the mean length of the SP in the cadavers examined was 22.54 ± 4.24 mm. In this cohort of patients, the prevalence of an elongated styloid process was 3.3%, with a statistically significant difference between subjects with an elongated but asymptomatic SP (36.06 ± 6.12 mm) and those affected by ES (40 ± 4.72 mm) [21].

Similar results were obtained from a study conducted using CT on 35 patients with unilateral ES, where Singh R et al. found that the mean length of the styloid process on the symptomatic side was 33.61 mm, while on the asymptomatic side, it was 31.11 mm. This finding was statistically significant and allowed the authors to conclude that the length of the SP is a relevant factor in determining ES [17].

10.2.2 Styloid Process Angulation

Similarly to what has been described for length, studies have also been conducted on the angulation of the styloid process to determine its correlation with ES.

For angulation, we refer again to the work of Singh R et al., who evaluated the transverse angle (between the line connecting the base of the SP and the long axis of the SP) and the sagittal angle (between the long axis of the SP and McRae's line—a line connecting the anterior and posterior lips of the foramen magnum) (Fig. 10.4). The results obtained showed that the mean transverse angle was 72.37° on the symptomatic side and 74.17° on the asymptomatic side, values that were not statistically significant [17].

On the other hand, in a study conducted on 23 patients affected by ES, Burulday V et al. concluded that there is a statistically significant correlation between the coronal angle (equivalent to what Singh R et al. refer to as the

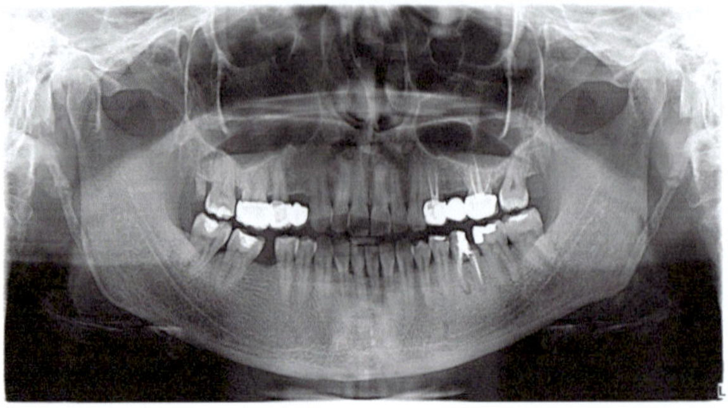

Fig. 10.4 Panoramic radiograph of our patient demonstrating bilaterally a styloid process, which is notably not calcified but is bony, with both cortex and medulla clearly distinguishable

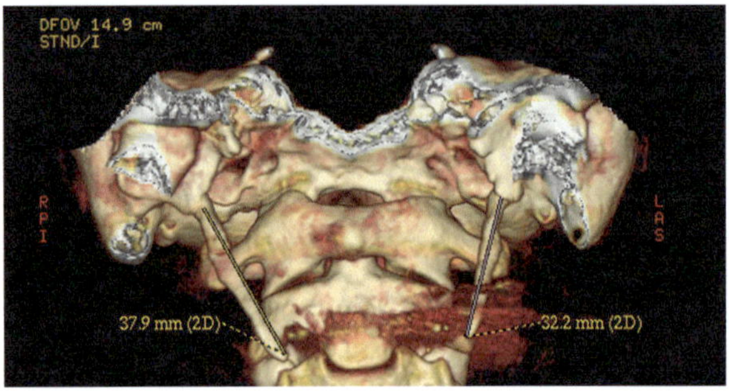

Fig. 10.5 Length of styloid process

sagittal angle) and ES. Specifically, the SPs on the side affected by ES had an average coronal angle of 69.4°, compared to an average angle of 65.6° on the unaffected side [22].

A similar study was conducted by Yavuz H et al. in 2008, based on lateral skull and Towne's X-rays acquired for 30 patients affected by ES and 31 patients in a control group. In this case, the medial angulation, measured on Towne's X-ray and defined as the angle between a vertical line passing through the base of the styloid process and the line passing through the long axis of the styloid process, and the anterior angulation, obtained from the lateral skull X-ray and defined as the angle present between a vertical line perpendicular to the Frankfurt line (Fig. 10.5), were evaluated. The authors concluded that the anterior angulation in patients was 33.6° ± 8.6° on the right and 36.7° ± 9.1° on the left, while in the control group, the anterior angulation was 21.4° ± 7.7° on the right and 18.5° ± 8.1° on the left, a statistically significant value that also allowed Yavuz H et al. to conclude that the angulation of the styloid process is relevant in ES [23] (Fig. 10.6, 10.7, and 10.8).

10.2.3 Distance from Tonsillar Fossa

The length and angulation of the SP are not the only anatomical parameters that have been taken into consideration but also its relationship with the surrounding

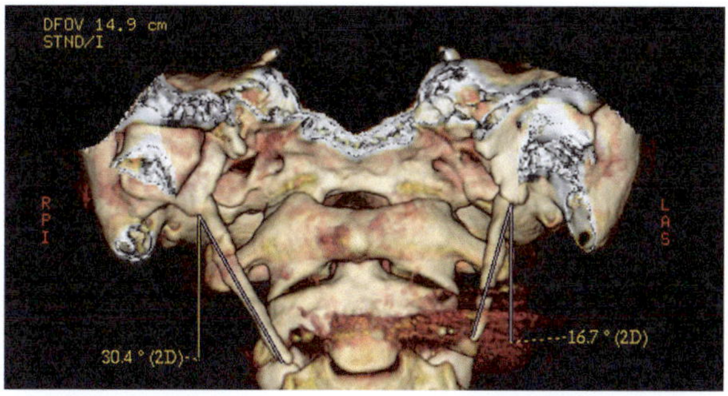

Fig. 10.6 Styloid process angulation

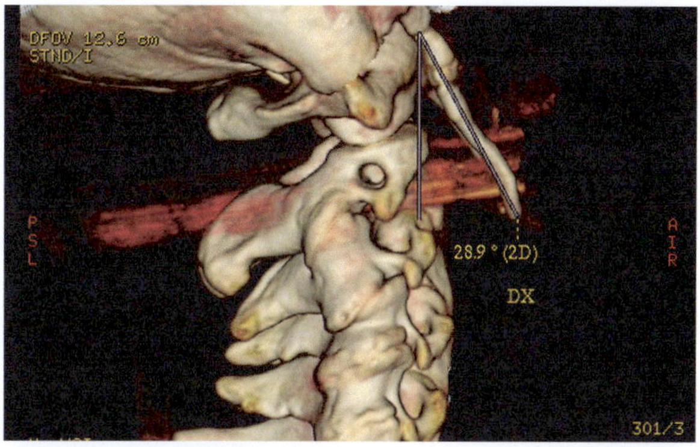

Fig. 10.7 Styloid process angulation

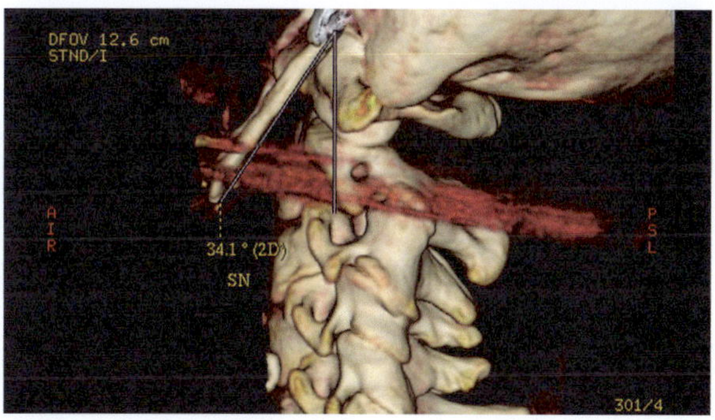

Fig. 10.8 Styloid process angulation

structures and soft tissues. In particular, an interesting parameter is the minimum distance between the SP and the surface of the tonsillar fossa. In their study, Kent DT et al., in addition to evaluating length and angulation, assessed "in the axial plane, the shortest distance between the SP tip to the soft tissue/air interface of the tonsillar fossa" [24]. Indeed, their data clearly show that, in patients affected by ES, this distance was significantly shorter compared to the control cases. Specifically, the SP was within 13 mm of the tonsillar fossa in 70% of the ES group compared with 3.3% of the asymptomatic patients. In our experience, this is the only author who has analyzed this aspect, although

Yavuz H et al. had nevertheless suggested that a greater anterior angulation corresponded to a closer proximity of the SP to the surface of the tonsillar fossa [23] (Fig. 10.9).

10.2.4 Distance between Styloid Basis and Tips

A final parameter we want to mention is the distance between the two SPs, specifically the distance between the bases of the right and left SPs, as well as the distance between their tips. This parameter was analyzed in the study by Patil S et al., who in 2014 examined 114 dry skulls, of which 98 had SPs within normal limits, while in 16 cases, they appeared elongated [26]. The authors, in addition to measuring length and angles of inclination, also assessed the distance between the bases of the styloid processes and the distance between the tips. These parameters were found to be statistically significantly different between the two groups, highlighting that both parameters were reduced in patients with elongated SPs. Notably, the distance between the tips changed significantly, measuring an average of 6.4 ± 0.61 mm in patients with normal SPs, while in patients with elongated SPs, the measurement reduced to just 2.9 ± 0.69 mm. Alongside these findings, the authors emphasize that there is a greater anterior angulation in patients with elongated SPs, reinforcing the findings of Yavuz H et al. regarding the correlation between increased anterior angulation and the reduced distance between the tips and the tonsillar fossa (Figs. 10.10 and 10.11).

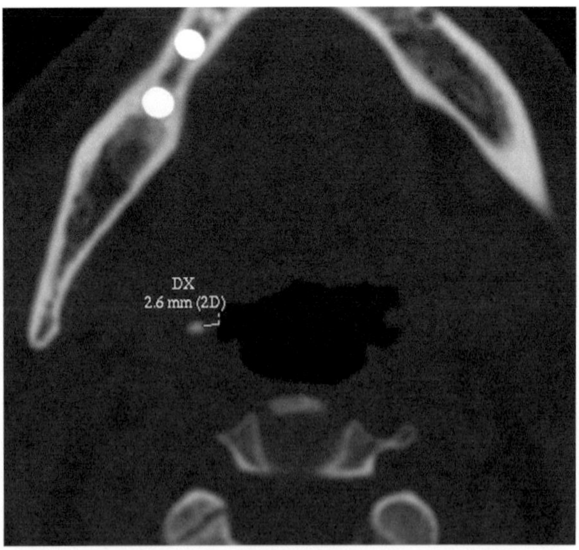

Fig. 10.9 Distance from tonsillar fossa, which was measured to be 2.6 millimeters at this point

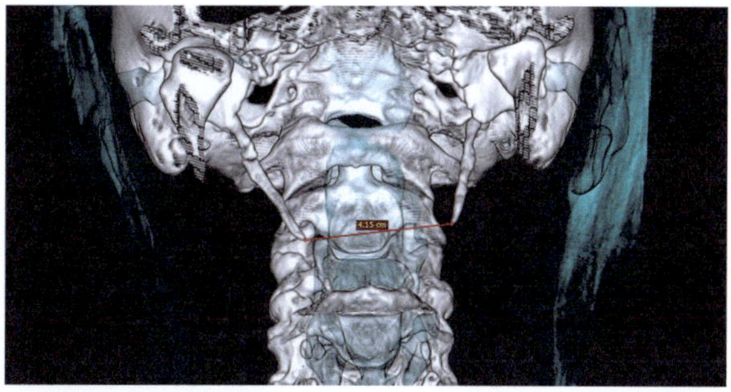

Fig. 10.10 Distance between styloid tips

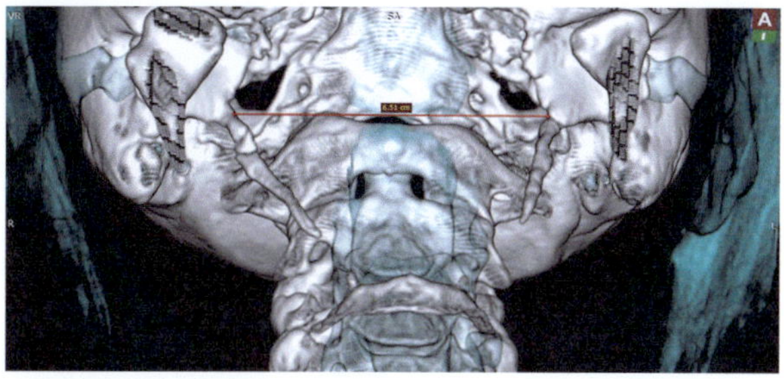

Fig. 10.11 Distance between styloid basis

The review of the existing literature has thus been useful in understanding how the evidence present in the literature, coming from cohort or retrospective studies conducted on radiological images acquired via CT, as well as from cadaver studies, has offered evidence that the length and angulation of the styloid process are significant variables in the development of ES. This leads us to understand how the 3D CT scan has become fundamental in the diagnostic pathway of ES. Specifically, the 3D CT does not suffer from errors in estimating the length of the SP, and in particular, Nayak DR et al. have shown that the length of the SP measured with the 3D CT scan differs by 1 to 10 mm compared to that measured by X-ray [2]. The same authors also highlighted that there is a difference of 1°–2° between the two methods.

10.3 Conclusions

In conclusion, the CT scan, and when available, 3D reconstruction, is now the reference method for diagnosing elongated SP and, therefore, ES. In our clinical practice, we have also used CT scans with 3D reconstruction as the reference diagnostic method. Specifically, in our case series, we found a mean length of the symptomatic SP of 39.28 ± 7.9 mm. Regarding angulation, in our case series, we calculated both the coronal angle, with an average value of 72.56° ± 3.81°, and the sagittal angle, with an average value of 91.34° ± 5.16°.

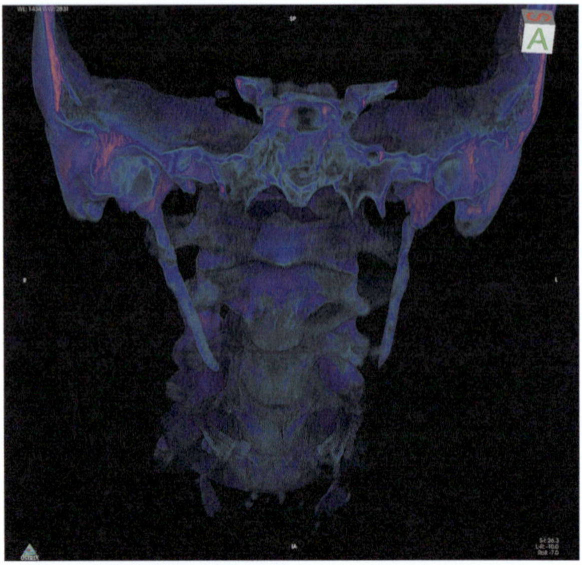

Fig. 10.12 CT 3D reconstructions from multiple perspectives

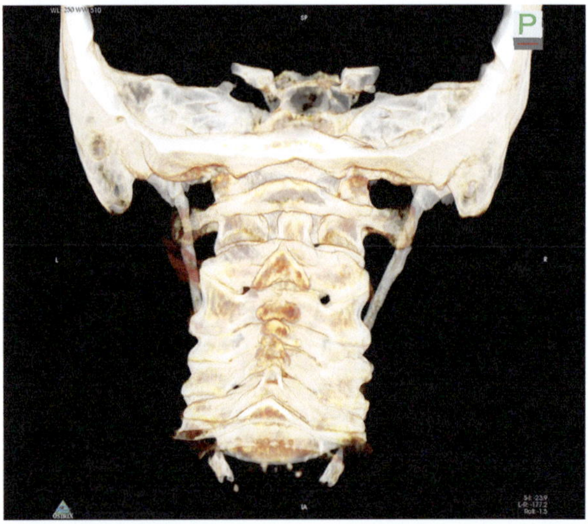

Fig. 10.13 CT 3D reconstructions from multiple perspectives

We will now review some examples of 3D reconstructions performed on patients we have treated (Figs. 10.12, 10.13, and 10.14).

Below, we present some details about the styloid process obtained from CT scans performed on our patients (Fig. 10.15, 10.16, 10.17, and 10.18).

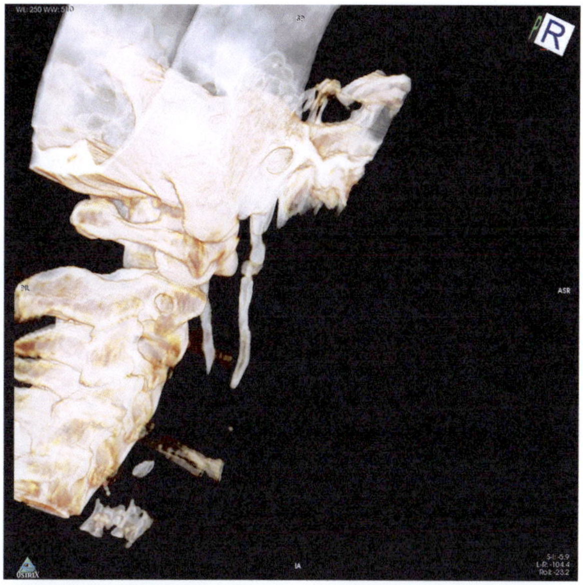

Fig. 10.14 CT 3D reconstructions from multiple perspectives

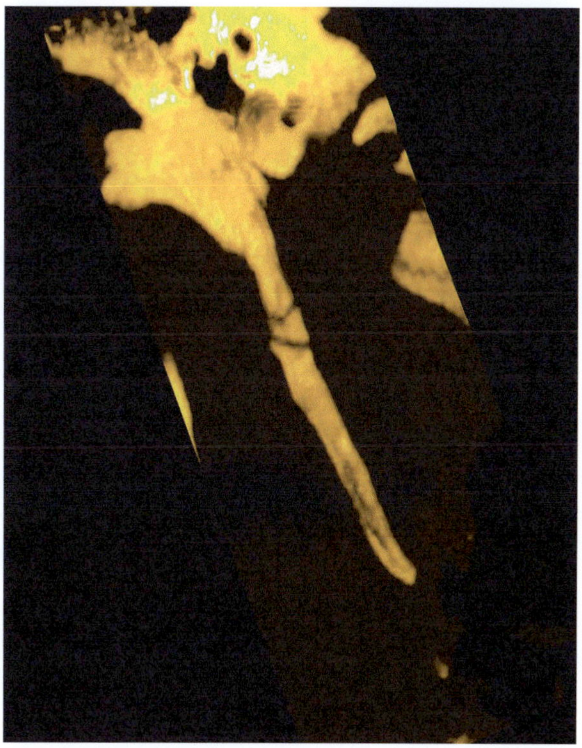

Fig. 10.15 Styloid process details obtained with CT scans

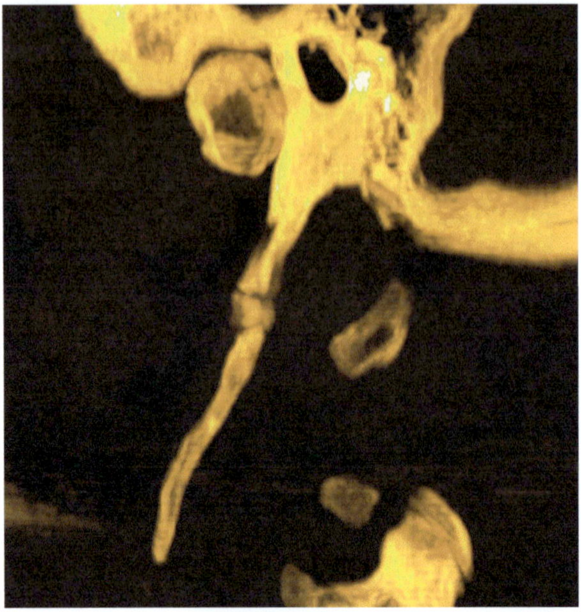

Fig. 10.16 Styloid process details obtained with CT scans

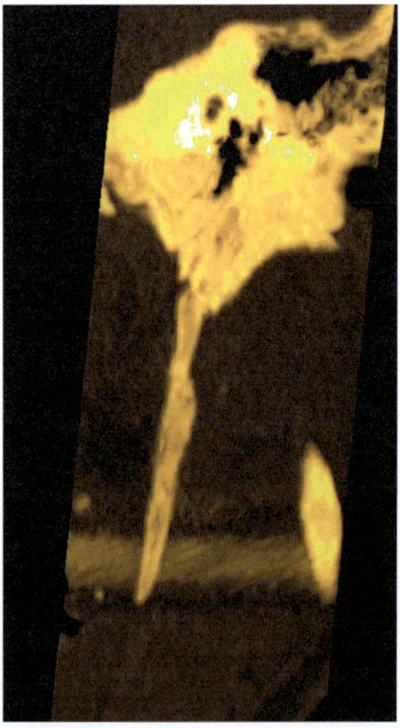

Fig. 10.17 Styloid process details obtained with CT scans

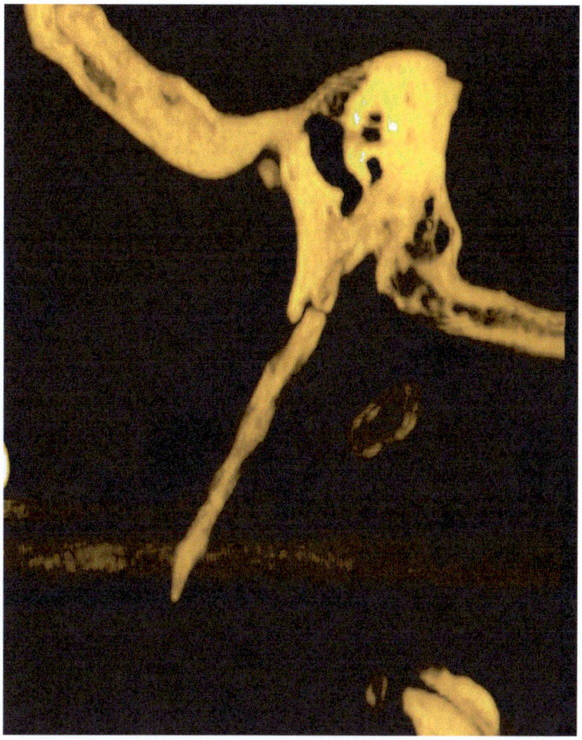

Fig. 10.18 Styloid process details obtained with CT scans

References

1. Eagle WW, Durham NC. Elongated styloid processes. Report of two cases. Arch Otolaryngol Head Neck Surg. 1937;25:584–7.
2. Nayak DR, Pujary K, Aggarwal M, Punnoose SE, Chaly VA. Role of three-dimensional computed tomography reconstruction in the management of elongated styloid process: a preliminary study. J Laryngol Otol. 2007;121(4):349–53. https://doi.org/10.1017/S0022215106003276.
3. Hardin FM, Xiao R, Burkey BB. Surgical management of patients with Eagle syndrome. Am J Otolaryngol. 2018;39(5):481–4. https://doi.org/10.1016/j.amjoto.2018.05.003.
4. Keur JJ, Campbell JP, McCarthy JF, Ralph WJ. The clinical significance of the elongated styloid process. Oral Surg Oral Med Oral Pathol. 1986;61(4):399–404. https://doi.org/10.1016/0030-4220(86)90426-3.
5. Gossman JR Jr, Tarsitano JJ. The styloid-stylohyoid syndrome. J Oral Surg. 1977;35(7):555–60.
6. Langlais RP, Miles DA, Van Dis ML. Elongated and mineralized stylohyoid ligament complex: a proposed classification and report of a case of Eagle's syndrome. Oral Surg Oral Med Oral Pathol. 1986;61(5):527–32. https://doi.org/10.1016/0030-4220(86)90400-7.
7. Stafne EC, Hollinshead WH. Roentgenographic observations on the stylohyoid chain. Oral Surg Oral Med Oral Pathol. 1962;15:1195–200. https://doi.org/10.1016/0030-4220(62)90154-8.
8. MacDonald-Jankowski DS. Calcification of the stylohyoid complex in Londoners and Hong Kong Chinese. Dentomaxillofac Radiol. 2001;30(1):35–9. https://doi.org/10.1038/sj/dmfr/4600574.
9. Carroll O, MK. Calcification in the stylohyoid ligament. Oral Surg Oral Med Oral Pathol. 1984;58(5):617–21. https://doi.org/10.1016/0030-4220(84)90089-6.

10. Öztaş B, Orhan K. Investigation of the incidence of stylohyoid ligament calcifications with panoramic radiographs. J Investig Clin Dent. 2012;3(1):30–5. https://doi.org/10.1111/j.2041-1626.2011.00081.x.
11. Ferrario VF, Sigurtá D, Daddona A, Dalloca L, Miani A, Tafuro F, Sforza C. Calcification of the stylohyoid ligament: incidence and morphoquantitative evaluations. Oral Surg Oral Med Oral Pathol. 1990;69(4):524–9. https://doi.org/10.1016/0030-4220(90)90390-e.
12. Sokler K, Sandev S. New classification of the styloid process length--clinical application on the biological base. Coll Antropol. 2001;25(2):627–32.
13. Badhey A, Jategaonkar A, Anglin Kovacs AJ, Kadakia S, De Deyn PP, Ducic Y, Schantz S, Shin E. Eagle syndrome: A comprehensive review. Clin Neurol Neurosurg. 2017;159:34–8. https://doi.org/10.1016/j.clineuro.2017.04.021.
14. Saccomanno S, Greco F, Corso EDE, Lucidi D, Deli R, D'Addona A, Paludetti G. Eagle's syndrome, from clinical presentation to diagnosis and surgical treatment: a case report. Acta Otorhinolaryngol Ital. 2018;38(2):166–9. https://doi.org/10.14639/0392-100X-1479.
15. Mantovani G, Zangrossi P, Flacco ME, Di Domenico G, Nastro Siniscalchi E, De Ponte FS, Maugeri R, De Bonis P, Cavallo MA, Zamboni P, Scerrati A. Styloid jugular nutcracker: the possible role of the styloid process spatial orientation-A preliminary morphometric computed study. Diagnostics (Basel). 2023;13(2):298. https://doi.org/10.3390/diagnostics13020298.
16. Sultan S, Acharya Y, Soliman O, Hynes N. Stylohyoid Eagle syndrome and EXTracranial INternal carotid arTery pseudoaneurysms (EXTINCT) with internal jugular vein nutcracker syndrome: a challenging clinical scenario. BMJ Case Rep. 2022;15(4):e249558. https://doi.org/10.1136/bcr-2022-249558.
17. Singh R, Sharma R, Sharma VK, Prajapati N, Rana AK. Styloid process; correlation between symptoms, palpability and measurements on three dimensional computed tomography. Indian J Otolaryngol Head Neck Surg. 2022;74(Suppl 3):5556–61. https://doi.org/10.1007/s12070-021-02901-5.
18. Eagle WW. Elongated styloid process: further observations and new syndrome. Arch Otolaryngol. 1948;47:630–40.
19. Onbas O, Kantarci M, Murat Karasen R, Durur I, Cinar Basekim C, Alper F, Okur A. Angulation, length, and morphology of the styloid process of the temporal bone analyzed by multidetector computed tomography. Acta Radiol. 2005;46(8):881–6. https://doi.org/10.1080/02841850500335085.
20. Ceylan A, Köybaşioğlu A, Celenk F, Yilmaz O, Uslu S. Surgical treatment of elongated styloid process: experience of 61 cases. Skull Base. 2008;18(5):289–95. https://doi.org/10.1055/s-0028-1086057.
21. Balcioglu HA, Kilic C, Akyol M, Ozan H, Kokten G. Length of the styloid process and anatomical implications for Eagle's syndrome. Folia Morphol (Warsz). 2009;68(4):265–70.
22. Buruldaу V, Akgül MH, Bayar Muluk N, Yağdiran B, Inal M. The importance of medial-lateral styloid process angulation/coronal plane angle in symptomatic eagle syndrome. Clin Anat. 2017;30(4):487–91. https://doi.org/10.1002/ca.22842.
23. Yavuz H, Caylakli F, Yildirim T, Ozluoglu LN. Angulation of the styloid process in Eagle's syndrome. Eur Arch Otorrinolaringol. 2008;265(11):1393–6. https://doi.org/10.1007/s00405-008-0686-9.
24. Kent DT, Rath TJ, Snyderman C. Conventional and 3-dimensional computerized tomography in Eagle's syndrome, glossopharyngeal neuralgia, and asymptomatic controls. Otolaryngol Head Neck Surg. 2015;153(1):41–7. https://doi.org/10.1177/0194599815583047.

11 Typical Eagle Syndrome

Claudio Vicini, Angelo Cannavicci, Michela Melegatti, Ruggero Campisi, and Alberto Caranti

Rare But Not Impossible

11.1 Introduction

The so-called classic or typical Eagle syndrome (TES) is the first form of elongated styloid-related cluster of complaints originally described by Watt Weems Eagle (1898–1980) in 1937, an American otolaryngologist who worked at Duke University, in North Carolina, USA [1].

Basically, TES includes prominent neuropathic, mainly pain, symptoms related to glossopharyngeal nerve entrapment and additional mechanical complaints, mainly dysphagia, related to pharynx impingement, both centered in the buccal-pharyngeal area with possible referred sites of irradiation in different head and neck areas [2, 3]. By definition, an "elongated styloid proccss" is demonstrated at the same side of the pain [1, 3]. Carotid artery and jugular vein problems are not strictly included in the profile of TES, but in some cases, a combination of some features of classic, carotid, and jugular variants is occasionally reported in the literature [4–7].

C. Vicini (✉) · R. Campisi
University of Ferrara, Cona, FE, Italy
e-mail: claudio@claudiovicini.com

A. Cannavicci
Morgagni-Pierantoni Hospital, Forlì, FC, Italy

M. Melegatti
Department of Otorhinolaryngology, Head and Neck Surgery, ASST Lariana, Ospedale Sant'Anna, Como, Italy

A. Caranti
University of Ferrara, Cona, FE, Italy

Otorinolaringoiatria, S. Pier Damiano di Faenza - GVM care & research, Faenza, Italia

C. Vicini et al. (eds.), *EAGLE Syndrome*,
https://doi.org/10.1007/978-3-031-92829-1_11

In the same way, by far less commonly, an elongated styloid may interfere with cranial nerves different from IX producing different varieties of "atypical" Eagle syndrome, which will be described in a different chapter of this monograph.

11.2 Epidemiology

From an epidemiological point of view, TES is an uncommon entity. If compared with better known head and neck pain syndromes, its prevalence is significantly lower. The prevalence of temporomandibular joint and muscle disorder (TMJD) is between 5% and 12% [8, 9]. The prevalence of trigeminal neuralgia ranges between 0.1% and 0.7%. The prevalence of stylohyoid syndrome may be roughly estimated at about 0.16% of the general population, and it is quite lower than the percentage of the symptom-free population with styloid process of more than 30 mm of length (4% of the general population) [4, 10]. There is a significant prevalence of females in most of the case series and case reports as well as in our personal experience [2, 3]. Even if the peak of incidence for age of presentation is between 30 and 50 years, cases were reported in teenage or elderly [10].

11.3 History of the Illness

The list of the possible symptoms of TES as reported in the literature is summarized in Table 11.1. At a glance, it is immediately evident the impressive variety of different complaints, usually in variable and unpredictable combination for each patient. In a very rough but practical way, all the complaints may be related to a couple of basic mechanisms:

1. Entrapment and/or irritation and/or damage of IX cranial nerve or its branches.
2. "Stabbing" of the pharynx by the tip of the elongated styloid process.

According to the literature, pain represents the main symptom in most patients suffering from TES, a fact also confirmed in our series (100% of our patients) [11]. For this reason, TES should routinely be considered in the differential diagnosis for any orofacial pain of unknown etiology and actively demonstrated or excluded. The onset of the problem is usually described many years before, very rarely of recent occurrence. The average number of previous consultations for the same problem in our experience is about ten.

In 41.5% of our patients, the previous diagnosis, if present, was temporomandibular joint disorder, and more than 30% of the cases were treated with oral devices without pain reduction. There is no clear acute or sudden onset, but the problem, after a gradual appearance without a defined date or time of onset, is usually described as progressive in intensity over months or years. The topographic distribution of the pain, as described in the literature, is the same as glossopharyngeal neuralgia: base of the tongue, angle of the mandible, ear, and mastoid [11]. It meets

Table 11.1 List of TES symptoms as reported in the literature

Nerve entrapment symptoms	Neuralgic pain secondary to the distribution of the glossopharyngeal nerve (tongue base, angle of mandible, ear, mastoid) Dull pain Pain varying in intensity Pain increased by head rotation Pain less intense and more constant, not induced by hot/cold food or tongue movements
Pharynx impingement symptoms	Nagging or aching pharyngodynia Foreign body sensation Gagging Bolus Sialorrea Taste complaints Dysphagia (and weight loss) Pharyngoesophageal spasm Voice change Glossodynia Swallowing Yawing Chew phonodynia Hardness in the tonsil bed Tenderness in the tonsil bed
ex adjuvant criterion	Local anesthetic injection reduces pain

the criteria of the so-called secondary glossopharyngeal neuralgia, pain attributed to a demonstrated lesion of the nerve.

In our personal series, the detailed distribution can be summarized as follows: in the cervical area (70.7%), in the maxillary/orodental region (61%), in the frontal area (24%), in the occipital region (17.1%), and in the auricular and/or TMJ area (46.3%). Probably due to the difficulties for many patients in accurately describing their pain distribution, and possibly because in some cases TES may coexist with some characteristics of carotid Eagle syndrome (compression of the sympathetic plexus of the adventitia of the carotid artery), the distribution of pain may be described somewhat differently.

If the external carotid artery is in the area of the elongated styloid process, more facial, peri−/retro-orbital pain is described [12]. In the case of internal carotid artery compression, the pain seems to spread to the vertex, parietal, and frontal areas [13]. In jugular Eagle syndrome, pain manifestations are usually described as generalized headaches [13, 14]. The quality and intensity of pain in TES seem to be somewhat different from the pain of idiopathic glossopharyngeal neuralgia. In most cases, it is more constant and dull in character, without paroxysms. But probably the most useful aspect for differential diagnosis is the quite different profile of precipitating factors. In TES, pain is not precipitated or worsened by hot/cold foods or tongue movements, but is more closely related to head rotation, which produces a sudden increase in nerve entrapment [12].

11.4 Lidocaine Infiltration Test

An *ex juvantibus* treatment can be useful to show evidence of a suspected role of the elongated styloid process in the production of pain. The lidocaine infiltration test (LIT) (Fig. 11.1) is among the diagnostic criteria included in the International Classification of Headache Disorders, third edition, classified at the same informational level as styloidectomy [15].

If the injection of a local anesthetic agent into the stylohyoid ligament can produce significant pain improvement, it is considered among the evidence of the styloid process's responsibility in the production of the described pain. It is one of the main diagnostic steps required for a solid diagnosis of TES. At the same time, LIT has traditionally been applied also as a selective tool to distinguish patients eligible for styloidectomy, to prevent unsuccessful surgeries and increase the success rate of an invasive approach [16]. In this application, LIT plays a role in surgical selection and as a prognostic tool. In the original description, "3 cc of 2% lidocaine were infiltrated into the tonsillar fossa on the side where the patient had pain and where the styloid process was. After 15 minutes, the patient was asked to indicate the intensity of the pain felt on the VAS. The change in intensity was recorded. A reduction in intensity to less than one-third of the original was considered positive."

A similar but different approach is the so-called lidocaine pain relief test described as in the authors' original proposal, "cotton soaked in 4% lidocaine placed on the palpation point of the styloid process for 10 seconds. The test is positive for

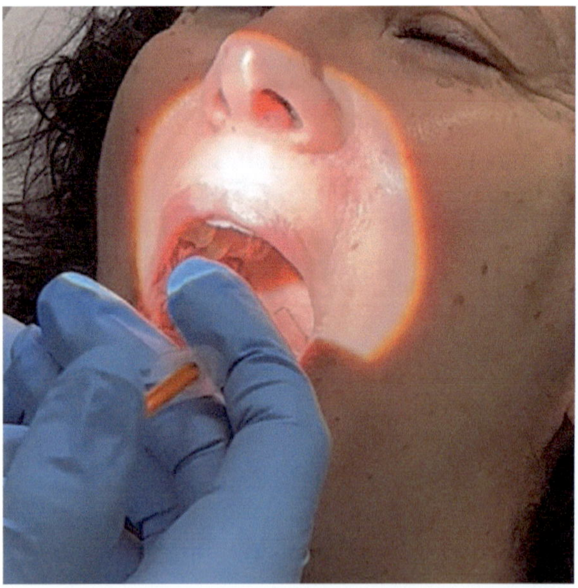

Fig. 11.1 Lidocaine infiltration test

stylalgia if there is no pain after the cotton is removed" [17]. Sharma N et al. suggest injecting a combination of steroid solution or long-acting anesthetic to the lesser horn of the hyoid bone or the lower aspect of the tonsillar fossa, without specific suggestions on pain monitoring after the injection [18].

It is also worth mentioning a special case of local injection in a "68-year-old man with a traumatic fracture of the ossified SHC complex, satisfactorily resolved with local steroid injections administered for cervical pain and odynophagia that persisted after complete fracture healing." "Five milligrams of dexamethasone at a concentration of 1 kg/m^3 were slowly injected into the painful point under ultrasound guidance. The patient reported immediate pain reduction, with pain intensity below 1 on the VAS. He was satisfied with the resolution and showed no recurrence during the 6-month follow-up after dexamethasone injection" [19].

This case also offers an example of the use of chemical infiltration of the styloid process as a therapeutic modality as well as a diagnostic tool. In our experience, all suspected patients are injected with 3–5 cc of a combination of a local anesthetic and methylprednisolone at the first consultation. After a preliminary spray of lidocaine on the affected side, an insulin syringe needle is inserted following palpation guidance if the tip of the styloid process is located, without any discomfort for the patient. If not palpable, the possible area of the styloid process tip is chosen through careful examination of the available images. The patient is asked to keep a diary of the pain course for a month after the injection. The pain VAS is required, but the true rule of success/failure has proven to be in our experience the comprehensive evaluation of the patient. The main question is: "Did the injection significantly change your symptoms?" If not, surgery is discouraged, or further injections may be proposed. Up to three injections at 30-day intervals can be useful in unclear cases. It also seems a way to reduce the placebo effect, which is quite common in any type of pain approach [20].

A second subset of symptoms is conceptually related to the chronic impingement of an elongated styloid on the pharynx and surrounding structures. We may also label them as mechanical symptoms, different from the neuropathic ones. If properly considered, they may lead the doctor to raise a suspicion of ES pointing the attention to the possible existence of an elongated styloid. Nagging or aching pharyngodynia and glossodynia are frequently described and were included in the historical description of Eagle [1, 11]. Sometimes the tip of the styloid bone, bulging out from the tonsil bed, is perceived by the patient as a foreign body, which may produce episodes of gagging in case of reduced threshold of vomiting. Bolus, sialorrhea, and more rarely taste disturbances are among the possible complaints, as expression of the same pathogenetic factors. Styloid bone may affect the proper pharyngoesophageal mechanics producing dysphagia and possibly reduced food intake and weight loss, as well as voice changes, sometimes pharyngoesophageal spasms [11]. Interestingly, swallowing, yawing, chewing, and speaking are sometimes felt as precipitating factors of pharyngeal pain and dysfunction [3].

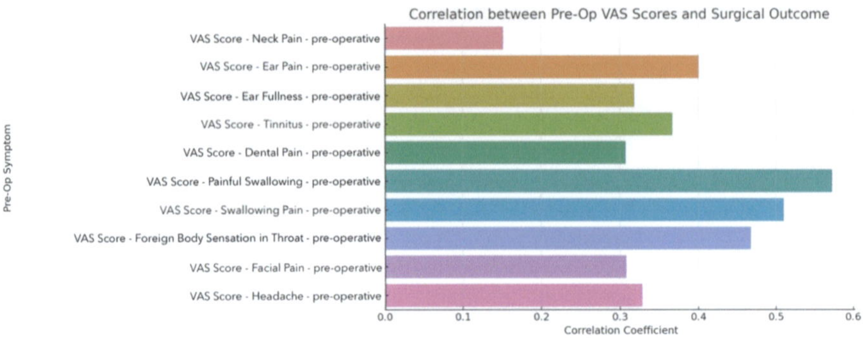

Fig. 11.2 Correlation between symptoms and surgical success

11.5 Psychological Profile

Another really important but frequently overlooked feature of TES is the psychological profile of many if not all the patients. Chronic pain is usually accompanied by psychological disturbance, in which anxiety and depression are the most commonly affected [21]. In the group reported by Xu and colleagues, eight out of ten patients were significantly anxious and/or depressed. It is interesting to note that after surgical treatment, most of them were normalized from the psychological point of view and did not recur.

Besides the role of the complaint profile for the ES diagnosis, a careful analysis of the main symptoms may be also useful for a better treatment planning. In Fig. 11.2 are listed the different symptoms' VAS scores and surgical outcomes. It is quite clear that a set of three mechanical high pain scores (odynophagia, painful swallowing, and foreign body sensation) and an elevated VAS score of ear referred pain may predict a better postoperative outcome and may help the surgeon to suggest and patient to accept styloidectomy for the higher expected success rate.

11.6 Family History

Family history is usually of minimal interest. Anyway, in one case, a clinical entity of familial ossification of the stylohyoid ligament in a three-generation family was described displaying autosomal dominant inheritance [22]. On the other hand, past history and comorbidity exploration are both very rich of information.

11.7 Past Medical History

Previous tonsillectomy was considered by Dr. Eagle in his first paper a prerequisite for diagnosis and probably the cause of the styloid process elongation, promoted by postoperative scarring [1]. This theory was reviewed by Dr. Eagle in his

Table 11.2 Data related to the clinical history of our patients

History of:
Tonsillectomy in 18 patients (*44%*)
Head concussion or previous head traumatic injury in ten (*25%*) at the mean age of 30 years old (range 10–50 years old)
15/27 (55,6%) female patients were in *menopause* at the time of surgery
4/41 (9,8%) had diagnosis of calcium metabolism disorder (vit. D or calcium deficiency)
1/41 (2,4%) had previous transient ischemic attack
17/41 (*41,5%*) were *previously diagnosed with TMJ disorder!!!*
15/41 (36,6%) were previously treated by oral appliance (bite) device
n. 9 (22,0%) patients had *endocrine disorders* (n.4 hypothyroidism)
n. 18 had comorbidities potentially relatable to ES, in particular:
n.4 (9,8%) diabetes mellitus
n.5 (12,2%) anxious SD
n. 2 (4,9%) facial or body dysmorphism or musculoskeletal impairment
n.2 (4,9%) rheumatologic disease
n.3 (7,3%) cervical hernia

second paper 11 years later [23]. In the last decade, the link between Eagle syndrome (ES) and tonsillectomy has been considered not so close in most reported cases or case series [24]. In our series, 44% of patients had undergone tonsillectomy. This percentage is still higher than the unselected adult population, where an average of 27% of operated patients was found in a recent Italian survey. A history of cranio-cervical trauma is probably the second most common historical event reported [25]. Trauma can cause a bone fracture of the stylohyoid complex, which sometimes can occur even without clear evidence of previous trauma (spontaneous fracture) [12]. The fracture of an elongated styloid process or an ossified stylohyoid ligament is rare in clinical practice as a cause of pain in Eagle syndrome, but it must be considered and checked by gentle palpation and evocation of pain at the bone interruption level [11]. Concussion with flexion-extension or rotation head movements with large indirect movements or direct injuries to the styloid process can induce fragmentation of the stylohyoid complex, sometimes including the hyoid bone. About 25% of our confirmed TES cases were positive for trauma. In Table 11.2, we report the data related to the clinical history of the patients in our case series.

11.8 Physical Examination

Last but not least are a couple of useful simple clinical signs that if routinely and properly checked may be of great importance for the final diagnosis. A systematic and gentle digital palpation of the lateral pharyngeal wall may reveal an unusual hardness in the depth or possibly the styloid tip may be clearly perceived (Fig. 11.3) [12]. Finally, if the pressure of the finger of the hardness may reproduce or somehow mimic the spontaneous pain of the patient, the suspicion of an ES became really strong [11].

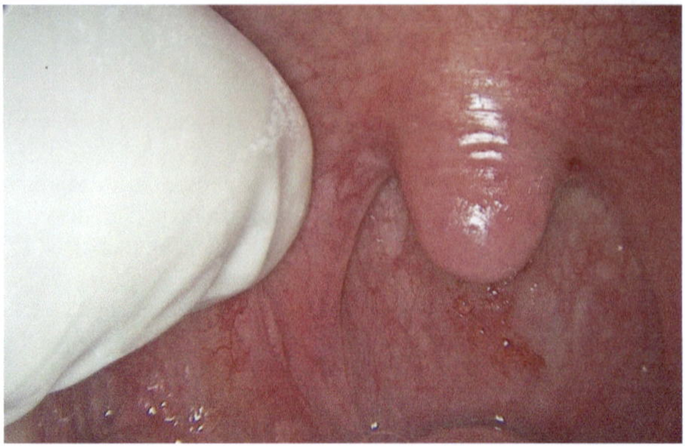

Fig. 11.3 Gentle finger palpation of the lateral pharyngeal wall

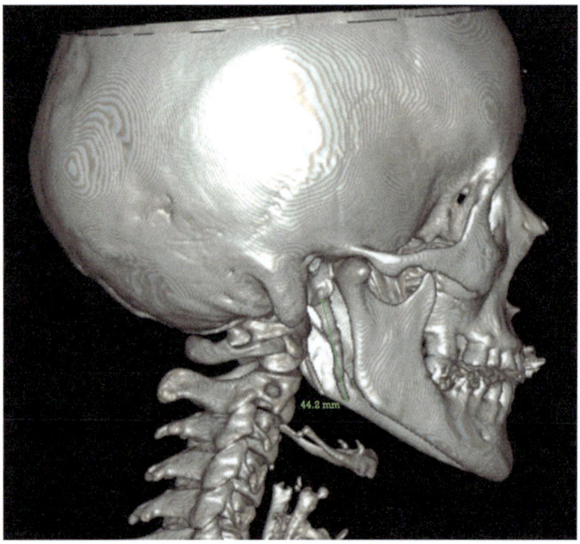

Fig. 11.4 A 3D CT of a styloid longer than 30 mm

11.9 Imaging

The confirmation of Eagle syndrome requires, after history and physical examination, evidence of a "pathological" styloid process by one of the many available imaging options (Fig. 11.4). A special chapter of this book is dedicated to a detailed discussion of the radiological semiology of the stylohyoid complex. Table 11.3 summarizes some of the pathological findings reported in ES patients.

By far the most common observation is an elongated styloid process defined as longer than 30 mm, which is considered by pure convention the limit of normality [26]. According to a large amount of data from anatomical and radiological studies in medical and forensic settings, it is well established that:

Table 11.3 Pathological findings associated with ES patients

Bone	Styloid elongation/angulation/medialized tip to tonsil bed Ossification of stylohyoid ligament (clinical elongation) Calcification Lengths of less than 3 cm in 15.4% of cases of ES styloid processes exceeding 3.5 cm in length in 34.2% of normal subjects Gender, age, ethnicity (pure anatomic elongation) Styloid fracture (trauma)
Muscle	Stylohyoid muscle hypertrophy/fibrosis/compression
Association with	Ponticulus posticus (or Kimmerle anomaly)

Table 11.4 Diagnostic criteria by the International Headache Society (IHS) Classification Committee in the International Classification of Headache Disorders, third edition

11.8 Headache or facial pain attributed to inflammation of the stylohyoid ligament
Previously used term: Eagle syndrome. Description: Unilateral headache, with neck, pharyngeal, and/or facial pain, caused by inflammation of the stylohyoid ligament and usually provoked or exacerbated by head turning
Diagnostic criteria:
Any head, neck, pharyngeal, and/or facial pain fulfilling criterion C1
Radiological evidence of calcified or elongated stylohyoid ligament
Evidence of causation demonstrated by at least two of the following:
Pain is provoked or exacerbated by digital palpation of the stylohyoid ligament
Pain is provoked or exacerbated by head turning
Pain is significantly improved by injection of local anesthetic agent into the stylohyoid ligament or by styloidectomy
Pain is ipsilateral to the inflamed stylohyoid ligament
Not better accounted for by another ICHD-3 diagnosis

A. The length of the styloid process (SP) is correlated with age, showing a slow increase over the years [27, 28].
B. A certain degree of asymmetry is normal [29, 30].
C. Gender is an additional differentiating factor, being longer in males [31].
D. Significant differences are also correlated with ethnicity [32].

11.10 TES Diagnosis

The diagnostic criteria for diagnosing TES, reported in Table 11.4, are well defined by the International Headache Society (IHS) Classification Committee in the International Classification of Headache Disorders, third edition [15].

The path to TES diagnosis is summarized in the following three levels of increasing accuracy, which can be defined with completely arbitrary terminology as possible/suspected, probable, and defined, according to different degrees of clinical evidence.

1. Possible or suspected Eagle syndrome
– Long-term pain in the face and/or neck (target complaint)
– Symptoms and pain profile fitting the Eagle syndrome description
– Radiological evidence of an elongated styloid process
– Exclusion of other differential diagnoses

It is the first level of diagnosis. It is simply observational, and the key is a compatible pain profile associated with a radiological pathologic styloid, provided that any possible differential diagnosis is excluded. In our personal opinion, it is just a provisional step, requiring in all the cases a second step of anesthetic infiltration of the affected side.

1. Probable Eagle syndrome
– Patients with possible ES who experienced a significant reduction in symptoms after local infiltration by anesthetic and corticosteroid

It is the second level of diagnostic accuracy, and it is based on the injection of a local anesthetic around the tip of the styloid process. In case of complete or partial pain control, the test is considered as positive, and TES may be labeled as probable. It is an interactive approach with some degree on invasiveness, and it requires the patient's consent. It is probably the most informative among the four IHS evidences of causation, and it is the most predictive of surgical success. False-negative responses are possible for technical errors, and false positive (pain relief) must be considered for placebo effect.

1. Confirmed Eagle syndrome
– Patients treated with surgical styloidectomy who experienced complete symptom reduction after surgery

In Fig. 11.5 are summarized in a flow chart the three levels of evidence.

The average pain control rate of styloidectomy is about 80%. A surgical success must be considered the final diagnostic confirmation at the best level of accuracy. Anyway, as in any kind of pain treatment even after surgery, some degree of placebo

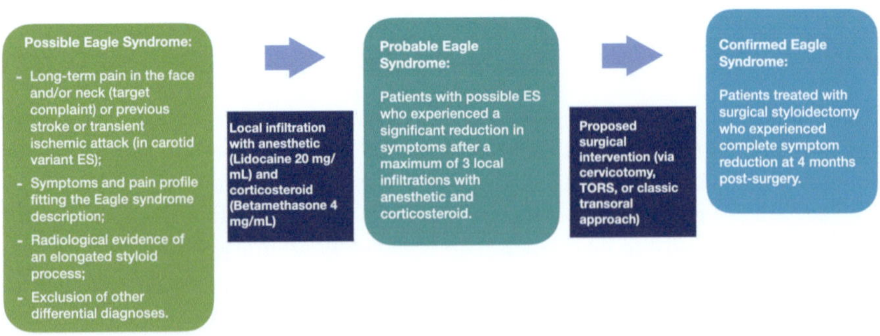

Fig. 11.5 The flow chart with the three levels of diagnostic probability

effect may play a role. In failed cases, many different explanations are possible (poor technique, insufficient resection, etc.), including wrong diagnosis of ES, which must be submitted to reevaluation.

11.11 Different Scenarios in the Practice

In daily clinical practice, more commonly in high-volume centers, different scenarios may be encountered and will be described into detail.

1. Patient referred for orofacial and neck pain of unknown origin requiring diagnosis (it poses the problem of ES underdiagnosis or delayed diagnosis). The main responsibility of the clinician is to rule out ES in any not yet clarified case of orofacial-neck pain, performing at least a proper tonsil fossa palpation. The second responsibility is to be aware of the special psychological frailty produced by a long story of chronic not controlled pain and by the frustration of a never-ending story of not diagnosis.
2. Patient with suspected TES requiring confirmation and treatment (it poses the problem of second opinion and taking charge). The key is to match the described clinical picture with the typical profile and to finalize the diagnostic pathway, very commonly missing of the lidocaine injection. If required, surgery may be offered, or the patient must be referred to a surgical center of reference.
3. Patient with elongated styloid but suffering from diseases different from TES claiming to be treated for TES (it poses the problem of the self- or overdiagnosis). It is an emerging and growing problem. In our series, patients with cricopharyngeal dysfunction, motor neuron disease, and oropharyngeal cancer with an elongated styloid self-referred themselves for ES treatment. A comprehensive differential diagnosis is mandatory.
4. Failures after previous treatments (it poses the problem of correct and not correct expectations). Keep in mind that not all the operated-on patients do respond. In few cases, an under-resected styloid may offer the opportunity to complete the resection, but revision styloidectomy may be very difficult and unsatisfactory.

References

1. Eagle WW, Durham NC. Elongated styloid processes. Report of two cases. Arch Otolaryngol Head Neck Surg. 1937;25:584–7.
2. Piagkou M, Anagnostopoulou S, Kouladouros K, Piagkos G. Eagle's syndrome: a review of the literature. Clin Anat. 2009;22(5):545–58. https://doi.org/10.1002/ca.20804.
3. Swanson D, Evensky CH, Yusuf S, et al. Eagle syndrome: pathophysiology, differential diagnosis and treatment options. Health Psychol Research. 2023;10(5) https://doi.org/10.52965/001c.67851.
4. Lee CJ, Chen HC. Eagle syndrome. Ear Nose Throat J. 2020;99(9):99–100. https://doi.org/10.1177/0145561320930059.
5. Baba A, Okuyama Y, Ojiri H, Nakajima T. Eagle syndrome. Clin Case Rep. 2017;5(2):201–2. https://doi.org/10.1002/ccr3.806.

6. Dabrowski DS, Ghali GE, Cotelingam JD. Bilateral Eagle syndrome. Ear Nose Throat J. 2022;101(10):645–6. https://doi.org/10.1177/014556132097355.
7. Montevecchi F, Caranti A, Cammaroto G, Meccariello G, Vicini C. Transoral robotic surgery (TORS) for bilateral Eagle syndrome. ORL J Otorhinolaryngol Relat Spec. 2019;81(1):36–40. https://doi.org/10.1159/000493736.
8. Ahmad M, Schiffman EL. Temporomandibular joint disorders and orofacial pain. Dent Clin N Am. 2017;96(3):270–6. https://doi.org/10.1177/0022034516679396.
9. Mueller D, Obermann M, Yoon MS, Poitz F, Hansen N, Slomke MA, Dommes P, Gizewski E, Diener HC, Katsarava Z. Prevalence of trigeminal neuralgia and persistent idiopathic facial pain: a population-based study. Cephalalgia. 2011;31(15):1542–8. https://doi.org/10.1177/0333102411424619.
10. Zammit M, Chircop C, Attard V, D'Anastasi M. Eagle's syndrome: a piercing matter. BMJ Case Rep. 2018;11(1):e226611. https://doi.org/10.1136/bcr-2018-226611.
11. Saccomanno S, Greco F, Corso EDE, Lucidi D, Deli R, D'Addona A, Paludetti G. Eagle's syndrome, from clinical presentation to diagnosis and surgical treatment: a case report. Acta Otorhinolaryngol Ital. 2018;38(2):166–9. https://doi.org/10.14639/0392-100X-1479.
12. Gupta M, Kumar Y, Vig H, Rizvi A. Classic Eagle's syndrome: Styloidectomy via the Transcervical approach. BMJ Case Rep. 2021;14(8):e244634. https://doi.org/10.1136/bcr-2021-244634.
13. Scerrati A, Norri N, Mongardi L, Dones F, Ricciardi L, Trevisi G, Menegatti E, Zamboni P, Cavallo MA, De Bonis P. Styloidogenic-cervical spondylotic internal jugular venous compression, a vascular disease related to several clinical neurological manifestations: diagnosis and treatment-a comprehensive literature review. Ann Transl Med. 2021;9(8):718. https://doi.org/10.21037/atm-20-7698.
14. Zamboni P, Scerrati A, Menegatti E, Galeotti R, Lapparelli M, Traina L, Tessari M, Ciorba A, De Bonis P, Pelucchi S. The eagle jugular syndrome. BMC Neurol. 2019;19(1):333. https://doi.org/10.1186/s12883-019-1572-3.
15. Headache classification Committee of the International Headache Society (IHS) the international classification of headache disorders, 3rd edition. Cephalalgia. 2018;38:1–211. https://doi.org/10.1177/0333102417738202.
16. Singhania AA, Chauhan NV, George A, Rathwala K. Lidocine infiltration test: an useful test in the prediction of results of Styloidectomy for Eagle's syndrome. Indian J Otolaryngol Head Neck Surg. 2013;65(1):20–3. https://doi.org/10.1007/s12070-012-0577-7.
17. Ravisankar M, Murugesan GS. Evaluation of Eagle's syndrome and assessment of post-operative outcome of excision of elongated styloid process: a prospective study, in tertiary care Centre, India. Indian J Otolaryngol Head Neck Surg. 2022;74(2):150–7. https://doi.org/10.1007/s12070-020-02255-4.
18. Sharma N, Ram R, Kamal R. Unusually elongated styloid process: a report of two cases with literature review. Ann Maxillofac Surg. 2016;6(2):297–9. https://doi.org/10.4103/2231-0746.200343.
19. Lee YW, Chung J. Eagle syndrome after a fracture of complete ossified stylohyoid ligament from indirect trauma treated using local steroid injection: a case report. Medicine (Baltimore). 2020;99(25):e20818. https://doi.org/10.1097/MD.0000000000020818.
20. Vase L, Wartolowska K. Pain, placebo, and test of treatment efficacy: a narrative review. Br J Anaesth. 2019;123(2):e254–62. https://doi.org/10.1016/j.bja.2019.01.040.
21. Xu Z, Shi P, Zhang P. Eagle syndrome: a rare neuropathic disorder affecting head and neck. Medicine (Baltimore). 2024;103(19):e38128. https://doi.org/10.1097/MD.0000000000038128.
22. Morrison PJ, Morrison RJ, McKinstry CS. Familial ossification of the stylohyoid ligament in a three generation family--a new clinical entity displaying autosomal dominant inheritance. Br J Radiol. 2012;85(1012):458–9. https://doi.org/10.1259/bjr/21631652.
23. Eagle WW. Elongated styloid process; further observations and a new syndrome. Arch Otolaryngol. 1925). 1948;47(5):630–40. https://doi.org/10.1001/archotol.1948.00690030654006.

24. Radak D, Tanaskovic S, Kecmanovic V, Babic S, Popov P, Gajin P. Bilateral Eagle syndrome with associated internal carotid artery kinking and significant stenosis. Ann Vasc Surg. 2016;34(271):e15–8. https://doi.org/10.1016/j.avsg.2016.01.015.
25. Fitzpatrick TH 4th, Lovin BD, Magister MJ, Waltonen JD, Browne JD, Sullivan CA. Surgical management of Eagle syndrome: A 17-year experience with open and transoral robotic styloidectomy. Am J Otolaryngol. 2020;41(2):102324. https://doi.org/10.1016/j.amjoto.2019.102324.
26. Eagle WW. The symptoms, diagnosis and treatment of the elongated styloid process. Am Surg. 1962;28:1–5.
27. Ceylan A, Köybaşioğlu A, Celenk F, Yilmaz O, Uslu S. Surgical treatment of elongated styloid process: experience of 61 cases. Skull Base. 2008;18(5):289–95. https://doi.org/10.1055/s-0028-1086057.
28. Raina D, Gothi R, Rajan S. Eagle syndrome. Indian J Radiol Imaging. 2009;19(2):107–8. https://doi.org/10.4103/0971-3026.50826.
29. Rath G, Anand C. Abnormal styloid process in a human skull. Surg Radiol Anat. 1991;13(3):227–9. https://doi.org/10.1007/BF01627991.
30. Natsis K, Repousi E, Noussios G, Papathanasiou E, Apostolidis S, Piagkou M. The styloid process in a Greek population: an anatomical study with clinical implications. Anat Sci Int. 2015;90(2):67–74. https://doi.org/10.1007/s12565-014-0232-3.
31. Gözil R, Yener N, Calgüner E, Araç M, Tunç E, Bahcelioğlu M. Morphological characteristics of styloid process evaluated by computerized axial tomography. Ann Anat. 2001;183(6):527–35. https://doi.org/10.1016/S0940-9602(01)80060-1.
32. Alkhabuli J, Zakaria H, Muayad A. Prevalence of stylohyoid complex elongation among patients attending RAK college of dental sciences clinic. Acta Stomatol Croat. 2020;54(1):60–8. https://doi.org/10.15644/asc54/1/7.

12 Stylo-Carotid Eagle Syndrome

Paolo Zamboni, Giulia Baldazzi, Francesco Stomeo, and Stefano Pelucchi

12.1 Introduction

The elongation of the styloid process was first described by the Italian surgeon Pietro Marchetti in 1652; however, the clinical syndrome and its subgroups (the classic and the vascular form) were clearly defined in 1937 only by Watt Weems Eagle [1].

The classic syndrome has already been clarified in the previous chapters of the book; in this section, we will explore the rarer second form of the Eagle syndrome named in multiple ways in the literature: "vascular syndrome, carotid artery syndrome, or stylo-carotid Eagle syndrome."

Quite recently, this entity has been recognized and inserted among the vascular compression syndromes in a consensus document written by the International Union of Angiology [2].

12.2 Pathogenesis and Clinical Features

As highlighted by the name itself, the stylo-carotid Eagle syndrome is caused by an abnormally elongated and/or angulated styloid process or by a calcified stylo-hyoid ligament, which causes compression on the vascular structures of the neck, particularly on the extracranial carotid axis, and the nervous plexus that surrounds them.

P. Zamboni (✉) · G. Baldazzi
Vascular Diseases Center, University Hospital of Ferrara, Ferrara, Italy
e-mail: zambo@unife.it; giulia.baldazzi@unife.it

F. Stomeo · S. Pelucchi
ENT & Audiology Unit, Department of Neurosciences, University Hospital of Ferrara, Ferrara, Italy
e-mail: francesco.stomeo@unife.it; stefano.pelucchi@unife.it

C. Vicini et al. (eds.), *EAGLE Syndrome*,
https://doi.org/10.1007/978-3-031-92829-1_12

The presence of an elongated styloid process has been found in approximately 4% of the general population; however, due to its rareness, the prevalence and incidence of the carotid artery syndrome are not available in the literature.

Frequently, as reported for the classic syndrome (Table 12.1), patients affected by vascular Eagle syndrome are mainly females, 50–60 years old, who present in their past medical history a traumatic event [3], consisting in car accidents, traumas, or previous surgery in the oropharyngeal or cervical region.

Usually, the Eagle syndrome results completely asymptomatic; however, when symptoms are present (4–10% of cases) [4], contralateral head rotational movements could exacerbate them.

The mechanical irritation of the perivascular nerve fibers could result in referred parietal or periorbital pain [5] or, in rare cases, in Horner's syndrome due to the compression on the sympathetic nervous system.

The compression of the cervical segment of arterial vessels, instead, could cause, on one hand, pain in the ipsilateral face and neck regions, when the external carotid artery branches are involved, and, on the other hand, the reduction or obstruction of the blood flow (Fig. 12.1), when the extracranial portion of the internal carotid artery (ICA) is affected, and consequent neurological symptoms such as headache, dizziness, transient visual loss, syncope, and/or other vascular and potentially severe symptoms [6].

In the literature, multiple vascular complications due to an elongated styloid process are reported: transient ischemic attacks (TIAs) [7, 8], stroke [9], vessel stenosis and occlusion (Fig. 12.1), pseudoaneurysm formation [10], and, rarely, blood leaks

Table 12.1 Differences in demographic and clinical data between classic and carotid Eagle syndrome

	Classic type	Carotid type
Sex	F > M	F > M
Age	Fifth and sixth decades (peak)	Fifth and sixth decades (peak)
History of tonsillectomy	Increased frequency	Increased frequency
Odynophagia	Frequent	Not observed
Dysphagia	Frequent	Not observed
Pain (absent/present)	Variable	Frequent
Pain (location)	Ipsilateral; parietal region to pectoral region	Ipsilateral: parietal region/superior periorbital region
Pain (quality)	Dull, constant	Variable (e.g., throbbing, stabbing)
Stridor	Rare (children)	Not observed
Dizziness	Not observed	Frequent
Syncope/TIA/stroke	Not observed	Frequent
Flexion/extension	Aggravates symptoms	Aggravates symptoms
Contralateral head rotation	Minimal effect	Aggravates symptoms
Tonsillar pillar palpation (exam)	Aggravates symptoms	Minimal effect

With kind permission of [1]

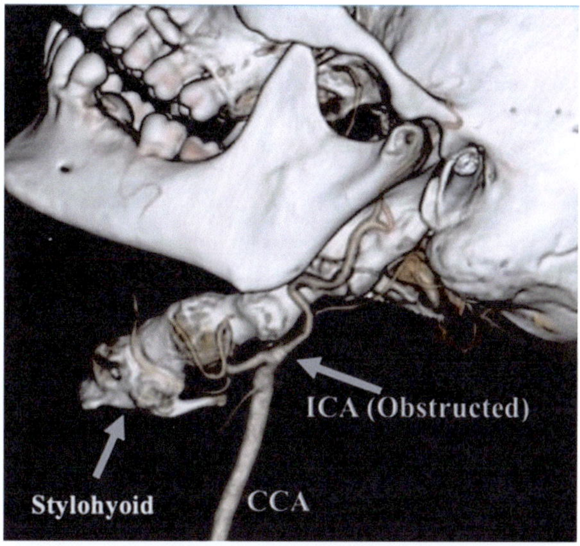

Fig. 12.1 3D reconstruction of an internal carotid artery (ICA) obstruction due to an elongated styloid process and concomitant ossification of the stylo-hyoid ligament. (Courtesy of Prof. Paolo Zamboni. Legend: common carotid artery (CCA))

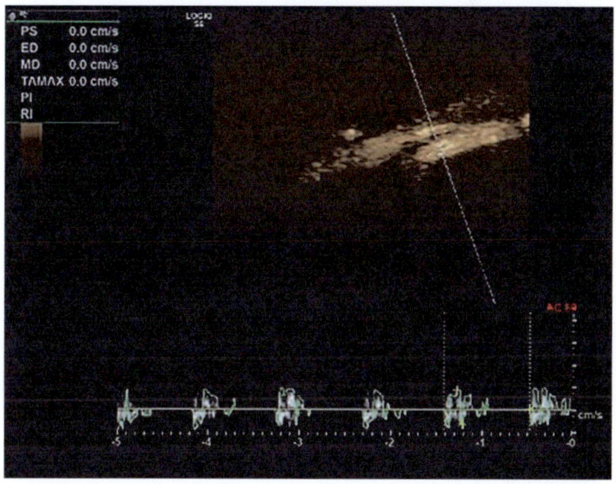

Fig. 12.2 Ultrasound scan in B-flow mode of an internal carotid artery (ICA) dissection due to an elongated styloid process. In the image, we could clearly distinguish the two lumens. The Doppler probe is positioned in the false lumen and documents the arterial flow in the dissected segment. (Courtesy of Prof. Paolo Zamboni)

in the cervical region that could express through hemoptysis, as described by Michiels et al. (2020) [11].

Another uncommon but significant vascular complication is determined by the ICA dissection; as described by Subedi et al. (2017) [12], the tip of an abnormally elongated styloid process could impact on the internal carotid artery, in particular during neck muscle contractions; this repeated trauma causes the vessel dissection that could result completely asymptomatic or symptomatic for cerebrovascular insults such as stroke or TIA [13, 14]. In Fig. 12.2, a case of ultrasound (US) accidentally finding ICA dissection due to an elongated styloid process (confirmed by a subsequent CT scan) is reported.

For these reasons, when vascular symptoms are present, performing a computed tomography angiography (CTA) of the supraortic and intracranial vessels is fundamental, and, in case of a patient that comes to our attention with ICA dissection, the presence of an elongated styloid process must occur to the examinator and to the radiologist, during imaging analysis. Moreover, most of the carotid dissections are usually evaluated by specialists in neurology, who could be unaware of this rare syndrome; therefore, we can hypothesize that a proportion of carotid dissection, induced by the styloid process, could not be properly diagnosed.

12.3 Treatment

There are several options of treatment that involve conservative medical therapy, as well as interventional and surgical procedures.

In case of both symptomatic (vessel stenosis, TIAs, stroke) and asymptomatic suspected stylo-carotid Eagle syndrome, it seems reasonable to equate this condition with a significant lesion of the ICA. Although there are no prospective and randomized studies evaluating the effectiveness of medical therapies with this particular indication, it is mandatory to protect the patient by the means of antiplatelet drugs, as applied for the atherosclerotic carotid disease [15]. Above all, medical therapy must be introduced when surgical interventions are not recommended, as reported by Qureshi et al. [16]; however, even after surgical procedures, the antiplatelet therapy must be started and continued for an undetermined period of time, as the literature lacks studies that define the duration of these therapies.

Open surgery is the only treatment that currently allows the removal of the "primum movens" of the syndrome, the styloid process. As described in the subsequent chapters, different techniques and ways of access (open transcervical or transoral styloidectomy) could be applied to remove this bone.

Otherwise, the mechanical compression of the styloid process on the ICA could determine vascular complications that usually need to be managed promptly. As suggested by Pagano et al. [5], treatment of symptomatic dissection of the carotid artery (TIAs or acute ischemic stroke) should be executed according to the ESO guidelines [17].

Pseudoaneurysms' formation, instead, could be faced either with surgical or endovascular approaches. In asymptomatic patients, it is not well defined whether this vascular complication should be addressed before, at the same time, or after performing the styloidectomy; however, aneurysmectomy and subsequent vascular anastomosis or substitution of the diseased carotid tract with an autologous or prosthetic graft are all available alternatives. The endovascular approach could be chosen when the operator wants to avoid cervical exposure (hostile necks due to previous surgery, radiotherapy, or traumas), reducing nerve injuries [18]. The deployment of a stent is the pillar of the endovascular pseudoaneurysm exclusion and could be applied to treat carotid stenosis also [19]; this procedure is usually realized gaining an arterial femoral access (humeral and radial accesses could represent alternatives) [15] and the lumen of the internal carotid artery, with the assistance long guidewires, sheets, and catheters, after performing serial angiograms of the aorta, the aortic arch, and the supraortic trunks to visualize the road to follow and navigate inside the vessels [19]. A proximal or distal protection device [20], based on the operator experience, could be applied to prevent migration and cerebral embolization of thrombus or plaques' pieces. Then, the stent [21, 22] is positioned and deployed in the diseased tract, and the final angiography is performed to check the correct stent positioning and the absence of cerebral embolization [23]. At the end, the endovascular devices are removed. The access site hemostasis could be achieved through manual compression or vascular closure devices [24, 25]. This approach, in theory, seems to be the easier way to simultaneously treat the vascular complication and to prevent the styloid process' compression and damage of the vascular axis. However, Hooker et al. (2016) published a case [4] describing the fracture of an ICA stent caused by the impingement of the styloid process against the carotid wall (Fig. 12.3). This report leads us to consider open surgery again as the possible best surgical treatment to remove the real cause of the syndrome.

For these reasons, further investigations and future research are warranted to identify the real prevalence of the stylo-carotid variant of the Eagle syndrome, its vascular complications' incidence, and best treatment options.

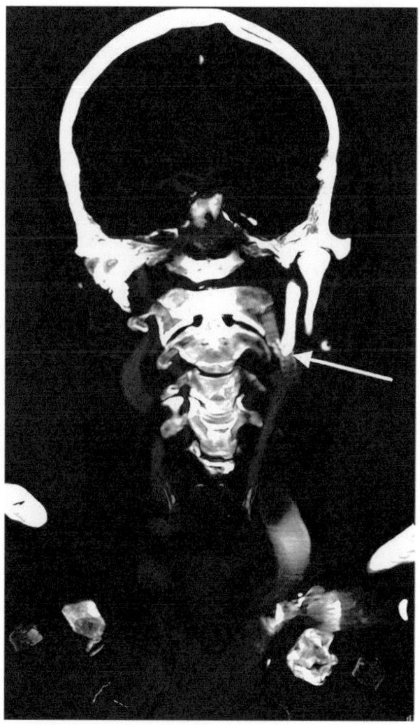

Fig. 12.3 Coronal CTA view that evidences the fracture of the stent positioned in the left internal carotid artery (pointed by the white arrow) due to an elongated styloid process. (Unchanged figure reproduction from [4])

References

1. Fusco DJ, Asteraki S, Spetzler RF. Eagle's syndrome: embryology, anatomy, and clinical management. Acta Neurochir. 2012;154(7):1119–26.
2. D'Oria M, Zlatanovic P, Anthony A, Dua A, Flores AM, Tanious A, Rodríguez Morata A, Scerrati A, Baccellieri D, Biscetti F, Baldazzi G, Mantovani G, Sen I, Peinado Cebrian J, Rocha-Neves J, Sousa J, Davidovic L, Juszynski M, Markovic M, Oller Grau M, Tessari M, Hynes N, Gloviczki P, Shaw P, Zamboni P, Hinchliffe R, Ricci R, Sultan S, Acharya Y, Troisi N, Antignani PL, Mansilha A, Komlos PP. International Union of Angiology consensus document on vascular compression syndromes. Int Angiol. 2023;42(4):282–309.
3. Saccomanno S, Quinzi V, D'Andrea N, Albani A, Coceani Paskay L, Marzo G. Traumatic events and Eagle syndrome: is there any correlation? A systematic review. Healthcare (Basel). 2021;9(7):825.
4. Hooker JD, Joyner DA, Farley EP, Khan M. Carotid stent fracture from stylocarotid syndrome. J Radiol Case Rep. 2016;10(6):1–8.
5. Pagano S, Ricciuti V, Mancini F, Barbieri FR, Chegai F, Marini A, Marruzzo D, Paracino R, Ricciuti RA. Eagle syndrome: an updated review. Surg Neurol Int. 2023;14:389.
6. Zamboni P, Scerrati A, Menegatti E, et al. The eagle jugular syndrome. BMC Neurol. 2019;19:333.
7. Farhat HI, Elhammady MS, Ziayee H, Aziz-Sultan MA, Heros RC. Eagle syndrome as a cause of transient ischemic attacks. J Neurosurg. 2009;110(1):90–3.
8. Varelas PN, Sinson G, Rand S, Book D. Clipping the Eagle's wings: treatment of an unusual cause of transient cerebral ischemia. Neurology. 2005;64(2):393–4.
9. Keshelava G, Kurdadze R, Tsiklauri D. Surgical management of a patient with an internal carotid artery stenosis, Eagle syndrome, and internal carotid artery tortuosity: a case of four pathologies of the carotid arteries. EJVES Vasc Forum. 2021;50:37–9. https://doi.org/10.1016/j.ejvsvf.2021.01.002.
10. Sayed AG, Aboloyoun H, Makarem YS, Elnaggar A. Internal carotid artery pseudoaneurysm after neck manipulation in a patient with Eagle syndrome. Clin Case Rep. 2024;12(5):e8814.
11. Michiels TD, Marsman MS, van Veen A, Vriens PWHE, Lauret GJ, Heyligers JMM. Eagle syndrome: a unique cause of carotid bleeding. JACC Case Rep. 2020;2(3):449–53.
12. Subedi R, Dean R, Baronos S. Dhamoon a: carotid artery dissection: a rare complication of Eagle syndrome. BMJ Case Rep. 2017;2017:bcr2016218184.
13. Baldino G, Di Girolamo C, De Blasis G, Gori A. Eagle syndrome and internal carotid artery dissection: description of five cases treated in two Italian institutions and review of the literature. Ann Vasc Surg. 2020;67:565.e17–24.
14. Todo T, Alexander M, Stokol C, Lyden P, Braunstein G, Gewertz B. Eagle syndrome revisited: cerebrovascular complications. Ann Vasc Surg. 2012;26(5):729.e1–5.
15. Naylor R, et al. European Society for Vascular Surgery (ESVS) 2023 clinical practice guidelines on the management of atherosclerotic carotid and vertebral artery disease. Eur J Vasc Endovasc Surg. 65:7. https://doi.org/10.1016/j.ejvs.2022.04.011.
16. Qureshi S, Farooq M, Gorelick PB. Ischemic stroke secondary to stylocarotid variant of Eagle syndrome. Neurohospitalist. 2019;9:105–8.
17. Debette S, Mazighi M, Bijlenga P, et al. ESO guideline for the management of extracranial and intracranial artery dissection. Eur Stroke J. 2021;6(3):XXXIX–LXXXVIII.
18. Sidawy AN, Perler BA. Rutherford's vascular surgery and endovascular therapy. Faculty Bookshelf; 2018. Volume I, Section 13, Chapter 89, p. 3925. https://hsrc.himmelfarb.gwu.edu/books/133
19. Speziale F, et al. Chirurgia Vascolare III Edizione. A cura di Società Italiana di Chirurgia Vascolare ed Endovascolare (SICVE). Torino: Edizioni Minerva Medica; 2022.
20. Texakalidis P, Letsos A, Kokkinidis DG, Schizas D, Karaolanis G, Giannopoulos S, Giannopoulos S, Economopoulos KP, Bakoyannis C. Proximal embolic protection versus

distal filter protection versus combined protection in carotid artery stenting: a systematic review and meta-analysis. Cardiovasc Revasc Med. 2018;19(5 Pt A):545–52.
21. Pini R, Faggioli G, Paraskevas KI, Campana F, Sufali G, Rocchi C, Palermo S, Gallitto E, Gargiulo M. Carotid artery stenting with double-layer stent: a systematic review and meta-analysis. J Endovasc Ther. 2024;31(3):339–49.
22. Mazurek A, Malinowski K, Sirignano P, Kolvenbach R, Capoccia L, de Donato G, van Herzeele I, Siddiqui AH, Castrucci T, Tekieli L, Stefanini M, Wissgott C, Rosenfield K, Metzger DC, Snyder K, Karpenko A, Kuczmik W, Stabile E, Knapik M, Casana R, Pieniazek P, Podlasek A, Taurino M, Schofer J, Cremonesi A, Sievert H, Schmidt A, Grunwald IQ, Speziale F, Setacci C, Musialek P, CArotid Revascularization systematic reviews and MEta-aNalyses (CARMEN) Collaborators. Carotid artery revascularization using second generation stents versus surgery: a meta-analysis of clinical outcomes. J Cardiovasc Surg. 2023;64(6):570–82.
23. Wodarg F, Turner EL, Dobson J, Ringleb PA, Mali WP, Fraedrich G, Chatellier G, Bequemin JP, Brown MM, Algra A, Mas JL, Jansen O, Bonati LH, Carotid Stenosis Trialists' Collaboration. Influence of stent design and use of protection devices on outcome of carotid artery stenting: a pooled analysis of individual patient data. J Neurointerv Surg. 2018;10(12):1149–54.
24. Reich R, Helal L, Mantovani VM, Rabelo-Silva ER. Hemostasis control after femoral percutaneous approach: a systematic review and meta-analysis. Int J Nurs Stud. 2023;137:104364.
25. Koziarz A, Kennedy SA, El-Karim GA, Tan KT, Oreopoulos GD, Jaberi A, Rajan DK, Mafeld S. The use of vascular closure devices for brachial artery access: a systematic review and meta-analysis. J Vasc Interv Radiol. 2023;34(4):677–684.e5.

Jugular Eagle Syndrome

13

Paolo Zamboni, Giulia Baldazzi, Francesco Stomeo, and Stefano Pelucchi

13.1 Introduction

The jugular Eagle syndrome represents the last described variant of the Eagle syndrome and, as underlined by the name itself, is characterized by the internal jugular vein (IJV) compression or obstruction due to an elongated styloid process. First traces of this entity could be found in 2008 and are correlated with the definition of an entity called chronic cerebrospinal venous insufficiency (CCSVI), which is characterized by extracranial narrowing of the IJV, compensated by substitute circles; CCSVI will be better discussed in a subsequent chapter. The initial description of this novel Eagle syndrome's variant has been followed by several confirmations, leading to a recognition of such novel nosological entity [1, 2].

13.2 Pathogenesis and Clinical Presentation

In this particular variant of the Eagle syndrome, the cause of primary obstruction of the IJV, just below its exit from the cranial base, at the level of its superior portion (defined as J3), is constantly represented by a bone nutcracker between the transverse process of C1 and the elongated styloid process, as shown in Fig. 13.1.

P. Zamboni (✉) · G. Baldazzi
Vascular Diseases Center, University Hospital of Ferrara, Ferrara, Italy
e-mail: zambo@unife.it; giulia.baldazzi@unife.it

F. Stomeo · S. Pelucchi
ENT & Audiology Unit, Department of Neurosciences, University Hospital of Ferrara, Ferrara, Italy
e-mail: francesco.stomeo@unife.it; stefano.pelucchi@unife.it

C. Vicini et al. (eds.), *EAGLE Syndrome*,
https://doi.org/10.1007/978-3-031-92829-1_13

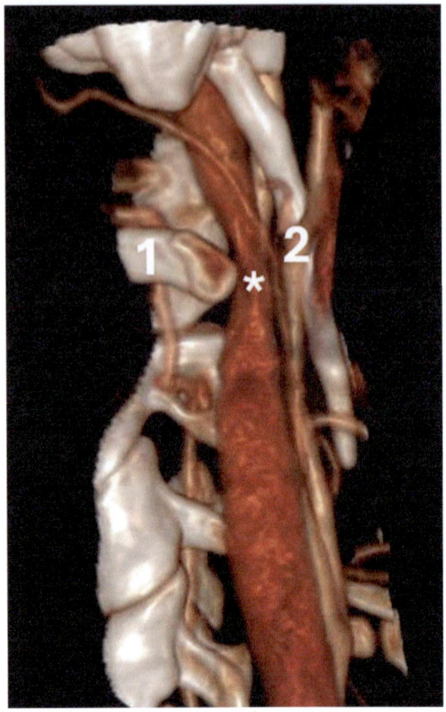

Fig. 13.1 3D reconstruction of an angio-computed tomography (CT) scan of an internal jugular vein nutcracker between the C1 transverse process (*1*) and the elongated styloid process (*2*). The area of venous compression is identified by the *

Mantovani et al. [3], in a quite recent paper, after developing an angio-CT software to process images, suggest that different angles and directions of this elongated bone could determine the variants of the Eagle syndrome. In particular, they highlight that the spatial orientation and the adherence between C1 and the styloid process are more important factors as compared to the length of the bone itself; in fact, considering the jugular variant of the Eagle syndrome, the authors suggest that patients with a more vertical and medial-directed styloid process may have a significant probability of developing jugular nutcracker.

The clinical presentation and the subjective symptoms of this variant significantly differ from the other Eagle syndromes, as highlighted in Table 13.1.

Headache results the most prevalent symptom, often associated with numbness and dizziness [2]. In another multicentre survey, headache was found in 46% of patients, tinnitus in 44% and insomnia in 40%, with monolateral and bilateral IJV stenosis present in 46% and 54% of patients, respectively [4]. Headache, numbness and dizziness have been constantly reported when the so-called CCSVI was demonstrated. As commonly known, the IJV represents the main pathway of drainage of the catabolites from the brain; however, the presence of jugular vein obstruction and concomitant vicariant circle leads to a significant increased transit time of the venous blood for the brain to the right atrium [5].

The theory of glymphatic system (brain's lymphatic system), detailing described by Minagar [6], allowed to at least partially explain the impairment of cerebral drainage due to IJV stenosis or obstruction: the cerebrospinal fluid (CSF) is generated by ultrafiltration from the arterial side of capillaries and flows in the interstitial space, throughout the brain parenchyma, thanks to arterial pulsatile transmission. After collecting all the catabolites, the CSF must reenter in the venous system, to drain useless and damaging substances in the general circulation. At the venous level, fluid exchange mainly depends on the transmural pressure (TMP), determined by the difference between the extravascular and the intravascular pressure. Focusing on the mechanism above described, it is evident how the IJV compression or obstruction determines an increased pressure at the level of intracranial veins (intravenous pressure), causing a reduced catabolite clearance and absorption in the venular system and fluid and waste stasis in the interstitial space; this situation could enhance neuroinflammation and lastly influence the correct brain blood inflow also. This significant reduction of the perfusion of the brain parenchyma, highlighted in multiple papers [7–10], may explain the reported impairment of working memory chronic fatigue, blurred vision and "cerebral fog" which ultimately affect the patient social relationships. Moreover, another interesting complication, explicated in Table 13.1, is the onset of perimesencephalic

Table 13.1 Comparison of symptoms described by patients affected by different variants of the Eagle syndrome (classic, carotid, and jugular one)

Symptoms and associated comorbidities	Classic syndrome	Carotid variant	Jugular variant	RR 95% CI	*p-value*
History of tonsillectomy	1/14	1/1	0/8	N.A.	0.43
Odynophagia	1/14	0/1	1/8	0.53 0.03–7.44	0.58
Dysphagia	4/14	0/1	0/8	N.A.	0.15
Ipsilateral pain (present/absent)	11/14	1/1	0/8	N.A.	0.0003
Stabbing pain	4/14	1/1	1/8	2.67 0.37–19.09	0.29
Periorbital pain extension	0/14	0/1	1/8	N.A.	0.35
Pain at contralateral head rotation	0/14	1/1	0/8	N.A.	0.65
Dizziness	1/14	1/1	3/8	0.35 0.07–1.71	0.21
Otalgia	3/14	0/1	0/8	N.A.	0.24
Ipsilateral facial oedema	0/14	0/1	1/8	N.A.	0.35
Numbness	0/14	0/1	3/8	N.A.	0.03
Headache	0/14	1/1	5/8	0.11 0.01–0.76	0.009
TIA/stroke	0/14	1/1	0/8	N.A.	0.65
Perimesencephalic haemorrhage	0/14	0/1	6/8	N.A.	0.0003
Multiple sclerosis	0/14	0/1	2/8	N.A.	0.011
Dilated ventricles-CS spaces	0/14	0/1	2/8	N.A.	0.011

With kind permission of [2]

haemorrhage, defined as "sine materia", because neither aneurysm nor other vascular malformations can be found, even during extensive imaging and analysis. In addition, a state of endocranial venous hypertension, provoked by the jugular compression/obstruction, has been evocated to explain the pathogenesis of the haemorrhagic stroke. This novel vision seems to be confirmed by a study [11] where a significant jugular stenosis was found in 52% of patients in the group with nonaneurysmal subarachnoid haemorrhage versus just 18% in the control group. At univariate and multivariate analysis, the difference was highly significant ($p < 0.0001$).

13.3 Management and Conclusion

In case of symptoms that could refer to Eagle syndrome jugular variant, Doppler ultrasound (DUS) scan is considered the first-line imaging to detect morphological and haemodynamical alterations of the IJV and the activation significant collateral circles at the level of the neck, as well described in the subsequent "Complex Vascular Cases" chapter. CT or magnetic resonance imaging (MRI) venography, instead, may characterize and localize the bone nutcracker and allow surgical planning [12]. The elimination of the compression represents the aim of surgical treatment for this syndrome: styloidectomy, procedure already described in previous chapters, and partial C1 lateral mass resection, analysed in a dedicated chapter, are the main approaches.

As for the stylo-carotid Eagle syndrome and even for the jugular variant, further investigations are warranted to identify its real prevalence and its impact on brain circulation and on neurological disease pathogenesis.

References

1. D'Oria M, Zlatanovic P, Anthony A, Dua A, Flores AM, Tanious A, Rodríguez Morata A, Scerrati A, Baccellieri D, Biscetti F, Baldazzi G, Mantovani G, Sen I, Peinado Cebrian J, Rocha-Neves J, Sousa J, Davidovic L, Juszynski M, Markovic M, Oller Grau M, Tessari M, Hynes N, Gloviczki P, Shaw P, Zamboni P, Hinchliffe R, Ricci R, Sultan S, Acharya Y, Troisi N, Antignani PL, Mansilha A, Komlos PP. International Union of Angiology consensus document on vascular compression syndromes. Int Angiol. 2023;42(4):282–309.
2. Zamboni P, Scerrati A, Menegatti E, et al. The eagle jugular syndrome. BMC Neurol. 2019;19:333.
3. Mantovani G, Zangrossi P, Flacco ME, Di Domenico G, Nastro Siniscalchi E, De Ponte FS, Maugeri R, De Bonis P, Cavallo MA, Zamboni P, et al. Styloid jugular nutcracker: the possible role of the styloid process spatial orientation—a preliminary morphometric computed study. Diagnostics. 2023;13(2):298.
4. Scerrati A, Norri N, Mongardi L, Dones F, Ricciardi L, Trevisi G, Menegatti E, Zamboni P, Cavallo MA, De Bonis P. Styloidogenic-cervical spondylotic internal jugular venous compression, a vascular disease related to several clinical neurological manifestations: diagnosis and treatment-a comprehensive literature review. Ann Transl Med. 2021;9(8):718.
5. Zamboni P, Galeotti R, Menegatti E, et al. Chronic cerebrospinal venous insufficiency in patients with multiple sclerosis. J Neurol Neurosurg Psychiatry. 2009;80:392–9.
6. Minagar A. Neuroinflammation. 2nd ed; 2018. English ISBN: 9780128117095

7. Malagoni AM, Galeotti R, Menegatti E, Manfredini F, Basaglia N, Salvi F, Zamboni P. Is chronic fatigue the symptom of venous insufficiency associated with multiple sclerosis? A longitudinal pilot study. Int Angiol. 2010;29(2):176–82.
8. Zamboni P, Menegatti E, Weinstock-Guttman B, Dwyer MG, Schirda CV, Malagoni AM, Hojnacki D, Kennedy C, Carl E, Bergsland N, Magnano C, Bartolomei I, Salvi F, Zivadinov R. Hypoperfusion of brain parenchyma is associated with the severity of chronic cerebrospinal venous insufficiency in patients with multiple sclerosis: a cross-sectional preliminary report. BMC Med. 2011;9:22.
9. Zhou D, Meng R, Zhang X, Guo L, Li S, Wu W, et al. Intracranial hypertension induced by internal jugular vein stenosis can be resolved by stenting. Eur J Neurol. 2018 Feb;25(2):365–e13. https://doi.org/10.1111/ene.13512.
10. Zhou D, Ding JY, Ya JY, Pan LQ, Yan F, Yang Q, et al. Understanding jugular venous outflow disturbance. CNS Neurosci Ther. 2018 Jun;24(6):473–482. https://doi.org/10.1111/cns.12859.
11. Scerrati A, De Bonis P, Zamboni P, Dones F, Fontanella M, Cenzato M, Visani J, Bianchi F, Zanin L, Cavallo MA, Sturiale CL. A new insight in nonaneurysmal subarachnoid hemorrhage: the potential role of the internal jugular veins. J Neurol Surg A Cent Eur Neurosurg. 2022;83(4):344–50.
12. Jayaraman MV, Boxerman JL, Davis LM, Haas RA, Rogg JM. Incidence of extrinsic compression of the internal jugular vein in unselected patients undergoing CT angiography. AJNR Am J Neuroradiol. 2012;33:1247–50.

Differential Diagnosis of Eagle Syndrome vs Head and Neck Pain Syndromes

14

Anna Alessandri-Bonetti

In order to plan effective therapy, accurate identification of the pain source is needed. Also, the clinician should remember that pain may be heterotopic; therefore, primary and secondary pain must be distinguished. Patients with Eagle syndrome (ES) may present with a large variety of clinical presentations and a multitude of nonspecific symptoms that can overlap with a wide range of other conditions, often resulting in a challenging diagnosis.

ES is described according to the third edition of the International Classification of Headache Disorders (IHCD-3) [1] as a unilateral headache, with neck, pharyngeal, and/or facial pain, caused by inflammation of the stylohyoid ligament and usually provoked or exacerbated by head turning. However, it is also noted that headache or facial pain attributed to inflammation of the stylohyoid ligament is generally perceived in the oropharynx, neck, and/or face, but some patients experience more diffuse headache.

Considering the constellation of symptoms that may characterize ES, and because these symptoms are nonspecific and can mimic other disorders, ES should be distinguished diagnostically from the following conditions:

14.1 Temporomandibular Disorders (TMDs)

According to the American Association of Orofacial Pain definition, TMD is a collective term that encompasses pain and dysfunction of the masticatory muscles, temporomandibular joint, and associated structures [2]. Recent

A. Alessandri-Bonetti (✉)
Department of Dental Clinic and Maxillofacial Surgery, A. Gemelli University Policlinic IRCCS, Catholic University of Sacred Heart, Rome, Italy

C. Vicini et al. (eds.), *EAGLE Syndrome*,
https://doi.org/10.1007/978-3-031-92829-1_14

literature reports TMD prevalence to be about 31% among adult population. Despite being much more frequent than ES, they share a higher prevalence observed in females and an age peak occurring between 30 and 60 years [3, 4]. Common TMD symptoms include headache, pain, or stiffness in the jaw, the temples, and the ear or in front of the ear. Pain is generally modified by emotional stress, chewing, jaw movements (i.e., opening the mouth or moving the jaw forward or to the site), jaw habits (i.e., clenching and/or grinding), or jaw activities (i.e., talking, kissing, or yawning). ES and TMDs share symptoms like headache and pain with jaw movements; however, throat and neck pain are not typical symptoms of TMDs. In regard to pain description, TMD pain is usually bilateral and reported as intermittent, long-lasting, achy, and dull, while ES pain is generally unilateral, more constant, and increased by head turning, swallowing, and jaw movements.

TMDs can also be associated with clicking or popping sounds during jaw movement and limited jaw opening, while no sounds are typical of ES.

There is no widely accepted standard test available to diagnose TMDs; therefore, a complete examination should be performed with the aim of reproducing the familiar pain and identifying the pain source. As of today, the diagnostic criteria for temporomandibular disorders are considered the gold standard for TMD diagnosis [5]. Local anesthetic injections can be performed in the painful area to confirm the pain source and obtain a diagnosis.

Diagnostic imaging such as panoramic X-rays, CT, or MRI can help differentiate between these conditions by visualizing the styloid process and the TMJ.

14.2 Glossopharyngeal Neuralgia (GPN)

GPN is a rare pain syndrome in the sensory distribution of the glossopharyngeal nerve. According to the ICHD-3, GPN is characterized by unilateral brief sharp, stabbing, shooting pain in the sensory distribution of the glossopharyngeal nerve as well as the auricular and pharyngeal branches of the vagus cranial nerve [1]. GPN most commonly affects adults older than 50, with no gender predilection, while ES is more common in females under the age of 50. In regard to GPN pain distribution, similar to that of ES, it includes the ear, base of the tongue, throat, tonsillar fossa, and/or beneath the angle of the jaw. Similar to ES, GPN is characterized by unilateral pain; however, unlike ES, the pain is generally described in paroxysms of severe episodes lasting from 2 s to 2 min, abrupt in onset and termination, with a complete cessation of pain between episodes. Pain in glossopharyngeal neuralgia follows a relapsing and remitting pattern. Hot/cold food, tongue movements, talking, swallowing, coughing, or yawning can easily precipitate or worsen GPN pain [6–8].

The diagnostic test for GPN involves touching a cotton swab to the back of the throat, which elicits severe pain that is then relieved with the application of a local anesthetic. A thorough neurological examination and diagnostic tests can help to differentiate between GPN and ES.

14.3 Trigeminal Neuralgia (TN)

TN is a chronic painful neurological condition [9]. It is characterized by recurrent unilateral, electric shock-like or stabbing pain along the distribution of any or all divisions of the trigeminal nerve, typically affecting the maxillary and mandibular branches. Similar to ES, TN is more common in females than in males; however, it tends to occur after the age of 50, therefore after the age peak for ES. Although the pain can be severe and may overlap with areas affected by ES, TN usually differs from ES as it presents with paroxysms generally lasting a few seconds, triggered by innocuous stimuli like facial movements or light touch, and abrupt in onset and termination. TN may develop without apparent cause or be a result of another disorder. Additionally, there may or may not be concomitant continuous pain of moderate intensity within the affected division(s) [8].

Furthermore, TN is limited to the distribution of one or more divisions of the trigeminal nerve and does not involve throat symptoms. Unlike ES, TN enters into periods of complete remission in up to 63% of patients, with periods lasting from weeks to years [10].

Brain MRI is needed to confirm the suspicion of TN by identifying vascular compression of the trigeminal nerve or other abnormalities; no abnormal brain MRI findings are observed in patients with ES.

14.4 Ernest Syndrome

Ernest syndrome is a rare head and neck pain disorder affecting the stylomandibular ligament. It is characterized by the presence of pain in the preauricular area and angle of the mandible, which can radiate to the neck, shoulder, and eye on the same side, and it is associated with familiar pain upon palpation of the affected ligament. Differential diagnosis is complex as no pathognomonic factors have been reported. Symptoms of Ernest Syndrome may overlap with those of ES; however, ES typically presents with more pronounced dysphagia or globus sensation than Ernest syndrome. Unlike ES, pain does not increase with cranial motion; also unlike ES, no abnormalities are observed on radiographic imaging, as no significant elongation of the styloid process is present [11].

The diagnosis of Ernest syndrome is confirmed by symptom relief after administration of a local anesthetic at the insertion of the affected ligament [12].

The pathogenesis of Ernest syndrome is related to inflammation of the ligament; therefore, treatment is achieved through injections of corticosteroids at the mandibular insertion of the stylomandibular ligament [13].

14.5 Chronic Tonsillitis and Pharyngitis

Chronic tonsillitis and pharyngitis are common causes of throat pain and discomfort, and their symptomatology may mimic that of ES. However, these conditions are due to tenacious infection of the tonsils triggered by one of the several types of bacteria or viruses, which may result in tonsil stones [17]. In most cases, pharyngitis is caused by either bacterial or viral infection; however, other less common causes include allergies, trauma, reflux, cancer, and toxins [18]. Due to their most common pathophysiology, both tonsillitis and pharyngitis are often accompanied by signs of infection, such as fever, lymphadenopathy, and erythema or exudates in the throat [19], which are absent in ES. A detailed clinical history, throat examination, and response to antibiotic therapy can help differentiate these conditions from ES.

Both children and adults can be affected by chronic tonsillitis, while ES has been very rarely described in children.

14.6 Cervical Spine Disorders

Neck pain from various cervical spine disorders ranks second among the leading causes of musculoskeletal disorders [14]. The most common cervical spine disorders are cervical spondylosis and cervical disk herniation [15]. Neck pain shares with ES the age peak between 40 and 60 years, as well as some symptoms. However, pain from spondylosis is mechanical and described as a deep, dull, throbbing ache with occasional stiffness and/or headaches and typically located posterior along the midline or paraspinal aspects [16]. Pain from disk herniation is similar to spondylosis but usually also involves radiating neuropathic pain with numbness, tingling, burning, shooting, stabbing, and/or electrical shocks in the upper extremities as well as weakness in the upper extremities [16].

Cervical spine imaging, including X-rays, CT scans, and MRIs, can help distinguish these conditions from ES.

14.7 Carotid Artery Dissection

Carotid artery dissection is a condition whereby the layers of the carotid artery are spontaneously separated, potentially compromising blood flow and leading to a stroke [20]. The most common symptoms of carotid artery dissection include unilateral headache or neck pain and facial or eye pain and may be associated with focal cerebral ischemic symptoms or visual disturbances and weakness [20, 21]. The neck pain may be mistaken for ES, but carotid artery dissection is often associated with a sudden onset of symptoms and a history of recent trauma to the neck with anterior neck pain or connective tissue disorders. Doppler carotid ultrasound, computed tomographic angiography, magnetic resonance angiography, or digital subtraction angiography can identify and demonstrate carotid artery dissection [22]. None of these imaging is positive in patients with ES.

14.8 Migraine and Cluster Headaches

Migraine and cluster headaches can cause severe head and/or face pain, most often unilateral, which may extend to the neck, mimicking ES.

Migraine is a common, disabling primary headache disorder, ranked as the third highest cause of disability worldwide in both males and females under the age of 50 years [23]. Migraine may present with or without aura; however, both types share the presence of recurrent headache episodes that last 4–72 h when untreated. Typical characteristics include unilateral location, pulsating quality, moderate or severe intensity, aggravation by routine physical activity, and association with nausea and/or photophobia and phonophobia [1].

Cluster headache is a type of trigeminal autonomic cephalalgia [1], characterized by attacks of severe, strictly unilateral pain located in the orbital, supraorbital, or temporal regions, or in any combination of these sites. The attacks last 15–180 min and occur from once every other day to up to eight times a day. The pain is associated with ipsilateral conjunctival injection, lacrimation, nasal congestion, rhinorrhea, forehead and facial sweating, miosis, ptosis and/or eyelid edema, and/or restlessness or agitation. These headaches can also be distinguished by their response to specific headache treatments. Unlike ES, no abnormalities are observed on radiographic imaging, as no significant elongation of the styloid process is present.

14.9 Eagle Syndrome Variants and Misdiagnosis

ES itself can present in variants, such as the carotid Eagle syndrome [24], where the elongated styloid process impinges on vascular structures like the internal carotid artery, causing symptoms related to vascular insufficiency or stroke, or the Eagle jugular syndrome [25], where the internal jugular vein gets compressed. Misdiagnosis is common due to the syndrome's varied presentation. Clinicians should maintain a high index of suspicion and use a combination of clinical examination and imaging studies, such as panoramic X-rays, CT scans, and 3D reconstructions, to accurately diagnose ES.

14.10 Conclusion

The differential diagnosis of ES is complex due to its overlapping symptoms with various head and neck pain syndromes, including TMD, GPN, TN, and others. Accurate identification of the pain source is essential for effective treatment, requiring a thorough understanding of the clinical presentation, careful history taking, and appropriate use of diagnostic imaging. While ES typically presents with unilateral throat pain, a foreign body sensation, and pain associated with neck movements, other conditions may exhibit similar symptoms but differ in pain characteristics, distribution, and associated signs. Accurate diagnosis is essential to guide effective treatment and prevent mismanagement. Awareness of the various differential diagnoses ensures that patients receive timely and appropriate care for their symptoms.

By considering the wide range of conditions that can mimic ES, clinicians can avoid misdiagnosis and improve patient outcomes through tailored therapeutic approaches. This comprehensive approach to differential diagnosis is crucial for the effective management of patients presenting with symptoms suggestive of ES (Table 14.1).

Table 14.1 Characteristics of the most common differential diagnosis for Eagle syndrome

Syndrome	Eagle syndrome	Temporomandibular disorders	Glossopharyngeal neuralgia	Trigeminal neuralgia	Ernest syndrome	Chronic tonsillitis and pharyngitis
Symptoms	Headache, persistent pharyngeal pain increased by head movements	Headache; pain or stiffness in the jaw, temples, and the ear or in front of the ear; increased jaw movements; chewing; emotional stress	Paroxysms of very severe pain of short duration, with a complete cessation of pain between episodes	Unilateral, electric shock-like pain, of very brief duration, along the distribution of the trigeminal nerve	Pain in the preauricular area and angle of the mandible, which can radiate to the neck, shoulder, and eye	Pain the throat often accompanied by fever, lymphadenopathy, and erythema or exudates in the throat
Radiography	Radiographic imaging shows lengthening of the styloid, further confirmed by CT	Radiographic imaging can present within normal limits or it may show condylar abnormalities	Radiographic imaging present within normal limits	Brain MRI shows vascular compression of the trigeminal nerve or other abnormalities	Radiographic imaging present within normal limits	Radiographic imaging present within normal limits
Treatment	Injections with local anesthetics and corticosteroids and/or surgical resection	Conservative treatment is indicated; however, it depends on the affected structure	Pharmacotherapy is the preferred first-line treatment	Pharmacotherapy; and/or surgical treatment	Injections of corticosteroids	Pharmacotherapy is the preferred first-line treatment

References

1. Headache Classification Committee of the International Headache Society (IHS). The international classification of headache disorders, 3rd edition. Cephalalgia. 2018; 38:1–211.
2. Klasser GD, Reyes MR. Orofacial pain: guidelines for assessment, diagnosis, and management (AAOP the American Academy of orofacial pain). 7th ed. New Malden: Quintessence Publishing; 2024.
3. Valesan LF, Da-Cas CD, Réus JC, Denardin ACS, Garanhani RR, Bonotto D, Januzzi E, de Souza BDM. Prevalence of temporomandibular joint disorders: a systematic review and meta-analysis. Clin Oral Investig. 2021;25(2):441–53.
4. Iodice G, Cimino R, Vollaro S, Lobbezoo F, Michelotti A. Prevalence of temporomandibular disorder pain, jaw noised and oral behaviours in an adult Italian population sample. J Oral Rehabil. 2019;46:1–8.
5. Schiffman E, Ohrbach R, Truelove E, et al. Diagnostic criteria for temporomandibular disorders (DC/TMD) for clinical and research applications: recommendations of the International RDC/TMD Consortium Network and Orofacial Pain Special Interest Group. J Oral Facial Pain Headache. 2014;28(1):6–27.
6. Tepper SJ. Cranial neuralgias. Continuum (Minneap Minn). 2018;24(4, Headache):1157–78.
7. Blumenfeld A, Nikolskaya G. Glossopharyngeal neuralgia. Curr Pain Headache Rep. 2013;17(7):343.
8. International classification of orofacial pain, 1st edition (ICOP). Cephalalgia 2020; 40(2):129–221.
9. Allam AK, Sharma H, Larkin MB, Viswanathan A. Trigeminal neuralgia: diagnosis and treatment. Neurol Clin. 2023;41(1):107–21.
10. Maarbjerg S, Gozalov A, Olesen J, Bendtsen L. Trigeminal neuralgia: a prospective systematic study of clinical characteristics in 158 patients. Headache. 2014;54:1574–82.
11. Frugone-Zambra R, Berzaghi A, Gómez-Álvarez J, Bianchi A, Bortolini S. Eagle and Ernest syndromes: a scoping review. Minerva Dent Oral Sci. 2024;73(2):119–30. https://doi.org/10.23736/S2724-6329.22.04724-6.
12. Peñarrocha-Oltra D, Ata-Ali J, Ata-Ali F, Peñarrocha-Diago MA, Peñarrocha M. Treatment of orofacial pain in patients with stylomandibular ligament syndrome (Ernest Syndrome). Neurologia. 2013;28(5):294–8. English, Spanish
13. Domínguez J, Bornhardt T, Wen S, Iturriaga V. Ernest syndrome: a systematic review of the literature. J Oral Facial Pain Headache. 2020;34(2):167–73.
14. Oral A, Sindel D, Ketenci A. Evidence-based physical medicine and rehabilitation strategies for patients with cervical radiculopathy due to disc herniation. Turk J Phys Med Rehab. 2014;60:47–53.
15. Metzger RL. Evidence-based diagnosis and treatment of cervical spine disorders. Nurse Pract. 2019;44(8):30–7.
16. Cohen SP. Epidemiology, diagnosis, and treatment of neck pain. Mayo Clin Proc. 2015;90(2):284–99.
17. Abu Bakar M, McKimm J, Haque SZ, Majumder MAA, Haque M. Chronic tonsillitis and biofilms: a brief overview of treatment modalities. J Inflamm Res. 2018;11:329–37.
18. Wolford RW, Goyal A, Belgam Syed SY, Schaefer TJ. Pharyngitis. 2023. In: StatPearls [Internet]. Treasure Island (FL): StatPearls Publishing; 2024.
19. Murray RC, Chennupati SK. Chronic streptococcal and non-streptococcal pharyngitis. Infect Disord Drug Targets. 2012;12(4):281–5.
20. Goodfriend SD, Tadi P, Koury R. Carotid artery dissection. 2022. In: StatPearls [Internet]. Treasure Island (FL): StatPearls Publishing; 2024.
21. Desfontaines P, Despland PA. Dissection of the internal carotid artery: aetiology, symptomatology, clinical and neurosonological follow-up, and treatment in 60 consecutive cases. Acta Neurol Belg. 1995;95(4):226–34.
22. Hakimi R, Sivakumar S. Imaging of carotid dissection. Curr Pain Headache Rep. 2019;23(1):2.

23. Steiner TJ, Stovner LJ, Vos T. GBD 2015: migraine is the third cause of disability in under 50s. J Headache Pain. 2016;17(1):104.
24. Ramachandra KK, Krishnan SA, Reddy SS. Carotid type of Eagle's syndrome. J Indian Soc Periodontol. 2015;19(3):336–8.
25. Zamboni P, Scerrati A, Menegatti E, Galeotti R, Lapparelli M, Traina L, Tessari M, Ciorba A, De Bonis P, Pelucchi S. The eagle jugular syndrome. BMC Neurol. 2019;19(1):333.

Atypical Neurological Presentation of Eagle's Syndrome

15

Manuele Casale, Antonio Moffa, and Iafrati Francesco

15.1 Introduction

Eagle's syndrome is a rare clinical condition that results from an elongated styloid process or a calcification of the stylohyoid ligament with compression of adjacent structures, including nerves, blood vessels, and soft tissues, leading to a wide range of symptoms. Styloid process is considered elongated when it is longer than 25 mm; generally, discomfort is seen in patients where it is 40 mm or longer [1, 2]. In 1937, the first case of symptoms related to an elongated styloid process was described by Watt W. Eagle [3]. Subsequently, clinical manifestations were further classified according to the prevalence of vascular or neurological structure involvement [4].

It is estimated that 4% of the population has an elongated styloid process and that only a fraction of them are symptomatic [5].

The classic symptoms of Eagle's syndrome are pharyngeal pain, cervical pain, pharyngeal foreign body sensation, dysphagia, otalgia/hearing impairments/tinnitus, temporomandibular or facial pain, odynophagia, and headache. Symptoms are often triggered or worsened by head rotation, tongue movements, and swallowing [6]. However, in some cases, the neurological manifestations of Eagle's syndrome may be atypical, making diagnosis challenging.

This chapter will describe the atypical neurological presentations of Eagle's syndrome involving the cranial nerves as reported in the literature.

M. Casale (✉) · A. Moffa · I. Francesco
Integrated Therapies in Otolaryngology, Fondazione Policlinico Università Campus Bio-Medico di Roma, Rome, Italy
e-mail: M.Casale@policlinicocampus.it; a.moffa@policlinicocampus.it

C. Vicini et al. (eds.), *EAGLE Syndrome*,
https://doi.org/10.1007/978-3-031-92829-1_15

15.2 Case Reports of Atypical Presentation

15.2.1 Facial Palsy and VII Cranial Nerve Involvement

Péus et al. [7] reported the case of a 39-year-old patient with periodical episodes of left-side peripheral facial palsy from 2012 to 2016 and diffuse pain in the left side of the neck. Initially, the infectious causes that could justify the symptoms were excluded. Electroneurography demonstrated a marked comparative amplitude reduction on the left side, compatible with axonal damage of the left facial nerve. On physical examination, a trigger point was found for pain at the base of the sternocleidomastoid muscle. The review of MRI and CT scan revealed a pseudoarthrosis of the fracture at the beginning of styloid process; the inflammatory callus and granulation tissue could have been responsible for the symptomatology. The enlarged styloid process was surgically removed by a transcervical approach. Six months after the surgery, the pain had disappeared but a slight paralysis of the facial nerve persisted.

Nunes et al. [8] published a case report of a 62-year-old female admitted to the emergency department with right peripheral facial palsy, grade 5 on the House-Brackmann facial paralysis scale. After 5 days of corticosteroid therapy, the symptoms disappeared; however, a foreign body sensation, odynophagia, and neck pain remained. A neck CT scan documented an elongated styloid process due to calcification of the stylohyoid ligament, and the patient was candidate to surgical treatment.

Furtado-Freitas et al. [9] described the case of a 55-year-old man who experienced headaches, difficulty to open his mouth, and pain upon palpation of the left masseter muscle for 6 months, with the development of left peripheral facial paralysis in the previous month. Radiological examinations revealed an elongated styloid process consistent with Eagle's syndrome. The patient underwent excision of the left styloid process by transcervical approach and the symptoms subsided.

15.2.2 Tongue Paresthesia and Lingual Nerve Involvement

A 59-year old man reported a 12-year history of neck pain radiating to the temporal and cervical regions especially during head rotation associated with paresthesia on the left side of the tongue. The computed tomography showed an elongated styloid process (81.7 mm), and the patient underwent surgical treatment with a transcervical approach. The lingual nerve was identified immediately near the styloid process. Pain completely regresses, and tongue paresthesia significantly improves after 1 week [10].

15.2.3 Horner's Syndrome and Sympathetic Plexus Involvement

Bensoussan et al. [11] reported the case of a 56-year-old woman with a 2-week history of right neck pain, right hemitongue atrophy with fasciculations, and right

Horner's syndrome. A CT scan revealed bilateral elongation of the styloid process; on the right side, it was medially deviated, compressing the internal carotid artery at the C2 level with 75% stenosis. The patient underwent a right styloidectomy by a cervical approach, which revealed inflammatory tissue surrounding the hypoglossal nerve. At the 6-month follow-up, no residual symptoms were documented.

Maamouri et al. described [12] two cases of Eagle's syndrome with unilateral and painful Horner's syndrome, characterized by ptosis of the upper eyelid, inverse ptosis of the lower eyelid, and anisocoria greater in darkness. CT scans showed elongated styloid processes compressing the sympathetic plexus. The patients were treated with analgesia, and one of them was candidate to surgery.

15.2.4 Spinal Accessory Nerve Involvement

Mitchell et al. [13] published two cases of "winged" Eagle's syndrome with spinal accessory nerve palsy due to compression by a posteriorly angulated or calcified styloid process. Both patients presented with lateral scapular winging and atrophy of the trapezius and sternocleidomastoid muscles. The first patient, a 71-year-old man, reported a 2-year history of unilateral shoulder weakness and fatigue while performing overhead tasks. The second patient, a 61-year-old man, experienced progressive shoulder pain and difficulty with overhead activities. Both patients underwent decompression of the spinal accessory nerve and styloidectomy via transcervical approach, which resulted in the resolution of symptoms.

15.2.5 Seizures in an Elderly Patient

A 62-year-old Indian woman presented with frequent drop attacks, somctimes leading to unconsciousness and rarely associated with seizures in the previous 10 years, along with slight pain on the medial part of the left gum. After detailed investigations, she was initially diagnosed with idiopathic epilepsy and started therapy with sodium valproate, which provided no benefit. A thorough review of the MRI revealed an elongated styloid process of the left temporal bone measuring 29.3 mm. It was hypothesized that the glossopharyngeal nerve was being irritated, causing neuralgia with syncopal attacks and seizures. Bimanual palpation of the tonsillar fossa triggered the symptoms. The patient was started on therapy with pregabalin and carbamazepine, resulting in complete regression of the symptoms [14].

15.2.6 Bilateral Presentation of Eagle's Syndrome

Bilateral Eagle's syndrome is a very rare condition. Lerra et al. [15] documented the case of a 35-year-old man who had been complaining of bilateral otalgia, intermittent tinnitus, and recurrent throat pain for 2 years. A CT scan revealed a bilateral styloid process measuring more than 3 cm. Surgical treatment was performed via a transoral approach with tonsillectomy, followed by partial styloidectomy.

A 40-year-old woman reported a 6-month history of throat pain and a foreign body sensation in the submandibular region. On bimanual palpation, tender bony prominences were found in both tonsillar fossae. CT scans confirmed bilateral elongated styloid processes. The patient was initially treated with conservative therapy, but subsequently underwent a bilateral transoral tonsillectomy with styloidectomy [16].

A 31-year-old female complained of bilateral neck pain worsening with head rotation and swallowing in the previous 4 years. On the examination, the styloid process could be easily felt both intraorally and extraorally. A transcervical resection of the bilateral styloid processes was performed, and 24 hours after surgery, the patient was already symptom-free [17].

15.2.7 Retroauricular Pain for Vagus Nerve Compression

A 48-year-old female complained of right retroauricular and occipital pain for several years, accompanied by occasional dysphagia and tinnitus. The symptoms worsened with lateral rotation of the head. Computed tomography revealed elongation of the styloid process. The patient was treated conservatively [18].

Pace et al. reported the case of a 20-year-old female with a history of pain in the left external ear (concha, antitragus, part of the tragus). The physical examination was normal. Computed tomography confirmed the presence of an elongated left styloid process compressing the vagus nerve. The patient underwent a styloidectomy via a transoral approach, resulting in complete resolution of the pain [19].

15.2.8 Multiple Cranial Nerve Involvement

A 38-year-old man underwent an extended intensive care unit stay (37 days) due to pneumonia. When he was extubated, he presented left-side IX, X, and XII cranial nerve palsy. CT scan showed bilateral elongated styloid process (50 mm) compressing the IX, X, and XII cranial nerves in the left side. Tapia syndrome is the eponym usually used to describe the concurrent paralysis of the X and XII cranial nerves. In this case, the prolonged bed rest and neck flexion potentially contributed to this condition [20].

Bedajit et al. [21] reported the case of a 45-year-old female with a clinical history of left-sided facial pain, earache, and hoarseness that occurred after a parotidectomy. The pain was aggravated by swallowing and coughing. On examination, she had left vocal cord paralysis, left palatal paresis, and deviation of the tongue toward the left due to the involvement of the IX, X, and XII cranial nerves. A CT scan revealed an elongated styloid process. She was treated conservatively with medication as she refused surgery.

A 60-year-old male was evaluated for cervical pain, dysphonia, and dysphagia for 5 months. On examination, he had left IX and X cranial nerve palsy. A neck CT scan revealed an elongated styloid process and stylohyoid ligament pseudoarthrosis [22].

15.3 Final Considerations

Eagle's syndrome is a rare and often underdiagnosed condition. This chapter emphasizes how critical it is to identify the unusual neurological presentations that can complicate diagnosis and delay appropriate treatment. The cases presented demonstrate that Eagle's syndrome can involve multiple cranial nerves with symptoms mimicking other neurological conditions. These atypical presentations underline the importance of thorough clinical evaluation and imaging studies, such as CT scans, in patients presenting with unexplained craniofacial or cervical symptoms. To obtain an accurate diagnosis and maximize treatment, frequently a multidisciplinary approach comprising otolaryngologists, neurologists, radiologists, and occasionally neurosurgeons is required.

While some patients may benefit from conservative management, such as analgesia or corticosteroid therapy, others with more severe or persistent symptoms may require surgical intervention, including styloidectomy via transoral or transcervical approaches.

References

1. Prasad KC, Kamath MP, Reddy KJ, Raju K, Agarwal S. Elongated styloid process (Eagle's syndrome): a clinical study. J Oral Maxillofac Surg. 2002;60(2):171–5.
2. Kaufman SM, Elzay RP, Irish EF. Styloid process variation. Radiologic and clinical study. Arch Otolaryngol. 1970;91(5):460–3.
3. Eagle WW. Elongated styloid processes: report of two cases. Arch Otolaryngol. 1937;25(5):584–7.
4. Eagle WW. Elongated styloid process; further observations and a new syndrome. Arch Otolaryngol (1925). 1948;47(5):630–40.
5. Farina R, Foti PV, Pennisi I, Conti A, Meli GA, Vasile T, Gozzo C, Tallamona E, Ini C, Palmucci S, Venturini M, Basile A. Stylo-jugular venous compression syndrome: lessons based on a case report. Am J Case Rep. 2021;22:e932035.
6. Hassani M, Gronlund EW, Albrechtsen SS, Kondziella D. Neurological phenotypes and treatment outcomes in Eagle syndrome: systematic review and meta-analysis. PeerJ. 2024;12:e17423.
7. Peus D, Kollias SS, Huber AM, Huber GF. Recurrent unilateral peripheral facial palsy in a patient with an enlarged styloid process. Head Neck. 2019;41(3):E34–7.
8. Nunes F, Fernandes MJ, Silva M, Porteiro B, Dutschmann R. Eagle's syndrome presenting as peripheral facial palsy. Cureus. 2022;14(2):e22499.
9. Furtado-Freitas L, Alves I, Dourado-Yoshioka-Toldo L, Curioni OA, Amaral-Carlotti F, Fontana-Velludo S, Duarte ML. Giant eagle syndrome with pseudoarthrosis and peripheral facial palsy. Rev Neurol. 2023;77(8):203–4.
10. Dong Z, Bao H, Zhang L, Hua Z. Eagle's syndrome associated with lingual nerve paresthesia: a case report. J Oral Maxillofac Surg. 2014;72, (5):886.e881–4.

11. Bensoussan Y, Letourneau-Guillon L, Ayad T. Atypical presentation of Eagle syndrome with hypoglossal nerve palsy and Horner syndrome. Head Neck. 2014;36(12):E136–8.
12. Maamouri R, Ouederni M, Oueslati Y, Mbarek C, Chammakhi C, Cheour M. Acute painful Horner's syndrome revealing Eagle's syndrome: a report of two cases. Neuroophthalmology. 2022;46(4):244–7.
13. Mitchell EC, Wu KY, Siddiqi F, Yoo J, Ohorodnyk P, Ross D, Miller TA. "Winged" Eagle's syndrome: neurophysiological findings in a rare cause of spinal accessory nerve palsy. Illustrative cases. J Neurosurg Case Lessons. 2023;6(24):CASE23358.
14. Malik Y, Dar JA, Almadani AA. Seizures with an atypical aetiology in an elderly patient: Eagle's syndrome—how does one treat it? BMJ Case Rep. 2015;2015:bcr2014206136.
15. Lerra S, Nazir T, Quadri S, Kirmani M. Eagle's syndrome: a rare presentation with bilateral otalgia and review of literature. Int J Otorhinolaryngol. 2008;9(2)
16. Sigdel B, Karn M, Sah K. Bilateral elongated styloid processes: Eagle syndrome. Lancet. 2021;397(10282):1387.
17. Anuradha V, Sachidananda R, Pugazhendi SK, Satish P, Navaneetham R. Bilateral atypical facial pain caused by Eagle's syndrome. Case Rep Dent. 2020;2020:3013029.
18. Paiva ALC, Araujo JLV, Lovato RM, Teixeira JAR, Miura FK, Guirado VMP, Veiga JCE. Retroauricular pain caused by Eagle syndrome: a rare presentation due to compression by styloid process elongation. Rev Assoc Med Bras (1992). 2017;63(3):213–4.
19. Pace A, Rossetti V, Iannella G, Magliulo G. Unusual symptomatology in Eagle syndrome. Clin Med Insights Case Rep. 2020;13:1179547620948728.
20. Paramalingam S, Kuok YJ. Eagle syndrome as a potential cause of Tapia syndrome. Med J Aust. 2015;202(9):491.
21. Bedajit R, Priyokumar O, Abhilash R, Kumar S. Eagle syndrome with multiple cranial nerve involvement. J Med Soc. 2014;28(2):117–9.
22. Albuquerque LC, Duarte JA, Klaes AI, Mota SM, Krammer BR, Bianchini L, Bianchin MM. Eagle's syndrome: a pain in the neck. Arq Neuropsiquiatr. 2017;75(2):130–1.

Eagle Syndrome and Insomnia

16

Claudio Vicini, Alberto Caranti, Ruggero Campisi, and Elena Briganti

16.1 Introduction

The real prevalence of insomnia is a matter of great debate in the worldwide literature since a long time. Depending on the specific definitions used (i.e., insomnia symptoms vs disorder, sleep dissatisfaction), prevalence rates have varied from as low as 5% to as high as 50%. In general, population-based data indicate that about one-third of adults (30–36%) reports at least one nocturnal insomnia symptom (i.e., difficulty initiating or maintaining sleep, non-restorative sleep), but this rate decreases to values between 10% and 15% when daytime consequences (e.g., fatigue) are added to the case definition. Rates of sleep dissatisfaction, without regard to specific sleep diagnosis, also vary widely (10–25%) in the adult population. When using more stringent and operational DSM-5 or ICSD-3 diagnostic criteria, prevalence rates tend to cluster between 6% and 10% [1]. Table 16.1 summarizes the major somatic and mental comorbidities of insomnia.

It is quite evident that many different medical conditions may predispose to insomnia, and the underlying conditions should be checked and treated in any patient seeking advice for insomnia. Among the many possible comorbidities of insomnia, a new clinical entity was recently described by an Italian group based in Ferrara [2]. More recently, Chaobo Bai et al. described in a very comprehensive review the clinical characteristics and neuroimaging findings of internal jugular

C. Vicini · A. Caranti · R. Campisi
University of Ferrara, Cona, FE, Italy
e-mail: claudio@claudiovicini.com

E. Briganti (✉)
Department of Medical and Surgical Sciences, University of Bologna, Bologna, Italy

Pediatric Neuromuscular Unit, Pediatric Neuropsychiatry Unit, IRCCS Institute of Neurological Sciences, Bologna, Italy
e-mail: elena.briganti4@unibo.it

C. Vicini et al. (eds.), *EAGLE Syndrome*,
https://doi.org/10.1007/978-3-031-92829-1_16

Table 16.1 Main comorbidities of insomnia [1]

Psychiatric	Medical	Neurological	Substance use/ dependence
Depressive disorders Bipolar disorders Generalized anxiety disorder Panic disorder Post-traumatic stress disorder Schizophrenia	Chronic obstructive pulmonary diseases Diabetes mellitus Chronic kidney diseases Human immunodeficiency virus infection Malignancy Rheumatic disorders Chronic pain Sleep apnea	Neurodegenerative diseases Fatal familial insomnia Cerebrovascular diseases Multiple sclerosis Traumatic brain injury Restless legs syndrome	Alcohol Nicotine Caffeine Marijuana Opioids Designer drugs Cocaine Amphetamine

vein stenosis (IJVS) induced by Eagle syndrome (ES) [3]. In this cohort, the top 3 symptoms were insomnia (22/27, 81.5%), tinnitus (17/27, 63.0%), and head noises (17/27, 63.0%), respectively.

16.2 Eagle Syndrome (ES) and Insomnia

One of the most common complaints in the vast majority of all variants of Eagle syndrome (ES) is pain. Chronic pain and insomnia are highly comorbid: approximately 50% of those with chronic pain experience insomnia or clinically significant sleep disturbances, and 50% of those with insomnia experience chronic pain and the severity of sleep disturbance is related to pain intensity [5, 6]. As stated by Ferini-Strambi (2017), "neuropathic pain is associated with sleep disturbances, and in turn poor sleep quality leads to increased pain sensitivity, so it is essential to assess sleep alongside neuropathic pain" [7].

Insomnia among individuals with chronic pain is highly prevalent and closely related to mechanisms of central sensitization [8]: there is a close interaction between central sensitization and sleep disturbances in people with chronic pain. A single night of total sleep deprivation has been shown to induce generalized hyperalgesia and increase state anxiety in healthy people [9, 10]. Likewise, sleep curtailment impairs endogenous nociceptive-inhibitory function and increases spontaneous pain in healthy people [11]. These findings suggest that sleep disturbances might not only perpetuate central nervous system hyperexcitability in people with chronic pain but may also serve as an etiological factor. This may in turn ensue a vicious cycle: poor sleep lowers pain thresholds, which then contributes to hyperalgesia and subsequent increased incidence and/or severity of insomnia [8]. The link between central sensitization and insomnia is underscored by various research findings: in particular, in people with temporomandibular joint disorder, insomnia is associated with hyperalgesia at a non-orofacial site, suggesting that insomnia may be linked with central sensitization [12]. The link between insomnia and central sensitization might imply overlapping mechanisms in the central nervous system, for instance, mesolimbic dopaminergic pathways playing a cardinal role in both sleep regulation and endogenous analgesia [13]. Hence, decreased dopamine availability may explain both sleep disturbances and dysfunctional endogenous analgesia in people with chronic pain. Serotoninergic pathways are also implicated in shared modulatory mechanisms of pain and sleep regulations. Serotonin is critical for top-down orchestration of endogenous analgesia [14], as well as of circadian rhythm control [15]. Serotoninergic dysfunction can result in altered patterns of circadian behavior or even contribute to a disruption of sleep-wake homeostasis along with dysfunctional endogenous analgesia. While it is unlikely that either of the two mentioned neurotransmitters is the sole factor underlying the links between pain and insomnia, both seem to play major roles in explaining sleep disturbances in people with chronic pain. Essentially, a possible dysfunction in either dopaminergic or serotonergic systems fits within the view that central sensitization is exacerbated or even initiated by sleep disturbances [8]. Preclinical studies support this view by revealing that selective melatonin MT2 receptor partial agonists hold analgesic properties through modulation of "on/off" cells of the brainstem descending antinociceptive systems in neuropathic pain models [16, 17].

An additional mechanism underlying insomnia in JES is more specifically related to the typical profile of this pathology as a cerebrovenous outflow disorder (COD). "Examples of severe sequelae of venous disorders abound, including Cerebral Venous Thrombosis (CVT)-mediated visual impairment, epilepsy, and intracranial hypertension; and non-thrombotic Cerebral Venous Sinus (CVS) stenosis and/or IJVS-induced long-term unbearable head noise, tinnitus, headache, dizziness, sleeping disorder, and severe intracranial hypertension" [18].

Tinnitus is an auditory sensation that is generated by aberrant activation within the auditory system. Sleep disturbances are a frequent problem in the tinnitus population [19]: they are known to worsen the distress caused by the tinnitus, which in turn worsens sleep quality (see Table 16.2). Beyond that, disturbed sleep is a risk factor for mental health problems, and distressing tinnitus is often associated with enhanced depressivity, anxiety, and somatic symptom severity. Moreover, the presence of one or more specific personality traits of high neuroticism, low extraversion, high stress reaction, higher alienation, lower social closeness, lower well-being, lower self-control, lower psychological acceptance, presence of a type D personality, and externalized locus of control was associated with tinnitus distress [20]. Besides, there is evidence that therapies that alleviate tinnitus-related distress have a positive influence on sleep quality and help interrupt this vicious cycle. This suggests that distressing tinnitus and insomnia may both be promoted by similar physiological mechanisms: one candidate mechanism is hyperarousal caused by enhanced activation of the sympathetic nervous system. There is much evidence for hyperarousal in insomnia patients, and animal models of tinnitus and insomnia show conspicuous similarities in the activation pattern of limbic and autonomous brain regions [21]: probably, the relationship between poor sleep and tinnitus is likely contributed by central processes without a major role of mediation via the peripheral auditory system; indeed, negative sleep characteristics were associated with tinnitus, while there was no clinically meaningful association between sleep and hearing loss [22].

Table 16.2 Correlations between sleep questionnaires and age, duration of tinnitus perception and Tinnitus Handicap Inventory in the study by Gallo et al. [4] about the effects of tinnitus on sleep quality and insomnia

	n	%	Age	Duration of tinnitus	Tinnitus handicap inventory
Insomnia Severity Index					
Absence of insomnia	7	38.9	*r* = 0,016 *p* = 0,095	*r* = 0,289 *p* = 0,244	*r* = 0,499 *p* = 0,035*
Sub-threshold insomnia	5	27.8			
Moderate insomnia	5	27.8			
Severe insomnia	1	5.6			
Total	18	100			
Pittsburgh Sleep Quality Index					
Good sleep quality	5	27.8	*r* = 0,039 *p* = 0,878	*r* = 0,056 *p* = 0,826	*r* = 0,582 *p* = 0,011*
Poor sleep quality	13	72.2			
Total	18	100			
Epworth Sleepiness Scale					
Yes	5	27.8	*r* = – 0,193 *p* = 0,442	*r* = – 0,457 *p* = 0,057	*r* = 0,227 *p* = 0,364
No	13	72.2			
Total	18	100			
STOP-BANG					
Low-risk OSA	12	66.7	*r* = 0,272 *p* = 0,276	*r* = 0,417 *p* = 0,085	*r* = 0,374 *p* = 0,127
Intermediate-risk OSA	4	22.2			
High-risk OSA	2	11.1			
Total	18	100			

Statistical test—Spearman's correlation coefficient
*Statistical difference ($p < 0.05$)
Abbreviation: *OSA* obstructive sleep apnea

16.3 Diagnosis of Insomnia in ES

Concerning the sleep disturbances in ES, the insomnia evaluation needs a careful patient history and examination addressing sleep and waking functions as well as common medical, psychiatric, and medication/substance-related comorbidities: sometimes the sleep assessment itself can lead to the diagnostic suspect of ES and in particular of JES; otherwise, if the patient arrives after a JES diagnosis, a careful sleep assessment is necessary to set up properly the treatment. International guidelines suggest evaluating insomnia symptoms using the Consensus Sleep Diary for at least 1 or 2 weeks to assess the insomnia day-to-day variability. In addition, the administration of questionnaires and survey instruments has been suggested to assess outcomes and guide treatment—the *Insomnia Severity Index (ISI)*, the *Sleep Condition Indicator (SCI)*, and the *Epworth Sleepiness Scale (ESS)*—which are the questionnaires that have been suggested for the evaluation of insomnia and of its daytime consequences. Additional evaluations have been suggested to include the assessment of predisposing, precipitating, and perpetuating factors: particularly for the evaluation of perpetuating negative behaviors and cognitive processes, the

Dysfunctional Beliefs and Attitudes About Sleep Scale (DBAS) is the most recommended scale. Both polysomnographic and actigraphic registrations are still not recommended for the routine evaluation of insomnia [23].

16.4 Treatment and Management of Insomnia in ES

Insomnia among individuals with chronic pain (condition where ES falls within) is characterized by low-grade neuroinflammation, associated with stress/anxiety, and does not respond effectively to pharmacological treatment. The Cognitive-Behavioral Therapy for Insomnia (CBT-I) is the internationally considered first-line treatment for chronic primary insomnia [23]: the advantage over sedative drugs or classical hypnotics mainly lies in the sustainability of treatment effects and a lower risk for side effects. The first report of a treatment trial targeted at sleep for people with chronic pain dates back to 2010: this study and the following ones demonstrate that CBT-I for comorbid insomnia and chronic pain induces clinically meaningful improvements in various sleep parameters (e.g., self-reported sleep onset latency, time spent awake after sleep onset, sleep efficiency, sleep quality), particularly in sleep continuity; also, it has been shown that CBT-I does not consistently improve pain severity, but appears to reduce pain interference with daily activities, depression, fatigue, and disability [24]. Furthermore, CBT-I shows long-term (six months) effects despite the presence of continued moderate-to-severe pain [25]. However, at this moment there is still relatively little evidence about optimal administration procedures (timing, simultaneous priming, or hierarchy) for the treatment of sleep disorders in contexts of chronic pain: however, a recent systematic review concluded with high-quality evidence that with additional training, cognitive-behavioral interventions are effective for low back pain, allowing implementation within the field [26]. CBT-I typically includes sleep (or bedtime) restriction recommendations, stimulus control instructions, psychoeducation regarding sleep and sleep hygiene, and cognitive therapy [23]. CBT-I may not be a stand-alone treatment for people with chronic pain and comorbid insomnia, but may preferentially be combined with other effective treatment interventions, such as CBT for pain (CBT-P) [27] and, in the specific case of JES, the conservative and surgical measures presented above.

About tinnitus (present in JES) and its association with sleep disorders, even though there are differences between distressing tinnitus and insomnia, there are striking similarities between the two conditions in which hyperarousal appears to play a major role [21]. Distressing tinnitus is often accompanied by insomnia, and even when occurring in separation, both conditions are associated with similar comorbidities such as depressivity and anxiety [28]. There are indeed therapeutic implications of this hypothesis: therapeutic interventions that specifically aim to reduce hyperarousal should ameliorate a distressing tinnitus, even more so if the tinnitus is accompanied by insomnia. For example, therapies such as neurofeedback, that has been applied promisingly to treat independently tinnitus and insomnia [29, 30] might be used to decrease arousal, resulting in therapies that demand less effort than the existing behavioral approaches.

16.5 A Descriptive Study of Insomnia in a Sample of Italian Patients with Classic ES

Although in the literature insomnia disorder is mainly reported in the jugular variant of ES [3], our study was conducted with intent to observe whether a significant prevalence of insomnia is also found in the classic variant of ES. In fact, classic ES has similar symptoms to JES and is also characterized by chronic pain and tinnitus, which frequently occur in comorbidity with insomnia, as we saw above.

Our descriptive study was therefore conducted by a retrospective analysis of patients affected by classic ES visited and operated by the surgical team of Dr. Claudio Vicini in Forlì (Italy), at the Morgagni-Pierantoni Hospital and at the Primus Forlì Medical Center.

Nineteen adults affected by classic ES were selected for the study: they were ten females and nine males, with an average age of 48,79 years (SD = 12,85). In these 19 adults, we studied the occurrence and the severity of insomnia before and after surgery in this sample of patients.

The seriousness of insomnia was evaluated by means of the Italian version of the *Insomnia Severity Index—ISI*: the *ISI* is a seven-item self-report questionnaire assessing the nature, severity, and impact of insomnia [31]. The usual recall period is the "last month," and the dimensions evaluated are severity of sleep onset, sleep maintenance and early morning awakening problems, sleep dissatisfaction, interference of sleep difficulties with daytime functioning, noticeability of sleep problems by others, and distress caused by the sleep difficulties. A 5-point Likert scale is used to rate each item (e.g., 0 = no problem; 4 = very severe problem), yielding a total score ranging from 0 to 28. The total score is interpreted as follows: absence of insomnia (0–7), sub-threshold insomnia (8–14), moderate insomnia (15–21), and severe insomnia (22–28).

First of all, in our case study we found 14 out of 19 patients affected by insomnia, corresponding to a prevalence of 73.68%, much higher than the prevalence of insomnia in the general population (which is around 30-50% in the most abundant estimates).

We also found a reduction in the total cases of insomnia and in the rate of severity of insomnia after surgery, as summarized in Table 16.3 and Figs. 16.1 and 16.2:

Table 16.3 Severity of insomnia pre- and post-surgery in our group of patients affected by classic ES

Classic Eagle syndrome—insomnia		
	Pre-surgery	Post-surgery
Absence of insomnia	5	8
Sub-threshold insomnia	4	6
Moderate insomnia	3	2
Severe insomnia	7	3
TOTAL PATIENTS WITH INSOMNIA	14	11

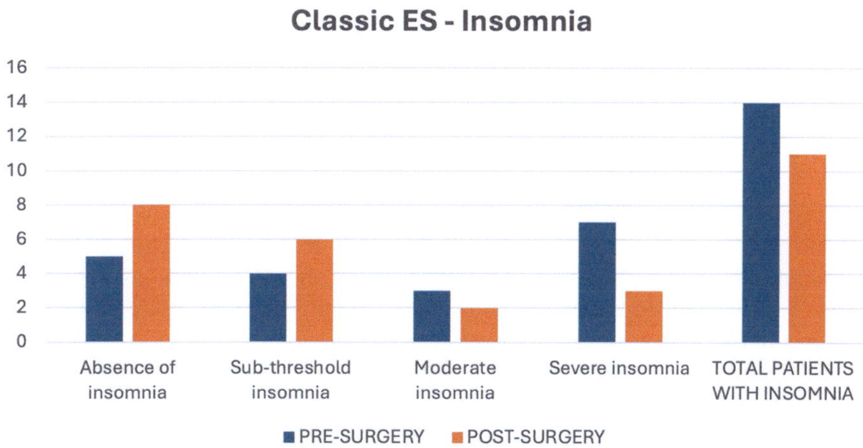

Fig. 16.1 Severity of insomnia pre- and post-surgery in our group of patients affected by classic ES

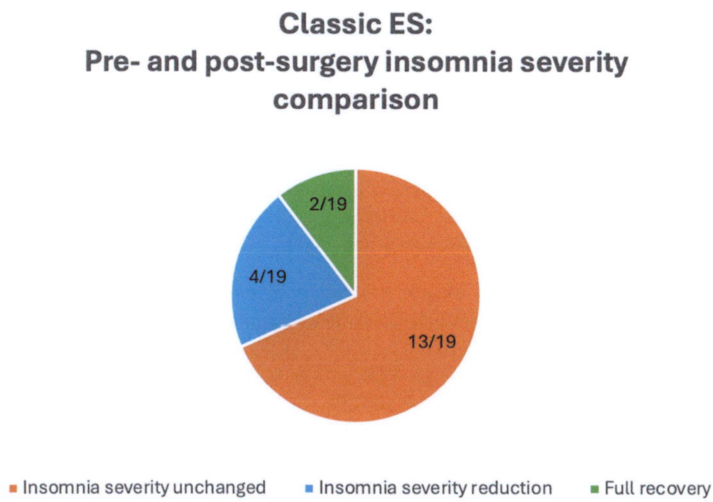

Fig. 16.2 Comparison between pre- and post-surgery insomnia severity in our group of patients affected by classic ES

however, it is a reduction of small amount, and, in most cases, insomnia persists, generally at the same level of severity, although the operation has completely resolved the painful symptoms of ES.

Although this one is a small case study, our finding should prompt reflection on the fact that insomnia may be present not only in the jugular variant of ES but also in the classic one.

Moreover, even when insomnia is secondary to an organic problem, it is a self-standing clinical entity, which deserves an ad hoc treatment. This is because, as explained by the 3P Model [32], insomnia develops and is maintained due to predisposing, precipitating, and perpetuating factors, which alter the brain mechanisms involved in hypnic regulation: hence, if chronic pain and tinnitus present in classic ES (as well as in JES) constitute the precipitating factors that determine the onset of the sleep disorder, however the patients then implement perpetuating behaviors that cause the insomnia to become chronic, maintaining it even after the operation and the resolution of the precipitating factors [33]. Furthermore, tinnitus (present in classic and jugular ES), as stated above, probably shares a neural substrate with insomnia and is generally associated with hyperarousal and anxious-depressive characteristics, aspects which are also found in insomniac patients and which contribute to the maintenance of the sleep disorder.

In conclusion, surgical treatment of ES should therefore be accompanied by a specific intervention on insomnia, which focuses on the perpetuating factors: in particular, the gold standard for the treatment of chronic insomnia, as mentioned, is represented by Cognitive-Behavioral Therapy for Insomnia (CBT-I).

Furthermore, it might be interesting as future prospect to expand the sample, also studying the carotid type of ES and analyzing the different prevalences of insomnia in the three subtypes of ES.

References

1. Riemann D, Baglioni C, Bassetti C, Bjorvatn B, Dolenc Groselj L, Ellis JG, et al. European guideline for the diagnosis and treatment of insomnia. J Sleep Res. 2017;26(6):675–700.
2. Zamboni P, Scerrati A, Menegatti E, Galeotti R, Lapparelli M, Traina L, Tessari M, Ciorba A, De Bonis P, Pelucchi S. The eagle jugular syndrome. BMC Neurol. 2019;19(1):333. https://doi.org/10.1186/s12883-019-1572-3.
3. Bai C, Wang Z, Guan J, Jin K, Ding Y, Ji X, Meng R. Clinical characteristics and neuroimaging findings in eagle syndrome induced internal jugular vein stenosis. Ann Transl Med. 2020;8(4):97. https://doi.org/10.21037/atm.2019.12.93.
4. Gallo KEB, Corrêa CDC, Gonçalves CGDO, Baran JBC, Marques JM, Zeigelboim BS, José MR. Effect of tinnitus on sleep quality and insomnia. Int Arch Otorhinolaryngol. 2023;27:197–202.
5. Todd J, Austin H, Clarke P, Notebaert L. Chronic pain, insomnia and their mutual maintenance: a call for cognitive bias research. J Pain. 2022;23(9):1530–42. https://doi.org/10.1016/j.jpain.2022.03.241.
6. Cheatle MD, Foster S, Pinkett A, Lesneski M, Qu D, Dhingra L. Assessing and managing sleep disturbance in patients with chronic pain. Anesthesiol Clin. 2016;34(2):379–93. https://doi.org/10.1016/j.anclin.2016.01.007.
7. Ferini-Strambi L. Neuropathic pain and sleep: a review. Pain Ther. 2017;6(Suppl 1):19–23. https://doi.org/10.1007/s40122-017-0089-y.
8. Nijs J, Mairesse O, Neu D, Leysen L, Danneels L, Cagnie B, et al. Sleep disturbances in chronic pain: neurobiology, assessment, and treatment in physical therapist practice. Phys Ther. 2018;98(5):325–35.
9. Onen SH, Alloui A, Gross A, Eschallier A, Dubray C. The effects of total sleep deprivation, selective sleep interruption and sleep recovery on pain tolerance thresholds in healthy subjects. J Sleep Res. 2001;10:35–42.
10. Schuh-Hofer S, Wodarski R, Pfau DB, et al. One night of total sleep deprivation promotes a state of generalized hyperalgesia: a surrogate pain model to study the relationship of insomnia and pain. Pain. 2013;154:1613–21.
11. Smith MT, Edwards RR, McCann UD, Haythornthwaite JA. The effects of sleep deprivation on pain inhibition and spontaneous pain in women. Sleep. 2007;30:494–505.

12. Smith MT, Wickwire EM, Grace EG, Edwards RR, Buenaver LF, Peterson S, Klick B, Haythornthwaite JA. Sleep disorders and their association with laboratory pain sensitivity in temporomandibular joint disorder. Sleep. 2009;32(6):779–90. https://doi.org/10.1093/sleep/32.6.779.
13. Finan PH, Smith MT. The comorbidity of insomnia, chronic pain, and depression: dopamine as a putative mechanism. Sleep Med Rev. 2013;17:173–83.
14. Millan MJ. Descending control of pain. Prog Neurobiol. 2002;66:355–474.
15. Whitney MS, Shemery AM, Yaw AM, Donovan LJ, Glass JD, Deneris ES. Adult brain serotonin deficiency causes hyperactivity, circadian disruption, and elimination of siestas. J Neurosci. 2016;36:9828–42.
16. Lopez-Canul M, Palazzo E, DominguezLopez S, et al. Selective melatonin MT2 receptor ligands relieve neuropathic pain through modulation of brainstem descending antinociceptive pathways. Pain. 2015;156:305–17.
17. Lopez-Canul M, Comai S, DominguezLopez S, Granados-Soto V, Gobbi G. Antinociceptive properties of selective MT2 melatonin receptor partial agonists. Eur J Pharmacol. 2015;764:424–32.
18. Bai C, Wang Z, Stone C, Zhou D, Ding J, Ding Y, Ji X, Meng R. Pathogenesis and management in cerebrovenous outflow disorders. Aging Dis. 2021;12(1):203–22. https://doi.org/10.14336/AD.2020.0404.
19. Wakabayashi S, Saito H, Oishi N, Shinden S, Ogawa K. Effects of tinnitus treatments on sleep disorders in patients with tinnitus. Int J Audiol. 2018;57(2):110–4.
20. Durai M, Searchfield G. Anxiety and depression, personality traits relevant to tinnitus: a scoping review. Int J Audiol. 2016;55(11):605–15. https://doi.org/10.1080/14992027.2016.1198966.
21. Wallhäusser-Franke E, Schredl M, Delb W. Tinnitus and insomnia: is hyperarousal the common denominator? Sleep Med Rev. 2013;17(1):65–74. https://doi.org/10.1016/j.smrv.2012.04.003.
22. Awad M, Abdalla I, Jara SM, Huang TC, Adams ME, Choi JS. Association of sleep characteristics with tinnitus and hearing loss. OTO Open. 2024;8(1):e117.
23. Palagini L, Manni R, Liguori C, De Gennaro L, Gemignani A, Fanfulla F, et al. Evaluation and management of insomnia in the clinical practice in Italy: a 2023 update from the insomnia expert consensus group. J Neurol. 2024;271(4):1668–79.
24. Jungquist CR, O'Brien C, Matteson-Rusby S, Smith MT, Pigeon WR, Xia Y, Lu N, Perlis ML. The efficacy of cognitive-behavioral therapy for insomnia in patients with chronic pain. Sleep Med. 2010;11(3):302–9. https://doi.org/10.1016/j.sleep.2009.05.018.
25. Jungquist CR, Tra Y, Smith MT, Pigeon WR, Matteson-Rusby S, Xia Y, Perlis ML. The durability of cognitive behavioral therapy for insomnia in patients with chronic pain. Sleep Disord. 2012;2012(1):679648.
26. Hall A, Richmond H, Copsey B, Hansen Z, Williamson E, Jones G, Fordham B, Cooper Z, Lamb S. Physiotherapist-delivered cognitive-behavioural interventions are effective for low back pain, but can they be replicated in clinical practice? A systematic review. Disabil Rehabil. 2018;40(1):1–9. https://doi.org/10.1080/09638288.2016.1236155.
27. McCrae CS, Curtis AF, Miller MB, Nair N, Rathinakumar H, Davenport M, et al. Effect of cognitive behavioural therapy on sleep and opioid medication use in adults with fibromyalgia and insomnia. J Sleep Res. 2020;29(6):e13020.
28. Durai M, Searchfield G. Anxiety and depression, personality traits relevant to tinnitus: a scoping review. Int J Audiol. 2016;55(11):605–15.
29. Güntensperger D, Thüring C, Meyer M, Neff P, Kleinjung T. Neurofeedback for tinnitus treatment–review and current concepts. Front Aging Neurosci. 2017;9:386.
30. Lambert-Beaudet F, Journault WG, Provençal AR, Bastien CH. Neurofeedback for insomnia: current state of research. World J Psychiatry. 2021;11(10):897.
31. Morin CM. Insomnia: psychological assessment and management. New York: Guilford Press; 1993.
32. Spielman AJ, Caruso LS, Glovinsky PB. A behavioral perspective on insomnia treatment. Psychiatr Clin N Am. 1987;10(4):541–53.
33. Palagini L, Biber K, Riemann D. The genetics of insomnia–evidence for epigenetic mechanisms? Sleep Med Rev. 2014;18(3):225–35.

An Indian Perspective on Eagle's Syndrome

17

Seemab Shaikh and Sukhvinder Bindra

17.1 Introduction

Eagle's syndrome, though not very common, is a condition that can significantly affect the quality of the life in affected individuals. This is characterized by the elongation of the styloid process or calcification of styloid ligament. It was traditionally considered as rare condition, but recent studies suggest that it might be more common than previously believed, particularly within the Indian population.

Eagle's syndrome is also known by various other names, including stylohyoid syndrome, elongated styloid process syndrome, stylalgia, styloid-stylohyoid syndrome, styloid dysphagia, chronic styloid angina, temporal rheumatic styloiditis, stylocarotid syndrome, and Garel-Bernfeld syndrome [1].

This chapter aims to explore Eagle's syndrome within the Indian context, drawing upon research findings and clinical experiences to shed light on its epidemiology, clinical presentations, diagnostic challenges, and therapeutic strategies.

17.2 Historical Background

The elongated styloid process and ossification of the styloid ligament were first documented in 1652 by Italian surgeon Pietro Marchetti [2].

It wasn't until later that the elongated styloid process was identified as a distinct clinical entity, with notable mentions in the medical literature by Lucke in 1870 and Weinlecher in 1872 [3].

S. Shaikh (✉)
Department of ENT, Inamdar Multispecialty Hospital, Pune, India

S. Bindra
Senior Consultant Oral and Maxillofacial Surgeon, Apollo Hospitals, Shenoy Hospitals, Rainbow Hospitals, Secunderabad, India

C. Vicini et al. (eds.), *EAGLE Syndrome*,
https://doi.org/10.1007/978-3-031-92829-1_17

In 1937, otolaryngologist Watt W. Eagle coined the term "stylalgia" to describe the pain associated with this anomaly. Eagle Syndrome encompasses a range of symptoms resulting from the compression of nearby structures, such as nerves and blood vessels [4–6].

17.3 Etiopathogenesis

The exact cause of Eagle Syndrome is still not fully understood. Dr. Watt Eagle initially theorized that surgical procedures like tonsillectomy or ongoing local irritation could lead to inflammation of the styloid process and stylohyoid ligaments, resulting in bone growth and hyperplasia [4–6]. Supporting this, Gli Aspetti in 1976 proposed that trauma or mechanical stress might lead to residual mesenchymal elements undergoing a process known as osseous metaplasia [7].

Epifanio, in 1962, suggested that ossification of the styloid process might be linked to hormonal changes in postmenopausal women, who often experience similar ossification in other body ligaments [8].

Steinmann [9] proposed three theories for the ossification of the stylohyoid ligament:

1. *Theory of Reactive Hyperplasia:* Trauma can lead to ossification starting at the end of the styloid process, extending down through the styloid ligament. Since the styloid ligament retains remnants of its connective tissue and fibrocartilaginous origins, there remains a potential for ossification.
2. *Theory of Reactive Metaplasia:* An abnormal healing response following trauma can trigger the calcification of the stylohyoid ligament.
3. *Theory of Anatomic Variance:* The early elongation of the styloid process and subsequent ossification of the stylohyoid ligament are considered anatomical variations that may occur without any identifiable trauma.

Gokce C et al., in 2008, observed that patients with end-stage renal disease, particularly those with imbalances in calcium, phosphorus, and vitamin D levels, showed abnormal calcification, which could lead to the elongation of the styloid process, thereby triggering Eagle Syndrome [10].

17.4 The Pathophysiology

The pathophysiology behind the pain associated with Eagle Syndrome (ES) can be attributed to several mechanisms:

1. *Compression of Nerves:* One of the key causes of pain is the compression of important nerves by the elongated styloid process. This includes the glossopharyngeal nerve and the lower branch of the trigeminal nerve. Such compression can lead to significant discomfort and neurological symptoms.

2. *Fracture of the Ossified Stylohyoid Ligament:* In some cases, a fracture in the ossified stylohyoid ligament may occur, leading to the growth of granulation tissue. This tissue can exert pressure on adjacent structures, which in turn results in pain.
3. *Carotid Vessel Impingement:* The elongated styloid process can impinge on carotid arteries, leading to irritation of the sympathetic nerves that are located within the arterial sheath. This can cause pain, particularly in the neck and head regions.
4. *Insertion Tendinosis:* Another contributing factor is the degenerative and inflammatory changes that can develop in the tendinous part of the stylohyoid insertion. This condition, known as tendinosis, can be quite painful.
5. *Irritation of Pharyngeal Mucosa:* Direct compression of the pharyngeal mucosa by the elongated styloid process can lead to irritation, resulting in discomfort and pain in the throat area.
6. *Post-Tonsillectomy Effects:* Finally, after a tonsillectomy, the stretching and subsequent fibrosis of certain cranial nerves, specifically the fifth, seventh, ninth, and tenth, can lead to chronic pain in patients suffering from Eagle Syndrome. This post-operative condition can be particularly challenging to manage [11].

17.5 Epidemiology

17.5.1 Incidence and Prevalence

In the broader population, it is estimated that between 4% and 10% of individuals have an elongated styloid process (SP). However, of these, only around 4% present with symptoms, resulting in a prevalence of Eagle Syndrome (ES) that is below 2% [12]. Among Indian patients experiencing orofacial pain or related symptoms, the occurrence of this condition ranges between 1.9% and 4% [13].

Indian studies demonstrate a wide range in the incidence of elongated styloid processes, from as low as 1.4% [14] to 3.3% [15], with a notably low occurrence of symptomatic cases in some studies [16]. However, higher rates of 19.4% [17] and 24.8% [18]. have also been documented, highlighting significant regional variations.

The Mathura region in Northern India reported the highest prevalence, with 52.1% [19] of individuals showing an elongated styloid process, both unilateral and bilateral. This high rate is possibly due to lifestyle factors specific to this region, such as carrying heavy loads [20] on the head and chewing hard substances like tobacco and areca nut, [21] which put additional stress on the ligaments, leading to ossification. Furthermore, racial characteristics and the natural aging process seem to predispose this population to higher rates of elongated styloid processes [22].

In our Retrospective Radiographic observational study, conducted across Pune and Hyderabad, involved a series of cases based on Orthopantomograph (OPG X-rays) of 1521 patients and styloid process measuring more than 3.0 cm was considered elongated. 108 cases (6.81%) were found to have elongated styloid process. Out of these, only four patients (3.70%) exhibited symptoms, which aligns with global trends indicating that symptomatic cases are relatively uncommon, even though the prevalence of elongated styloid processes might be higher.

These variations in incidence and prevalence can be attributed to differences in healthcare access, diagnostic facilities, and levels of awareness across different regions. Urban centres, with their advanced diagnostic facilities, typically report higher detection rates compared to remote and rural areas.

Most studies examining the prevalence of Eagle Syndrome (ES) in India have employed Orthopantomographs (OPG X-rays) and dry skull specimens to assess elongated styloid processes and their calcification. These methods, however have certain limitations, as they may not offer a precise understanding of the symptoms or true incidence of Eagle Syndrome. This underscores the necessity for further research to obtain a more accurate picture.

17.6 Age

In Indian population, Eagle Syndrome is reported to predominantly affect the 30 to 50-year age group [23, 24].

The aforementioned study by the authors of this chapter encompassed patients aged 16 to 76 years, with the majority falling within the 40 to 50-year age group (40%), followed by those in the 30 to 40-year age group. This distribution is consistent with other studies conducted in India,

We observed a mean age of 47.5 years for male patients and 46.8 years for female patients, which is in line with findings reported by other Indian researchers [16, 25].

17.7 Gender

The literature on Eagle Syndrome reveals considerable variability in gender predilection within the Indian context. Many studies indicate a higher prevalence in females [24, 26].

Male patients showed a greater tendency for styloid process elongation in another group led by More CB et al. [18].

No significant gender differences in unilateral or bilateral elongation of the styloid process were observed in a study conducted in Mathura, which analysed 2706 panoramic radiographs [19].

Among our symptomatic cases, female patients outnumbered the male patients with a ratio of 3:1. The reasons behind this higher prevalence in females remain unclear, it is hypothesized that hormonal changes during the peri-menopausal period, along with ossification of other ligaments such as the iliolumbar and thyrohyoid ligaments, might play a role [8]. Further investigation is needed to elucidate these factors.

17.8 Average Length of the Styloid Process and Gender Variation

Eagle reported that the normal styloid process measures 2.5–3 cm. Studies across India show a wide range in styloid process length, typically between 1.78 and 6.2 cm [25, 27, 28].

Average length of the styloid process in our patients was in the range from 3.67 ± 0.68 cm to 4.89 ± 0.66 cm with a higher prevalence noticed among females.

Research indicates that styloid process lengthens with age [25, 29] and our case series concurs.

17.9 Unilateral vs Bilateral Elongation of Styloid Process

Bilateral elongation of styloid process is found to be more prevalent than unilateral elongation in numerous studies by Indian Authors [18, 23, 29].

Bagga et al., also reported a high prevalence of bilateral elongation at 79.5%, with only 20.5% showing unilateral elongation [19]. They also suggested that the high rate of bilateral elongation could be attributed to factors such as strenuous exercise and chewing habits, which lead to contraction of the masticatory muscles. This increased weight loading on the styloid processes bilaterally promoting ossification. Numerous studies by Indian authors have shown that bilateral elongation of the styloid process is more prevalent than unilateral elongation.

Majority of the patients included in the present case series (74.73%) exhibited bilateral elongation, while 25.27% had unilateral elongation of the styloid process. Among the patients with bilateral elongation of styloid Process, Right side styloid process was found to be longer than left side in 54.56% of the cases (lateralisation to the right).

However, despite the higher incidence of bilateral elongation, symptomatic cases are predominantly unilateral, This pattern underscores the complexity of styloid process elongation, where bilateral elongation is frequent, but symptoms may predominantly present unilaterally and elongated styloid process may not be symptomatic [30, 31].

17.10 Clinical Signs and Symptoms

Some cases of styloid process elongation are asymptomatic, others present with a range of symptoms [25]. The syndrome typically presents with nonspecific neck pain, a foreign body sensation in the pharynx, odynophagia (painful swallowing), otalgia (ear pain), temporomandibular joint pain, and trismus (restricted mouth opening). Additional symptoms can include changes in voice and hypersalivation (increased saliva production) [32]. The characteristic dull and nagging pain that worsens during deglutition and can be reproduced by palpation of the tonsillar fossa is a hallmark of the condition [33].

Eagle Syndrome is generally classified into two types:

17.11 Classic Eagle Syndrome

This condition often follows pharyngeal trauma or tonsillectomy. Patients report a foreign body sensation in the throat, dull and persistent pharyngeal pain localized to the ipsilateral tonsillar fossa, which may radiate to the ear and worsen with head rotation. Other symptoms include dysphagia, tinnitus, and cervicofacial pain. A palpable mass or bulge in the tonsillar fossa can exacerbate these symptoms.

17.12 Stylocarotid Syndrome

Stylocarotid Syndrome results from the elongated styloid process irritating the sympathetic nerve tissue in the internal and external carotid arteries. Symptoms include pain along the artery's distribution, which is aggravated by neck rotation and compression. Patients might experience supraorbital pain and parietal headache if the internal carotid is involved, or pain radiating to the infraorbital region if the external carotid is affected [5, 34]. Although both syndromes share a common aetiology, their symptoms differ significantly [35].

We exclusively encountered patients presenting with Classic Eagle Syndrome and our patients exhibited characteristic symptoms of Eagle syndrome.

Needle pricking sensation and pain on the right side of the mouth persisting for 2–3 years was reported by a 38-year-old female patient.

Another common symptom of Eagle Syndrome, sensation of a foreign body in the throat and pain during swallowing which was persisting for the past 7–8 months was observed in another female patient (Fig. 17.1). Pain on the right side of the neck worsening during neck rotation from the past 1.5 years was experienced by another patient. The male patient had difficulty in swallowing, and pain radiating to the left ear (Fig. 17.2).

None of our patients had a history of tonsillectomy. Our findings are in accordance with the other studies in literature results [20, 36–39].

The symptomatology of Eagle Syndrome often overlaps with other conditions and may remain masked, leading patients to consult multiple specialists. Due to the orofacial pain, dentists frequently play a pivotal role in diagnosing this condition. However, patients may also present to ENT surgeons or neurologists, depending on their predominant symptoms. The variable and sometimes obscure clinical presentation of Eagle Syndrome can result in either under- or over-investigation, contingent upon the expertise and clinical acumen of the consulting specialist.

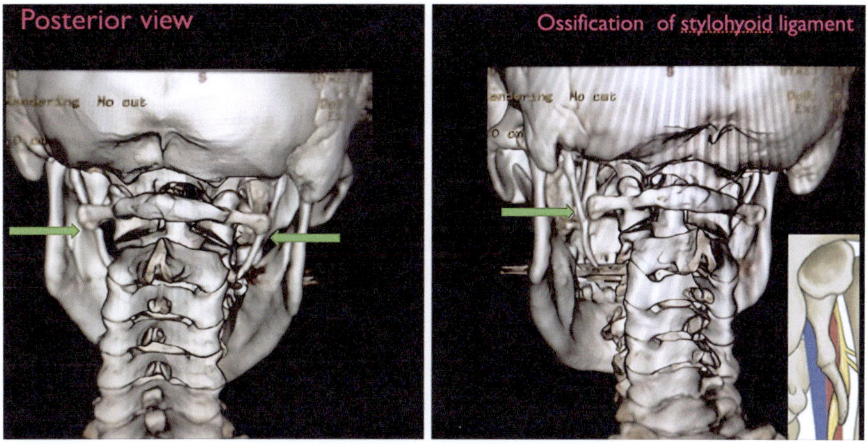

Fig. 17.1 3D-CT Scan image of the bilaterally elongated styloid process

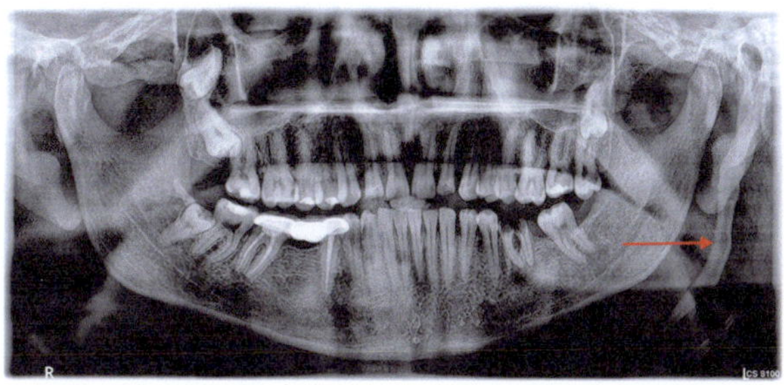

Fig. 17.2 OPT image of a markedly elongated left styloid process

17.13 Clinical Examination

The initial diagnosis of Eagle Syndrome begins with a detailed case history and a systematic clinical examination. A thorough and holistic approach is crucial, as this condition is often overlooked or misdiagnosed.

During history taking, patients are encouraged to provide comprehensive details about the onset, duration, and specific triggers of symptoms such as oropharyngeal pain, otalgia (ear Pain), odynophagia and dysphagia (difficulty in swallowing), allodynia, and facial pain. These symptoms should be correlated with the patient's daily activities, dietary habits, and previous medical interventions, particularly in the Indian context, where traditional treatments may have been attempted.

A comprehensive dental and ENT examinations are essential to exclude any specific odontogenic or ear issues before evaluating for the styloid process.

The physical examination involves positioning the patient comfortably with the head slightly tilted back and the mouth opened wide to access the tonsillar fossa.

The clinician, using a gloved dominant hand, gently inserts the index finger along the lateral pharyngeal wall towards the tonsillar fossa, palpating for a hard, bony protrusion indicative of an elongated styloid process. Pain response and radiating pain to the jaw, ear, or throat are assessed, with bilateral examination performed to check for asymmetry or elongation. Clear communication with the patient about pain and discomfort is maintained throughout, with reassurance provided afterward.

A meticulous examination of the neck and mandible, including the muscles of mastication, is conducted to detect any signs of tenderness, swelling, or radiating pain. This examination is essential for identifying any associated musculoskeletal or vascular involvement.

A detailed neurological assessment is also performed to identify any neurological deficits or referred pain patterns, particularly involving the glossopharyngeal or trigeminal nerves. In India, where patients may present at varying stages of the disease, it is vital to determine whether neurological symptoms are primary or secondary to Eagle Syndrome.

The manoeuvres that reproduce or exacerbate symptoms, such as swallowing, head rotation, or neck palpation, can provide valuable information and help establish a correlation with the anatomical abnormality of the styloid process. These manoeuvres offer a cost-effective method to strengthen the diagnosis before resorting to advanced imaging modalities.

Verma et al. [24] categorised the elongated styloid process based on its position relative to the tonsillar fossa as follows:

- *Grade I:* The tip of the styloid process is palpable in the upper pole.
- *Grade II:* The tip of the styloid process is palpable in the middle of the tonsillar fossa.
- *Grade III:* The tip of the styloid process is palpable in the lower pole and at the base of the tongue.

Three patients exhibited Grade III elongation, while one patient were found to have Grade II elongation.

The administration of 2% lignocaine with adrenaline provides immediate relief and serves as a confirmatory diagnostic tool.

17.14 Differential Diagnoses

The diagnosis of Eagle Syndrome should be distinguished from various other conditions that can present with similar symptoms, such as temporomandibular joint disorders, chronic tonsillitis, and trigeminal neuralgia. The clinical presentation must also be carefully differentiated from glossopharyngeal neuralgia, which may exhibit overlapping symptoms. Comprehensive clinical evaluation and appropriate imaging studies are essential in ruling out these conditions and confirming the diagnosis of Eagle Syndrome.

17.15 Imaging

Radiographic imaging plays a crucial role in diagnosing Eagle's syndrome. Panoramic radiographs (OPG) are commonly used due to their cost-effectiveness, particularly in rural and semi-urban populations in India. (Fig. 17.3). However, OPGs have limitations in the accurate determination of the exact length and anatomical relationship of the styloid processes. It is important to note that an elongated styloid process observed on an OPG does not necessarily indicate Eagle's syndrome, as approximately 4% of the population may have an elongated styloid without any symptoms.

While OPG and ultrasound help in screening [40, 41], CT (spiral CT with 3D reconstruction), (Figure 17.4a, b) imaging is preferred diagnostic tool.

As it provides more precise localization and measurement of the styloid processes, direction, angulation and anatomical relation of the styloid process to adjacent tissues [42]. This vital for patient counselling and surgical planning [41].

Goldstein and Scopa [43] have established criteria for the radiographic evaluation of the elongated styloid process:

1. *Not Observable:* Indistinct stylohyoid or stylomandibular ligament.
2. *Normal Range:* Radiopacity of the styloid process is less than one-third of the mandibular ramus length.
3. *Partially Calcified:* Radiopacity extends beyond one-third but does not reach the angle of the mandible.
4. *Completely Calcified:* Radiopacity reaches or touches the angle of the mandible.

Additionally, Langlais's classification (Fig. 17.5) based on radiographic appearance is as follows [44]:

- *Type I:* Uninterrupted and elongated styloid process.
- *Type II:* Styloid process joined to the stylohyoid ligament via a pseudoarticulation.
- *Type III:* Interrupted segments of the mineralized ligament, appearing as multiple calcified sections.

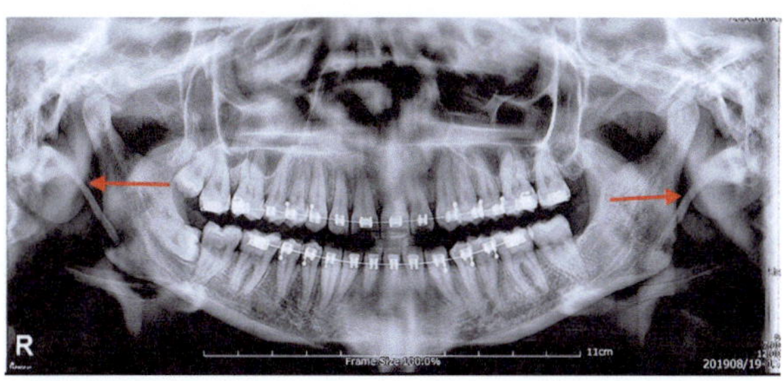

Fig. 17.3 OPT image of a markedly bilaterally elongated styloid process

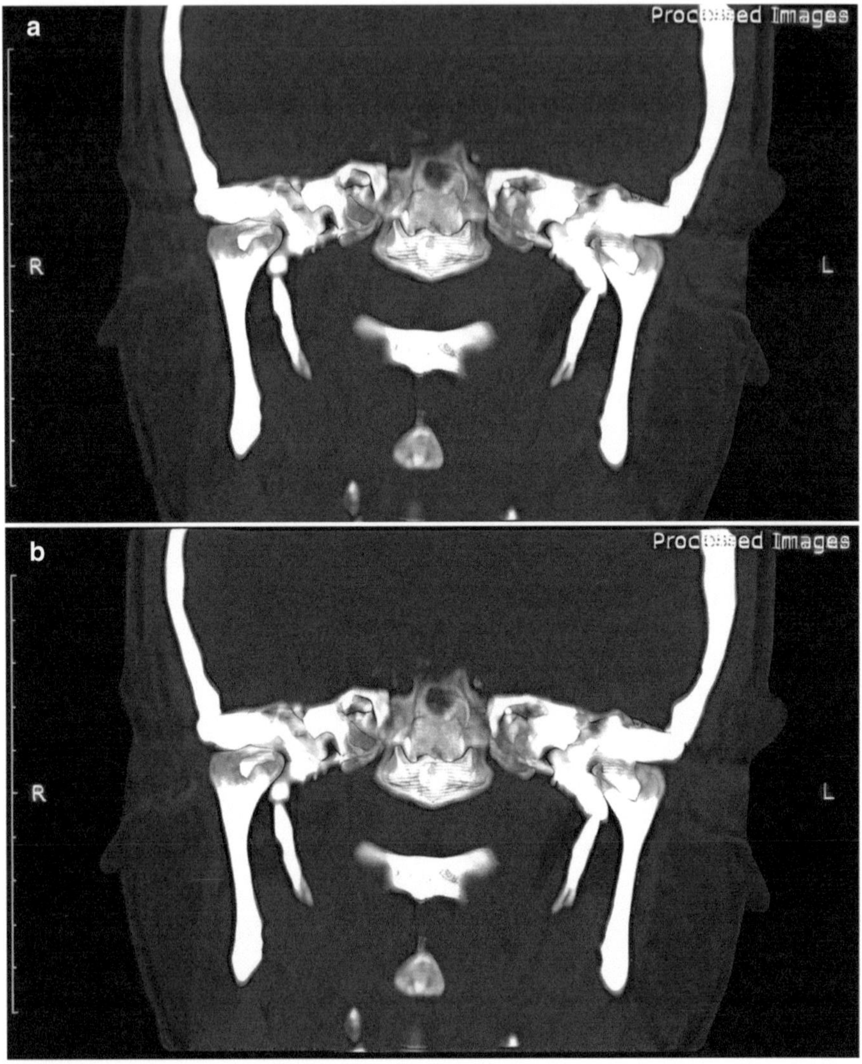

Fig. 17.4 In images (**a**) and (**b**), an example of the detail provided by the 3D reconstruction of CT scans performed for the diagnosis of Eagle Syndrome

Our assessment system was based on these criteria in mind while evaluating our radiographs and CT images.

Type 1 bilateral elongation of the styloid process was the most common finding in our patients followed by type 2 on the right and type 1 on the left side. This has also been observed by Shah et al. [31]. All our symptomatic patients had type 1 elongated styloid process.

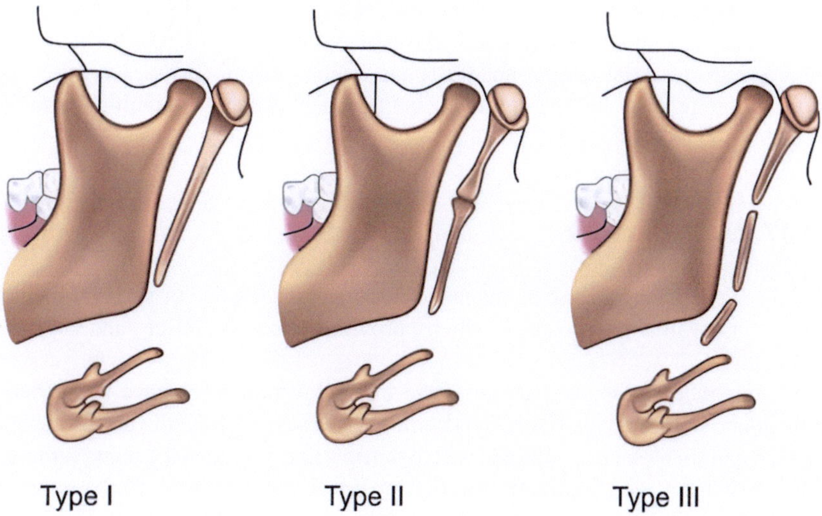

Fig. 17.5 Langlais's classification

Evaluating both the sagittal and transverse angles of the styloid process, alongside its length, is essential as it corresponds with the manifestation of symptoms. Even a slight medial deviation can trigger severe atypical facial pain [36].

However, merely detecting an elongated styloid process or mineralization of the stylohyoid complex on radiographs does not definitively indicate Eagle's syndrome due to the following reasons:

A. Many individuals with an ossified stylohyoid complex do not exhibit any symptoms.
B. There is no direct correlation between the intensity of pain and the degree of ossification.
C. Most patients who show symptoms do not have a history of tonsillectomy or cervicopharyngeal trauma [45].

For an accurate diagnosis of an elongated styloid process, a thorough clinical and radiological examination is necessary.

17.16 Diagnosis

The accurate diagnosis of Eagle Syndrome is predominantly clinical, with confirmation provided by imaging studies. It relies on the intraoral digital palpation of the tonsillar fossa, where the identification of a sharp, hard structure, accompanied by the exacerbation of symptoms, serves as a definitive sign of styloid process elongation. This clinical technique is the most vital diagnostic tool for identifying Eagle Syndrome. Radiographs and CT scans are instrumental in assessing the length of the styloid process and in guiding the management specially planning the surgical procedure.

17.17 Management

Eagle's Syndrome (ES) can be managed through conservative or surgical methods, with conservative approaches often providing initial relief and symptom management.

Various medications and conservative treatment modalities have been tried by Indian doctors to manage Eagle Syndrome (ES). These include the use of gabapentin, Gabapentin alone or combined with Amitriptyline to reduce the pain. Temporary relief has been demonstrated through medications such as Carbamazepine,, Diclofenac, and Pregabalin, sometimes supplemented with Deflazacort [15, 26, 36].

Use of Glucocorticoids have also been used by few doctors as they reduce the pain and discomfort by decreasing the inflammation and swelling [46–48]. Transpharyngeal injections of hydrocortisone with lignocaine, as recommended by Han et al., have been effective in reducing pharyngeal swelling and discomfort [49].

Other non-pharmacological approaches, like local heat application and innovative techniques such as digital fracturing of the styloid process [50], have also been explored, offering minimally invasive alternatives to surgery. Complementary therapies, including lidocaine infiltration, anxiolytics, TENS therapy [51], and percutaneous thermal radiofrequency ablation [52], have been tried for symptom relief in Indian clinical practice.

In our case series, a female patient was initially prescribed Diclofenac Sodium 75 mg twice daily, along with antibiotic (a combination of Amoxicillin 500 mg and Clavulanic Acid 125 mg) for 10 days. Additionally, she was given a combination of Pregabalin 75 mg and Amitriptyline 25 mg at night for 3 months. Although she experienced temporary relief, her symptoms recurred, leading to the administration of Carbamazepine 300 mg thrice daily for 2 months.

Other patients who received conservative medical treatment continued to experience persistent symptoms. Consequently, these patients were referred for further management. All patients were evaluated both clinically and radiographically to confirm the diagnosis, and it was determined that surgical intervention was necessary, as medical management did not provide adequate relief.

17.18 Surgical Approaches

The surgical management of Eagle's Syndrome typically involves shortening the elongated styloid process, which can be performed through either an intraoral or external approach. The selection of technique depends on various factors, including the severity of symptoms, the extent of elongation, and the anatomical positioning of the styloid process. Each method has its own advantages and limitations [53, 54].

Several transoral and extraoral surgical techniques have been documented, such as retromolar, paratonsillar, trans-tonsillar, transcervical, preauricular, and endoscopic-assisted styloidectomy, with or without navigation, as noted by Maryu [55].

Intra oral Trans tonsillar approach was carried out in all our cases for styloidectomy. All patients in our study were treated using the intraoral approach. Surgery was performed under general anesthesia with uneventful nasotracheal intubation. A Boyle-Davis mouth gag was used to keep the mouth open. Intraoral palpation identified the styloid process in the tonsillar fossa to check the bulge. Tonsillectomy was done using coblation, followed by identification of the superior constrictor muscle. Dissection was carried out along the fibres of the muscle, which was separated at the point where the styloid process was prominent and palpable. The internal jugular vein and internal carotid artery were identified and preserved. The periosteum was incised and elevated. A ring curette was passed across the styloid process, and the necessary amount of bone was resected. The styloid process was then broken and removed with a bone nibbler or curette. After excision, the superior constrictor muscle was closed with 3–0 vicryl sutures, and hemostasis was achieved either by cauterizing or ligating any blood vessels.

Postoperatively, patients were kept on clear fluids for 7–10 days. Parenteral antibiotics, including amoxicillin and clavulanic acid (1.2 gm twice daily) and metronidazole (500 mg thrice daily), were administered for 3 days. Analgesics included intravenous diclofenac sodium (75 mg) for the first day, followed by paracetamol (1000 mg twice daily) for the second day. Patients were discharged after 3 days with oral antibiotics and analgesics to be continued for next 5 days and followed up for 1 year.

The intra oral approach was preferred for the following advantages

- The procedure can be performed under local anesthesia.
- Dissection is limited to the tip of the process, avoiding blind dissection.
- Inadvertent exposure of the fossa is minimized.
- Bleeding is minimal.
- Healing is faster due to the elasticity of the tonsillar bed.
- The risk of neck space infection is low.
- Operative time is shorter.
- Postoperative complications and pain are reduced, leading to faster recovery [30].
- Postoperative morbidity and complications are low.
- The procedure is easy to perform, leaves no external scar, and has a shorter operating and recovery time [26].
- Less risk of injury to carotid artery as compared to the external approach.

Intraoral approach has been a choice of approach for many Indian sugeons. Lambor DV et al. reviewed 101 patients treated by the intraoral approach in Goa, with none found to have any intraoperative or postoperative complications [26]. Similar results have been documented by other Indian surgeons [13, 15, 23, 36–38, 56, 57].

17.18.1 Complications Associated with Intra Oral Approach

Despite the overall effectiveness and preference for the intraoral approach, certain complications may arise. These include pain and trismus, speech problems, which are immediate but manageable postoperative complications, and the necessity for careful dissection to avoid persistent symptoms.

2 patients in our study had trismus for 7–10 days which eventully improved over a period of 3 weeks. None of our patients encountered any major complications.

17.19 Extraoral Approach

The transcervical approach, an extraoral technique, involves making an incision that extends from the mastoid process along the sternocleidomastoid muscle to the level of the hyoid bone and then across the neck to the midline of the chin.

Only few cases India have been treated by extra oral approach. Jose et al. treated 12 patients using this approach, with the median duration of the procedure being 81 min [58].

17.20 Advantages of the Extraoral Approach

The extraoral approach offers several advantages, including excellent visualization and accessibility during the procedure, as well as a reduced risk of deep neck space infection.

17.21 Disadvantages of the Extraoral Approach

However, this method also has its drawbacks, such as requiring more surgical time, higher morbidity compared to the intraoral approach, and the presence of a visible scar [59].

17.21.1 Complications Associated with the Extraoral Approach

Reported complications include diffuse swelling behind the angle of the mandible, extending to the submandibular area, which typically subsides within a week. Murthy et al. observed this in 10% of their patients, while Strauss et al. reported it in 25% of cases. The other complications include increased surgical time, possible paraesthesia of greater auricular nerve, and elaborate plane of dissection [59]. The external approach necessitates a neck incision, and in rare instances, there is a risk of facial nerve palsy.

17.22 Challenges and Considerations in India

In India, socio-economic factors, cultural beliefs and practices, significantly impact the diagnosis and treatment of Eagle Syndrome. Delay in proper diagnosis and management is attributed to many factors like Financial constraints especially for those without insurance or from lower socio-economic backgrounds and many patients may first seek treatment from traditional or alternative medicine practitioners. Cultural attitudes towards surgery, including fear and concerns about risks, may also discourage patients from opting for necessary surgical interventions.

There is a notable disparity between urban and rural healthcare, with urban areas having better resources and rural areas often lacking essential facilities. Public healthcare is more affordable but overcrowded, while private healthcare, though better equipped, remains expensive for many. Regular follow-ups are difficult for patients in rural areas who may have to travel long distances, and socio-economic factors also affect adherence to postoperative care and rehabilitation.

- Increased awareness campaigns are needed to educate both healthcare professionals and the public about Eagle Syndrome, aiding in early recognition and treatment.
- Effective communication about the condition and treatment options is crucial for informed decision-making and compliance.
- Establish standardized diagnostic and treatment protocols and to encourage genetic and molecular research seeks to uncover hereditary patterns and potential biomarkers.
- Innovations in minimally invasive surgical techniques and non-surgical treatments, including advanced imaging and pain management protocols, are also being explored to shift to patient centric interdisciplinary approach to provide better patient care and outcomes.
- Enhance the screening in the rural areas of India, where there is limited or no access to dental and other medical services. Reaching the last mile is the key as it will help women to improve their quality of life and contribute better to the livelihoods.
- Ensuring that qualified surgeons equipped with both the training and knowledge to perform the procedure.

17.23 Conclusion

Eagle Syndrome is crucial in the medical field due to its diagnostic challenges, impact on quality of life, interdisciplinary relevance, and the need for appropriate management. Its rarity and nonspecific symptoms often lead to misdiagnosis and delayed treatment, affecting patient well-being. The condition's debilitating symptoms can significantly impair daily activities and mental health, making early recognition and treatment essential for improving quality of life. Additionally, understanding Eagle Syndrome is important for healthcare providers across various specialties, such as otolaryngology, dentistry, neurology, and pain management, to ensure accurate diagnosis and effective treatment, whether conservative or surgical.

References

1. Czako L, Simko K, Thurzo A, Galis B, Varga I. The syndrome of elongated styloid process, the Eagle's syndrome-from anatomical, evolutionary and embryological backgrounds to 3D printing and personalized surgery planning. Report of five cases. Medicina (Kaunas). 2020;56(9):458. https://doi.org/10.3390/medicina56090458.
2. Fini G, Gasparini G, Filippini F, Becelli R, Marcotullio D. The long styloid process syndrome or Eagle's syndrome. J Cranio Maxillofac Surg. 2000;28:123–7.
3. Kulvin MM. Elongated styloid processes; their formation and clinical significance. Laryngoscope. 1949;40(12):907–9.
4. Eagle WW. Elongated styloid process. Report of two cases. Arch Otolaryngol. 1937;25:584–7.
5. Eagle WW. Elongated styloid process; further observations and a new syndrome. Arch Otolaryngol. 1948;47(5):630–40. https://doi.org/10.1001/archotol.1948.00690030654006.
6. Eagle WW. Symptomatic elongated styloid process; report of two cases of styloid process-carotid artery syndrome with operation. Arch Otolaryngol. 1949;49:490–503.
7. Gli Aspetti LA. Clinici e radiologici delle anomalie dell' apparato stilo-joideo. Radiol Med. 1975;61:337–640.
8. Epifanio G. Processi stiloidea lunghi e ossificazione della catena stiloidea. Rad Prat. 1962;12:127–32.
9. Steinmann EP. A new light on the pathogenesis of the styloid syndrome. Arch Otolaryngol. 1970;91:171–4.
10. Gokce C, Sisman Y, Sipahioglu M. Styloid process elongation or Eagle's syndrome: is there any role for ectopic calcification? Eur J Dent. 2008;2:224–8.
11. Khandelwal S, Hada YS, Harsh A. Eagle's syndrome—a case report and review of the literature. Saudi Dent J. 2011;23(4):211–5. https://doi.org/10.1016/j.sdentj.2010.10.006.
12. Pagano S, Ricciuti V, Mancini F, Barbieri FR, Chegai F, Marini A, Marruzzo D, Paracino R, Ricciuti RA. Eagle syndrome: an updated review. Surg Neurol Int. 2023;14:389. https://doi.org/10.25259/SNI_666_2023.
13. Prasad KC, Kamath MP, Reddy KJ, Raju K, Agarwal S. Elongated styloid process (Eagle's syndrome): a clinical study. J Oral Maxillofac Surg. 2002;60(2):171–5. https://doi.org/10.1053/joms.2002.29814.
14. Kannan R, Thenmozhi MS. Morphometric study of styloid process and its clinical importance on Eagle's syndrome. Res J Pharm Technol. 2016;9:1137. https://doi.org/10.5958/0974-360X.2016.00216.X.
15. Kumar PS, Singh DK, Gupta SK, Raina S, Prasad BK. Of Eagle's syndrome and finding some clarity on its management. Indian J Otolaryngol Head Neck Surg. 2022;74(Suppl 2):2184–9. https://doi.org/10.1007/s12070-020-02079-2.

16. Sudhakara Reddy R, Sai Kiran C, Sai Madhavi N, Raghavendra MN, Satish A. Prevalence of elongation and calcification patterns of elongated styloid process in South India. J Clin Exp Dent. 2013;5(1):e30–5. https://doi.org/10.4317/jced.50981.
17. More CB, Asrani MK. Evaluation of the styloid process on digital panoramic radiographs. Indian J Radiol Imaging. 2010;20:261–5.
18. Phulambrikar T, Rajeshwari A, Rao BB, Warhekar A, Reddy P. Incidence of elongated styloid process: a radiographic study. J Indian Acad Oral Med Radiol. 2011;23:S344–6.
19. Bagga MB, Kumar CA, Yeluri G. Clinicoradiologic evaluation of styloid process calcification. Imaging Sci Dent. 2012;42(3):155–61. https://doi.org/10.5624/isd.2012.42.3.155.
20. Yadav SP, Chanda R, Gera A, Yadav RK. Stylalgia: an Indian perspective. J Otolaryngol. 2001;30:304–6.
21. Crowley LV. An introduction to human diseases: pathology and pathophysiology correlations. 8th ed. Sudbury: Jones and Bartlett Publishers; 2009. p. 719–20.
22. Srivastav A, Saraswat PK, Agarwal SK, Gupta P. A study of wrist ossification for age estimation in pediatric group in Central Rajasthan. J Indian Acad Forensic Med. 2004;26:132–5.
23. Salam RTA. A clinical analysis of Eagle's syndrome by its clinical features and therapeutic response to surgical treatment. Int J Sci Stud. 2017;5(10):97–104.
24. Verma R. Stylalgia. Indian J Otolaryngol Head Neck Surg. 1996;48:312–4. https://doi.org/10.1007/BF03048664.
25. Sridevi K, Mahesh N, Krishnaveni B, Deepika ADN, Thejasri V, Leninson BHD. Evaluation of styloid process and its anatomical variations: a digital panoramic study with systematic review. J Int Soc Prev Community Dent. 2019;9(3):256–62. https://doi.org/10.4103/jispcd.JISPCD_8_19.
26. Lambor DV, Shetgaunkar RR, De Sa C. Stylalgia: our experience of 101 cases treated by intraoral styloidectomy. Indian J Otolaryngol Head Neck Surg. 2022;74(Suppl 2):2198–204. https://doi.org/10.1007/s12070-020-02074-7.
27. Vadgaonkar R, Murlimanju BV, Prabhu LV, Rai R, Pai MM, Tonse M, Jiji PJ. Morphological study of styloid process of the temporal bone and its clinical implications. Anat Cell Biol. 2015;48(3):195–200.
28. Rathva A, Kubavat DM, Nagar SK. Study of styloid process: anatomical variations in length, angulation and distance between the two styloid processes. Int J Recent Trends Sci Technol. 2013;8:109–12.
29. Roopashri G, Vaishali MR, David MP, Baig M, Shankar U. Evaluation of elongated styloid process on digital panoramic radiographs. J Contemp Dent Pract. 2012;13(5):618–22.
30. Taneja S, Chand S, Dhar S. Stylalgia and styloidectomy: a review. J Maxillofac Oral Surg. 2023;22(1):60–6. https://doi.org/10.1007/s12663-022-01720-7.
31. Shah SP, Praveen NB, Syed V, Subhashini AR. Elongated styloid process: a retrospective panoramic radiographic study. World J Dent. 2012;3(4):316–9.
32. Olszewski J, Miłoński J, Jałocha-Kaczka A. A rare case of late diagnosis of elongated styloid process syndrome. J Hear Sci. 2019;9(4):33–6. https://doi.org/10.17430/1003481.
33. Pierrakou ED. Eagle's syndrome. Review of the literature and a case report. Ann Dent. 1990;49(1):30–3.
34. Eagle WW. Elongated styloid process: symptoms and treatment. AMA Arch Otolaryngol. 1958;67(2):172–6. https://doi.org/10.1001/archotol.1958.00730010178007.
35. Breault MR. Eagle's syndrome: review of the literature and implications in craniomandibular disorders. J Craniomandibular Pract. 1986;4(4):323–37.
36. Sham E, Reddy TJ, Menon PS, Kumar V, Nathan AS, Mathews S, Gowda KV, Dhanush CV. Anterior tonsillar fossa approach to elongated styloid process. Ann Maxillofac Surg. 2020;10(1):203–9. https://doi.org/10.4103/ams.ams_189_19.
37. Mishra A, Dabholkar J, Lodha MSJ, Mhashal S. Stylalgia—a missed diagnosis. Otolaryngol Pol. 2015;69(2):34–7. https://doi.org/10.5604/00306657.1131148.
38. Shedge Swapna A, et al. Stylalgia – glossopharyngeal neuralgia: outcome of management. Int J Approx Reason. 2017;5:3952–7.

39. Malik JN, Monga S, Sharma AP, Nabi N, Naseeruddin K. Stylalgia revisited: clinical profile and management. Iran J Otorhinolaryngol. 2018;30(101):335–40.
40. Müderris T, Bercin S, Sevil E, et al. Surgical management of elongated styloid process: intraoral or transcervical? Eur Arch Otorrinolaringol. 2013;271(6):1709–13. https://doi.org/10.1007/s00405-013-2664-0.
41. Nayak DR, Pujary K, Aggarwal M, et al. Role of three-dimensional computed tomography reconstruction in the managementof elongated styloid process: a preliminary study. J Laryngol Otol. 2007;121(4):349–53.
42. Matsumoto F, Kase K, Kasai M, et al. Endoscopy-assisted transoral resection of the styloid process in Eagle's syndrome. Head Face Med. 2012;8:21. https://doi.org/10.1186/1746-160X-8-21.
43. Goldstein GR, Scopp IW. Radiographic interpretation of calcified stylomandibular and stylohyoid ligaments. J Prosthet Dent. 1973;30(3):330–4. https://doi.org/10.1016/0022-3913(73)90192-3.
44. Langlais RP, Miles DA, Van Dis ML. Elongated and mineralized stylohyoid ligament complex: a proposed classification and report of a case of Eagle's syndrome. Oral Surg Oral Med Oral Pathol. 1986;61(5):527–32. https://doi.org/10.1016/0030-4220(86)90400-7.
45. Camarda AJ, Deschamps C, Forest D. Stylohyoid chain ossification: a discussion of etiology. Oral Surg Oral Med Oral Pathol. 1989;67:508–14.
46. Martin TJ, Friedland DR, Merati AL. Transcervical resection of the styloid process in Eagle syndrome. Ear NoseThroat J. 2008;87:399–401.
47. Gervickas A, Kubilius R, Sabalys G. Clinic, diagnostics, and treatment peculiarities of Eagle's syndrome. Stomatol Balt Dent Maxillofac J. 2004;6:11.
48. Glogoff MR, Baum SM, Cheifetz I. Diagnosis and treatment of Eagle's syndrome. J Oral Surg. 1981;39:941–4.
49. Han M, Kim D, Yang J. Nonsurgical treatment of Eagle's syndrome: a case report. Korean J Pain. 2013;26:169–72. https://doi.org/10.3344/kjp.2013.26.2.169.
50. Maity K, Misra S. Stylalgia: a novel approach to treatment. Bangladesh J Otorhinolaryngol. 2012;18(2):133–7. https://doi.org/10.3329/bjo.v18i2.11990.
51. Sowmya GV, Singh MP, Manjunatha BS, Nahar P, Astekar M. A case of unilateral atypical orofacial pain with Eagle's syndrome. J Cancer Res Ther. 2016;12(4):1323. https://doi.org/10.4103/0973-1482.144558.
52. Swain BP, Vidhya S, Kumar S. Eagle's syndrome managed successfully by pulsed radiofrequency treatment. Cureus. 2020;12(9):e10574. https://doi.org/10.7759/cureus.10574.
53. Beder E, Ozgursoy OB, Karatayli Ozgursoy S. Current diagnosis and transoral surgical treatment of Eagle's syndrome. J Oral Maxillofac Surg. 2005;63:1742–5.
54. Chrcanovic BR, Custódio AL, de Oliveira DR. An intraoral surgical approach to the styloid process in Eagle's syndrome. Oral Maxillofac Surg. 2009;13:145–51.
55. Maru YK, Patidar K. Stylalgia and its surgical management by intra oral route clinical experience of 332 cases. Indian J Otolaryngol Head Neck Surg. 2003;55(2):8790.
56. Ghosh LM, Dubey SP. The syndrome of elongated styloid process. Auris Nasus Larynx. 1999;26(2):169–75. https://doi.org/10.1016/s0385-8146(98)00079-0.
57. Naik SM, Naik SS. Tonsillo-styloidectomy for Eagle's syndrome: a review of 15 cases in KVG Medical College Sullia. Oman Med J. 2011;26(2):122–6. https://doi.org/10.5001/omj.2011.30.
58. Jose A, Arya S, Nagori SA, Roy ID, Tokas O. Styloid-stylohyoid syndrome: a rare cause of cranio-facial pain-a retrospective case series of 12 patients. Oral Maxillofac Surg. 2019;23(1):47–51. https://doi.org/10.1007/s10006-018-0736-4.
59. Vanza B, Khare N. Eyes don't see what mind doesn't know-study of 750 cases on Eagle's syndrome. Medical science. Indian J Appl Res. 2016;6:291–2.

18 Conservative Treatments in Eagle Syndrome

Alberto Caranti, Ruggero Campisi, and Claudio Vicini

18.1 Introduction

Conservative treatment can be employed, as discussed in other chapters of this monograph, as an ex adiuvantibus treatment strategy to provide a key element in predicting the successful surgical outcome of styloidectomy.

Conservative therapy can also serve as a valuable tool in many situations:

- For patients with ES on the waiting list for surgery who seek to alleviate symptoms caused by the condition.
- For fragile patients with ES who face high anesthetic risk and thus require an alternative to surgical intervention.
- For patients with ES who choose not to undergo surgery.

We have already extensively described the etiopathogenesis of the classic variant of ES. Therefore, it is not surprising that some conservative treatments are common to other types of neuralgias, whether primary or secondary.

Conservative methods of medical management can further be divided into first-line analgesics such as non-steroidal anti-inflammatory drugs (NSAIDs) and a multi-drug approach consisting of anticonvulsants, antidepressants, local injections, and manipulation. NSAIDs provide analgesia in Eagle syndrome and will likely

A. Caranti · R. Campisi · C. Vicini (✉)
University of Ferrara, Cona, FE, Italy
e-mail: claudio@claudiovicini.com

C. Vicini et al. (eds.), *EAGLE Syndrome*,
https://doi.org/10.1007/978-3-031-92829-1_18

provide the most benefit to patients suffering from symptoms that are inflammatory in nature [1]. Targeting of the styloid ligament and surrounding inflammation has been shown to decrease painful symptoms associated with Eagle syndrome.

Antiepileptic drugs, on the other hand, are used for neuropathic pain, such as that caused by primary neuralgias like trigeminal or glossopharyngeal neuralgia [2].

18.2 Medical Management

At the forefront, we have a range of drugs aimed at reducing pain rather than providing an outright cure [3]. In this regard, there is a wide selection of medications recommended by the International Association for the Study of Pain (IASP) for the treatment of glossopharyngeal nerve (GFN) neuralgia pain, which are summarized in Table 18.1 with their respective dosages [4].

The rationale for using these drugs should be to ensure, with the lowest possible dose, pain relief sufficient to conduct daily activities without issues [5]. Therefore, the algorithm to follow is to progressively reach the lowest effective dose to achieve this result, considering the possibility of increasing the dosage again in case of pain recurrence. This strategy typically allows for symptom control for intervals ranging from several months to several years. If the first-line drug no longer proves effective, one might opt for either a change in medication or a combination of two or more drugs [5].

In this case, the first-line therapeutic choice includes membrane stabilizers such as carbamazepine (acting on Na^+ channels), gabapentin and pregabalin (acting on $Ca2^+$ channels), and selective serotonin and norepinephrine reuptake inhibitors (SSNRI) like duloxetine, as well as valproic acid (Grade A evidence) [5, 6].

In the second line, the use of opioids such as morphine, oxycodone, methadone, levorphanol, and tramadol is indicated. In the third line, we have drugs such as serotonin reuptake inhibitors (SSRI) like citalopram or paroxetine, as well as mexiletine and NMDA receptor antagonists [6].

Taheri et al. demonstrated an 80% reduction in severity of pain with pain-free intervals 6–months post-treatment report of treating a patient with only oral medications (amitriptyline and pregabalin) [7].

Table 18.1 The International Association for the Study of Pain (IASP) recommended drugs with their dosages used in glossopharyngeal neuralgia

Drug	Dose (mg/day)
Carbamazepine	100–2000
Gabapentin	100–5000
Duloxetine	20–90
Valproic acid	125–2500
Clonazepam	0,5–8
Lamotrigine	50–500
Baclofen	10–80
Phenytoin	200–600
Pregabalin	75–500
Topiramate	50–1000

18.3 Stellate Ganglion Block

Similar cases, with similar results, used oral medications in conjunction with local injections and/or a stellate ganglion block.

The stellate ganglion block (SGB) is employed to treat various medical conditions, such as complex regional pain syndrome and peripheral vascular disease. Traditionally, the anesthetic is administered at the C6 or C7 vertebral level, using anatomical landmarks like Chassaignac's tubercle, the cricoid cartilage, and the carotid artery to guide the procedure. Due to a significant risk of complications, including pneumothorax and vascular puncture, it is highly recommended to use an image-guided approach, even with the relatively safer C6 method. Therefore, ultrasound or fluoroscopic guidance is currently utilized [8, 9].

For instance, as reported by Kawasaki M et al. [10], in a case of glossopharyngeal neuralgia secondary to ES, after informing the patient about the surgical benefits for resolving the condition and recording the patient's refusal to undergo surgery, a therapy regimen was proposed. This regimen combined an anticonvulsant medication, typically used for primary glossopharyngeal neuralgia [2], with a stellate ganglion block and a topical therapy using 8% lidocaine applied to the tonsillar fossa daily, every 8 hours (three times a day continuously).

In this study, a synergy between gabapentin and the topical therapy is hypothesized to enhance the half-life of the topical medication, as the authors observed an almost total and longer-lasting benefit compared to the expected half-life of the topical drug.

18.4 Ultrasound-Guided Injection of Steroids or Long-Lasting Anesthetics

Conservative treatment of Eagle syndrome also includes ultrasound-guided injection of steroids or long-lasting anesthetics [1] as described in a different chapter of this monograph.

Local injections, administered near the affected tonsillar fossa, are usually composed of a local anesthetic combined with a corticosteroid. These procedures can be performed effectively in an outpatient clinic without the need for advanced equipment, or they can be executed with the aid of ultrasound guidance to include a preliminary identification of important neurovascular structures adjacent to the styloid process [11].

Local infiltration with anesthetic and steroid is a component of our patient selection algorithm for surgery, which has helped us to outline a process for selecting patients who could truly benefit from surgical styloidectomy, with the aim of minimizing surgical failures as much as possible.

We proceed with a local anesthetic infiltration, composed of lidocaine (200 mg/10 mL) and corticosteroid (betamethasone 4 mg/2 mL), all in a single syringe with a thin insulin needle, which is administered in the region of the tonsillar fossa on the side under examination. The very first infiltration is carried out already at the first visit, so as not to waste the patient's time, also because our clinic is often visited by patients who come from very distant places both within Italy and from foreign countries. In the 30 days following the procedure, the patient will inform us about any changes in symptoms related to the infiltration. This, in the protocol we have adopted in clinical practice, is followed by three cycles of infiltration, spaced 1 month apart. We propose surgical treatment only to patients who have had a very tangible benefit from the cycle of infiltrations.

An important detail is relevant: it is clear that it would be complicated to set a cutoff for improvement based on subjective questionnaires, which would advise whether or not to proceed with surgical intervention. It also seemed unfair to propose surgical intervention aiming for the complete and definitive elimination of all subjective indicators of the pain symptom. We have, therefore, decided that the styloidectomy intervention should be exclusively proposed to patients who have determined, with the cycle of local infiltrations, a subjective improvement in symptoms satisfactory for them. Thus, the patient, properly and scrupulously informed about the methods, risks, and benefits of the surgical intervention, will inform us if the changes due to the local infiltration were appreciable compared to the pre-existing condition.

18.5 Pulsed Radiofrequency

Pulsed radiofrequency treatment in a case of classic Eagle syndrome was described by Fernando T. Mollinedo in 2012 [12].

In pulsed radiofrequency, short bursts of radiofrequency energy are applied to nervous tissue in order to produce a targeted neurolysis. It has been used by pain practitioners as a non- or minimally neuro-destructive technique, alternative to radiofrequency heat lesions. In 2020, one more case was reported: an elderly male who presented with features of glossopharyngeal neuralgia secondary to an elongated styloid process was managed successfully with pulsed radiofrequency treatment of the glossopharyngeal nerve [12]. There are anecdotal reports that radiofrequency thermoneurolysis is effective in treating symptoms of Ernest syndrome. The effectiveness of radiofrequency ablation for treatment of glossopharyngeal neuralgia was discussed in a systematic review of the current literature by Kenny Do and colleagues in 2024 [13].

Studies included in this systematic review encompassed idiopathic cases and secondary causes, such as an elongated styloid process, oropharyngeal cancers, and postsurgical/post-traumatic pain. Of the 288 patients treated with RFA, 231 experienced relief or complete resolution of pain, yielding an efficacy rate of 80.2%. Most of the patients experienced immediate pain relief after RFA; however, some patients reported numbness, dysphagia, and changes in taste. Further studies are mandatory [13].

Regarding vascular forms, which are not necessarily painful as in the case of secondary neuralgias, the use of antiplatelet and anticoagulant medications is documented to prevent major cardiovascular events such as stroke. Occasionally, as we will see shortly, these medications are also combined with physical or behavioral therapy [14].

18.6 Pulsed Radiofrequency

Physical therapists often treat patients for craniocervical pain. Wong et al. describe a case of a patient with a typical form of Eagle syndrome (ES) associated with lateral neck pain, which was treated with physical therapy [15].

Patient's craniocervical symptoms included the sensation of a lump in her throat, pain with swallowing, paresthesia and pain over the left maxillary and mandibular areas, occipital pain, and a sensation of mental cloudiness.

The therapy involved manual therapy interventions and concluded with gentle exercises aimed at enhancing neuromuscular control and recruitment of the deep cervical flexors. Counseling was provided for recommended ergonomic and postural adjustments. The goal was to advance the treatment program by progressively incorporating exercises with increasing demands on endurance, strength, and coordination of the upper quadrant.

Outcome measures included the craniocervical flexion test (CCFT—it is a method of evaluating weakness of the deep cervical flexors through the use of a biofeedback device [16]), Neck Disability Index (NDI) [17], and subjective complaints. The patient was evaluated at the initial visit, at discharge, and at a 3-month follow-up. At discharge, the patient reported complete cessation of craniofacial symptoms, her CCFT score had improved by 4 mmHg, and her NDI score had improved by 10%. At the 3-month follow-up, the patient's CCFT had improved an additional 4 mmHg, and her NDI score had declined by 4% [15].

18.7 Conservative Behavioral Therapy

A unique case of conservative behavioral therapy was described by Shindo T et al. [18], involving a patient with an embolic stroke due to extracranial internal carotid artery (ICA) dissection from the ipsilateral elongated styloid process, managed successfully without surgical intervention for more than 1.5 years.

Further imaging work-up included a three-dimensional computed tomography angiogram, which indicated cervical ICA dissection in proximity to an ipsilateral elongated styloid process measuring 3.1 cm. While the proximity of the elongated styloid process to the ICA was confirmed, direct evidence of impingement on the ICA could not be demonstrated as they avoided overextending the patient's neck to prevent cervical ICA compression.

Reviewing the patient's recent medical history revealed that the acute episode occurred during prolonged neck extension in an unnatural position. Consequently, they managed this patient conservatively with anticoagulation therapy using argatroban, followed by oral antiplatelet therapy. Additionally, they educated the patient to avoid excessive neck extension ("educated him and emphasized not to look up too much to avoid neck extension") to prevent mechanical ICA compression by the elongated styloid process [18].

From a pharmacological perspective, we do not have sufficient evidence to determine the effect of cannabinoids on the pain caused by this condition, although their use appears promising for other pain syndromes with neuropathic pain [19, 20].

18.8 Final Considerations

In conclusion, to provide an overview of the pharmacological and conservative treatment in patients with ES, a recent meta-analysis by Hassani et al., conducted on 497 patients, revealed that one-fourth of the patients ($n = 92$, 24.9%) were medically managed. The most prevalent medications were non-steroidal anti-inflammatory drugs ($n = 39$, 42.4%), analgesics ($n = 36$, 39.13%), and anticonvulsants ($n = 27$, 29.4%). Among the anticonvulsants, carbamazepine ($n = 17$) and gabapentin ($n = 9$) were the most widely used. Additionally, 11 patients tried physical therapy.

In the vascular subgroup, a significantly larger proportion ($n = 57$, 48.7%) received medical treatment, including 40 individuals (70.2%) on antiplatelet or anticoagulant medication and an additional 12 (21.1%) on non-steroidal anti-inflammatory drugs [14].

One factor that we absolutely cannot overlook when referring to medical therapy is the placebo effect. There is now well-established literature indicating that the perception of receiving treatment for pain can lead to an actual reduction in pain [21]. Additionally, we know that the placebo effect is also influenced by emotional factors, such as the patient's previous experiences and the verbal suggestion accompanying the administration of the treatment [22]. This can result not only in an initial benefit due to expectations but also in maintaining the therapeutic effect through a reinforcement loop. In this loop, the administration of the placebo generates a suggestion and thus an expectation, the expectation reduces pain perception, and the reduced pain perception reinforces the expectation, creating a self-sustaining cycle [23].

This can be particularly relevant in ES, especially when using medical therapy whose favorable outcome on pain becomes a deciding factor for whether or not to candidate the patient for surgery [24]. The patient's suggestion toward a treatment that, if successful, will lead to surgery promising to resolve their symptoms could thus translate into a placebo effect. This, in turn, could partly explain some of the long-term surgical failures.

References

1. Swanson D, Evensky CH, Yusuf S, et al. Eagle syndrome: pathophysiology, differential diagnosis and treatment options. Health Psychol Res. 2023;10(5). https://doi.org/10.52965/001c.67851.
2. Moretti R, Torre P, Antonello RM, Bava A, Cazzato G. Gabapentin treatment of glossopharyngeal neuralgia: a follow-up of four years of a single case. Eur J Pain. 2002;6(5):403–7. https://doi.org/10.1016/s1090-3801(02)00026-5. PMID: 12160515

3. Park JS, Ahn YH. Glossopharyngeal neuralgia. J Korean Neurosurg Soc. 2023;66(1):12–23. https://doi.org/10.3340/jkns.2022.0178.
4. International Association for the Study of Pain. Classification of chronic pain. Descriptions of chronic pain syndromes and definitions of pain terms. Pain Suppl. 1986;3:S1–226.
5. Singh PM, Kaur M, Trikha A. An uncommonly common: glossopharyngeal neuralgia. Ann Indian Acad Neurol. 2013;16(1):1–8. https://doi.org/10.4103/0972-2327.107662.
6. Dworkin RH, O'Connor AB, Backonja M, Farrar T, Finnerup NB, Jensen TS. Pharmacologic management of neuropathic pain: evidence-based recommendations. Pain. 2007;132:237–51.
7. Taheri A, Firouzi-Marani S, Khoshbin M. Nonsurgical treatment of stylohyoid (Eagle) syndrome: a case report. J Korean Assoc Oral Maxillofac Surg. 2014;40(5):246–9. https://doi.org/10.5125/jkaoms.2014.40.5.246.
8. McLean B. Safety and patient acceptability of stellate ganglion blockade as a treatment adjunct for combat-related post-traumatic stress disorder: a quality assurance initiative. Cureus. 2015;7(9):e320.
9. Piraccini E, Munakomi S, Chang KV. Stellate ganglion blocks. [Updated 2023 Aug 13]. In: StatPearls [Internet]. Treasure Island (FL): StatPearls Publishing; 2024. Available from: https://www.ncbi.nlm.nih.gov/books/NBK507798/
10. Kawasaki M, Hatashima S, Matsuda T. Non-surgical therapy for bilateral glossopharyngeal neuralgia caused by Eagle's syndrome, diagnosed by three-dimensional computed tomography: a case report. J Anesth. 2012;26(6):918–21. https://doi.org/10.1007/s00540-012-1437-z.
11. Maher T, Shankar H. Ultrasound-guided peristyloid steroid injection for eagle syndrome. Pain Pract. 2017;17(4):554–7. https://doi.org/10.1111/papr.12497.
12. Mollinedo FT, Esteban SL, Vega CG, Orcasitas AC, Maguregi AA. Pulsed radiofrequency treatment in a case of Eagle's syndrome. Pain Pract. 2013;13(5):399–404. https://doi.org/10.1111/j.1533-2500.2012.00592.x.
13. Do K, Kawana E, Zhitny V, Wajda MC, Zou S, Do J, Singh N, Pratasava V, Dannapaneni H, Stewart R, Gualtier RT. Effectiveness of radiofrequency ablation for treatment of glossopharyngeal neuralgia: a systematic review of the current literature. Pain Physician. 2024;27(3):97–110.
14. Hassani M, Grønlund EW, Albrechtsen SS, Kondziella D. Neurological phenotypes and treatment outcomes in Eagle syndrome: systematic review and meta-analysis. PeerJ. 2024;12:e17423. https://doi.org/10.7717/peerj.17423.
15. Wong ML, Rossi MD, Groff W, Castro S, Powell J. Physical therapy management of a patient with Eagle syndrome. Physiother Theory Pract. 2011;27(4):319–27. https://doi.org/10.3109/09593985.2010.498036.
16. Chiu TT, Law EY, Chiu TH. Performance of the craniocervical flexion test in subjects with and without chronic neck pain. J Orthop Sports Phys Ther. 2005;35(9):567–71. https://doi.org/10.2519/jospt.2005.35.9.567.
17. Vernon H, Mior S. The neck disability index: a study of reliability and validity. J Manip Physiol Ther. 1991;14(7):409–15.
18. Shindo T, Ito M, Matsumoto J, Miki K, Fujihara F, Terasaka S, Isu T, Isobe M. A case of juvenile stroke due to carotid artery dissection from an elongated styloid process-revisiting conservative management. J Stroke Cerebrovasc Dis. 2019;28(10):104307. https://doi.org/10.1016/j.jstrokecerebrovasdis.2019.104307.
19. Mastrofini GF, McFadden BA, Chandler AJ, Lints BS, Cintineo HP, Rhoades ND, Vincenty CS, Stray-Gundersen SO, Lane AD, Arent SM. The effects of a brand-specific, hemp-derived cannabidiol product on physiological, biochemical, and psychometric outcomes in healthy adults: a double-blind, randomized clinical trial. J Int Soc Sports Nutr. 2024;21(1):2370430. https://doi.org/10.1080/15502783.2024.2370430.
20. Medeiros AC, Medeiros P, Pigatto GR, Maione S, Coimbra NC, de Freitas RL. Cannabidiol in the dorsal hippocampus attenuates emotional and cognitive impairments related to neuropathic pain: the role of prelimbic neocortex-hippocampal connections. Prog Neuro-Psychopharmacol Biol Psychiatry. 2024;134:111039. https://doi.org/10.1016/j.pnpbp.2024.111039.
21. Vase L, Wartolowska K. Pain, placebo, and test of treatment efficacy: a narrative review. Br J Anaesth. 2019;123(2):e254–62. https://doi.org/10.1016/j.bja.2019.01.040.

22. Vase L, Robinson ME, Verne GN, Price DD. The contributions of suggestion, desire, and expectation to placebo effects in irritable bowel syndrome patients. An empirical investigation. Pain. 2003;105(1–2):17–25. https://doi.org/10.1016/s0304-3959(03)00073-3.
23. Jepma M, Koban L, van Doorn J, Jones M, Wager TD. Behavioural and neural evidence for self-reinforcing expectancy effects on pain. Nat Hum Behav. 2018;2(11):838–55. https://doi.org/10.1038/s41562-018-0455-8.
24. Singhania AA, Chauhan NV, George A, Rathwala K. Lidocine infiltration test: an useful test in the prediction of results of styloidectomy for Eagle's syndrome. Indian J Otolaryngol Head Neck Surg. 2013;65(1):20–3. https://doi.org/10.1007/s12070-012-0577-7.

Transoral Surgery

19

Claudio Vicini, Giuseppe Meccariello, Alberto Caranti, Ruggero Campisi, Giulio Gasparini, and Pierfrancesco Bettini

> …scarless surgery is the Holy Grail of surgery and the very purpose for this surgery was the reduction of scars and thereby pain and suffering of patients…

The common goal of all the transoral options for the treatment of ES is to interact with the elongated styloid process in order to address the neuropathic and mechanical effects without external incisions. Among them, the most simple option may be considered the infiltration of an anesthetic agent as described in the chapter dealing with typical Eagle syndrome (lidocaine infiltration test, LIT). In few and very selected cases, a repeated infiltration strategy may be adopted as provisional treatment modality, but in our personal practice, it was never used for long period of time, and we do not consider it a recommended treatment modality.

19.1 Transoral Styloid Out-Fracture (SOF)

It is a planned iatrogenic fracture of the elongated styloid produced by a strong digital pressure on the tonsillar fossa at the level of the palpable styloid tip. The pressure is aimed to displace and reposition the bone more laterally, possibly far from the affected nerves and vessels as well from the pharyngeal wall [1]. The maneuver is

C. Vicini (✉) · A. Caranti · R. Campisi · P. Bettini
University of Ferrara, Cona, FE, Italy
e-mail: claudio@claudiovicini.com

G. Meccariello
Morgagni-Pierantoni Hospital, Forlì, FC, Italy

G. Gasparini
Maxillo-Facial Department of the University of Rome, La Sapienza, Rome, Italy
e-mail: giulio.gasparini@policlinicogemelli.it

C. Vicini et al. (eds.), *EAGLE Syndrome*,
https://doi.org/10.1007/978-3-031-92829-1_19

possible in a complete outpatient setting with no or local anesthesia, and sometimes the patient may be instructed to perform the maneuver by himself. SOF is the most simple and easy surgical option for Eagle, but there is no evidence of its efficacy in the literature. Healing is absolutely unpredictable, and for those reasons, its application remains anecdotal [2]. It is difficult to know if the final lateralized position of the styloid will remain far from the nerves and vessels. In our personal experience, we performed SOF in just one ASA 3 patient with temporary (6 months) reduction of the symptoms.

19.2 Transoral Styloidectomy (TOS)

It was anecdotally reported in the last couple of centuries by few authors, but it was really described into detail in a significant series of patients by Eagle in his original papers [3, 4].

The rationale of the technique is to shorten the elongated styloid process by removing a distal segment in order to "normalize" its length and remove or reduce the mechanical effect of pressure or real damage on the nervous, vascular, and pharyngeal structures in strict relation with the styloid. There is a common agreement that surgery should be a second line of treatment if pain is not really controlled by a conservative approach applied for at least 6 months [5–7].

Moreover, according to a frequent statement and anyway in our routine, we do not offer surgery if lidocaine test injection was not effective. On the other hand, surgery may be a first-line option in the vascular types of ES, in order to relieve compression and prevent vascular accidents [8–12].

But a preliminary key point is how to choose a TOS instead of an open approach? It is quite clear that TOS is a "scar-free" procedure, avoiding any cosmetic issue. It is unusual but possible that the patient may refuse any external approach. In our experience, it happened just in one case (a young Brazilian lap dancer). TOS is also a natural orifice surgery, basically less invasive than open approach, with less tissue manipulation. Any general ENT is familiar with the required setting and with the tonsillectomy approach of TOS. From the strictly anatomical point of view in most of the cases, the distance of the styloid from the pharyngeal mucosal surface is inferior to the distance of the styloid from the neck skin. More direct approach and less tissue manipulation together means less operative time [13, 14].

In our experience, TOS may be carried on both sides much easier and faster than bilateral open styloidectomy, even if someone warns about a much more difficult post-op in case of bilateral TOS. We cannot confirm this experience, at least for transoral robotic styloidectomy. Last but not least, no drain or skin suture removal is required. On the other hand, TOS requires a minimal mouth opening, at least more than 20 mm, possibly more than 25 mm, as for any affordable and "safe" pharyngeal surgical procedure [7, 13, 15, 16].

A second and more debated issue is the need to be able to intraoperatively locate the styloid tip by finger palpation. In our experience, it is usually recommended in order to allow a targeted, quick, and safe dissection close to the styloid periosteum.

An intraoperative blind search of the bone is possible by a careful and progressive step-by-step blunt dissection, but this procedure is by far more time-consuming and risky. According to the single-case surgical field visualization, there is a different degree of intraoperative complication risk, especially of arterial bleeding, anyway more difficult to manage in TOS than in open [7, 13–16]. It is worth to mention that in TOS, internal carotid artery may be encountered between the mucosal incision and the styloid. "This risk of harming anatomical structures in the parapharyngeal area such as the carotid artery rises when using internal assessment procedures, due to the difficulty in full visualization of the area" [17]. This could lead to complications in the form of excessive or catastrophic bleeding during surgery and postoperative or disorders of orthostatic regulation [18]. Last point, surgical site infection, even if really unusual, is more probable in TOS than in open approach [13, 14]. There is no real agreement about the amount of bone resection requested to achieve the complete solution of the problem [19]. In most of the surgical case report, the resected bone is about 2 or 3 cm in length according to the size of the elongated bone, but sometimes a complete styloid removal is reported [20]. There is no evidence that a longer bone resection may be related to better outcomes. It could be logical to expect that if the residual bone is of no more than 2 or 3 cm long as in normal subjects, the clinical problem could be considered as addressed. The complete amputation of the process at the level of the skull base, sometimes impossible, always challenging, potentially dangerous may be considered as a "not necessary surgical virtuosity" in our opinion. A recent contribution by Kent and colleagues could demonstrate "that a post hoc power analyses of the tested variables related to ES revealed that distance to the tonsillar fossa was the only variable sufficiently powered to show a significant difference between ES and not ES [21]."

Translating this observation to the surgical practice, it seems reasonable to aim to increase the distance between elongated styloid and pharyngeal wall, without a complete ablation of the styloid, which seems to be useless. According to the literature, TOS may be carried out in outpatient setting and in local anesthesia by infiltration [22, 23]. Anyway, in most of the cases, the preferred setting is general anesthesia with nasal or orotracheal intubation. The basic patient position, also for the robotic approach, is the classic "tonsillectomy" position. In most of the surgical reports is not detailed the surgeon position (at patient side vs at patient head), which probably reflects the personal preferences. TOS setting will be described into detail later on in a special chapter. In case of endoscopic approach, the side position seems to be the most logical. Working with a head lamp or loupe, side or head position is probably equivalent. In our experience, according to the 3D anatomy of the styloid process (from the skull base, pointing down, medially and anteriorly), the side position allowing an easier looking up is more logical than the head position allowing the surgeon to visualize the styloid in the depth with smaller incisions. A routine tonsillectomy mouth gag (Crowe-Davis, Boyle-Davis, etc.) with tongue blades and cheek retractors are routinely used (Fig. 19.1). In orotracheal intubation, a blade with a groove for the tube may be preferred (more room for surgery). Additional retractors of different types are described in many surgical case reports in order to get a better exposure [13, 14].

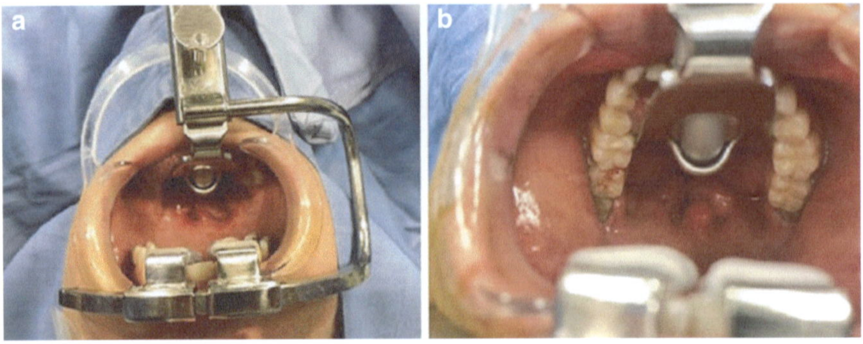

Fig. 19.1 Transoral styloidectomy setting: mouth gag, grooved blade, cheek retractors, orotracheal intubation

Fig. 19.2 An example of head loupe with LED lamp and 2.5× magnification

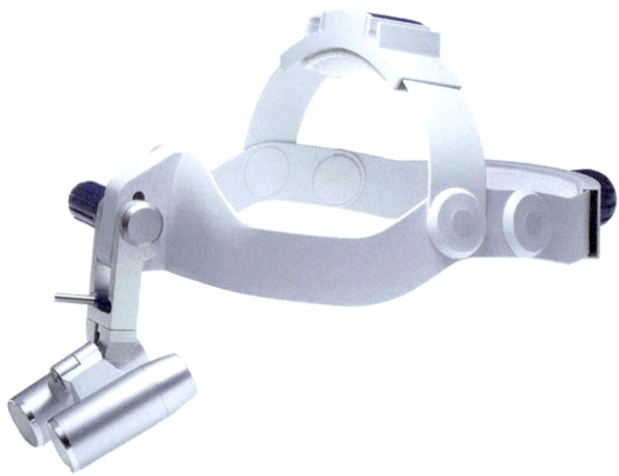

A special topic in TOS is the type of illumination and visualization of the surgical field. In the literature is reported a wide range of solutions. The most classic ones are the traditional naked eye observation assisted by traditional, halogen, or LED head lamps. In our personal experience, a magnifying halogen or LED loupe 2.5× may increase the surgical field detail with enhanced precision and safety (Fig. 19.2). 2D endoscopes and more recently 3D exoscope were described in the literature [24].

Angulated endoscopes share the interesting property of an "around the corner view," but all of them requires a head assistant who held the scope in order to allow the surgeon to operate in a bimanual way. 3D exoscopes offer a great view, which is sometimes defined as "better than live," but they do not offer an angulated view around the corner.

In all the cases of the first Eagle series, the patients were already tonsillectomized, and at that time, previous tonsillectomy was considered as responsible of the syndrome. The main feature of TOS in already tonsillectomized patients is the different degree of pharyngeal wall scarring, which may increase the difficulties for locating the styloid and/or the dense tissue dissection. Healing is also delayed in fibrous areas. More recently, in not tonsillectomized patients, a tonsil-sparing group of solutions was described.

In patients with palatine tonsils still in place, at least three different routes are described (Fig. 19.3).

1. **Trans-tonsillar approach (after preliminary tonsillectomy)**
2. **Extra-tonsillar—tonsil-sparing anterior or medial approach**
3. **Extra-tonsillar—tonsil-sparing lateral approach (retromolar, paratonsillar)** [25]

According to our personal opinion, the prerequisite for any TOS is the possibility to locate the tip of the styloid process by finger palpation (Fig. 19.4). The styloid tip is the crucial reference for entering the parapharyngeal space, which is cautiously dissected by blunt dissection after gentle spreading of the superior pharyngeal muscle fibers. Before proceeding with the surgical incision, we usually infiltrate the mucosa with a local anesthetic with adrenaline (Fig. 19.5). The mucosal incision site, with a vertical direction, is dictated basically by the location of the styloid tip

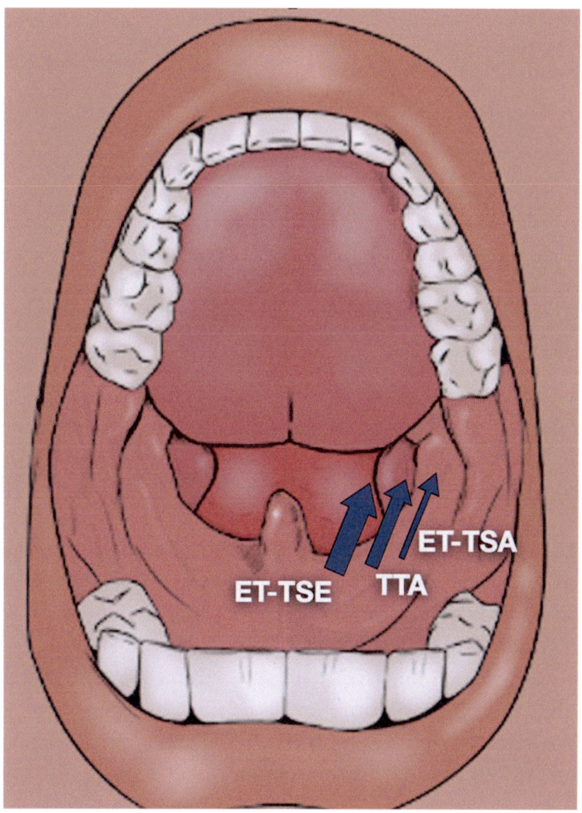

Fig. 19.3 The three blue arrows represent the three different TOS approaches: *ET-TSA* extra-tonsillar—tonsil sparing anterior, *TTS* trans-tonsillar approach, *ET-TSL* extra-tonsillar—tonsil sparing lateral

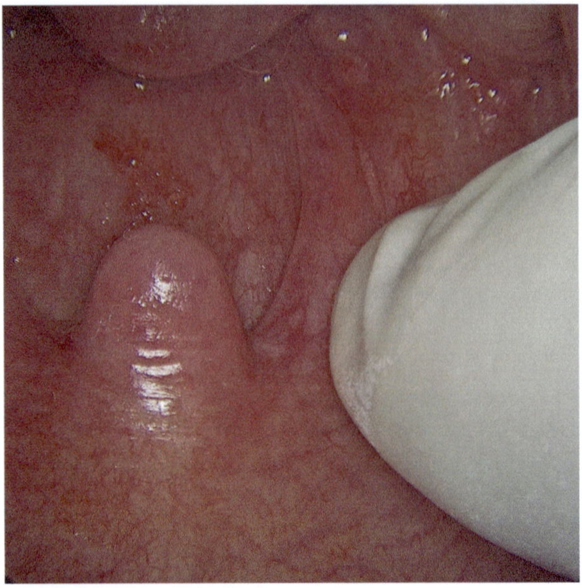

Fig. 19.4 Styloid tip digital palpation

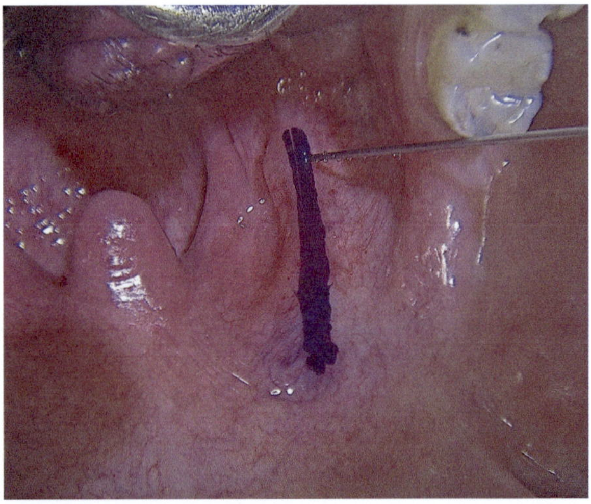

Fig. 19.5 Submucosal layer infiltration with local anesthetic and adrenaline

as defined by the intraoperative digital palpation of the styloid tip (Fig. 19.6). The extent of the incision is usually less than 3–4 cm and may be marked and injected by a vasoconstrictor solution according to the surgeon preferences. A cold knife or a bowie may be used as preferred.

Usually, a small Kelly forceps and the tip of the index finger are the most affordable and effective tools for dissecting the parapharyngeal fat. Dissection is carried out primarily under palpatory and visual control. Repeated gentle digital palpations are key to guiding the dissection directly to the mucosal and submucosal plane of

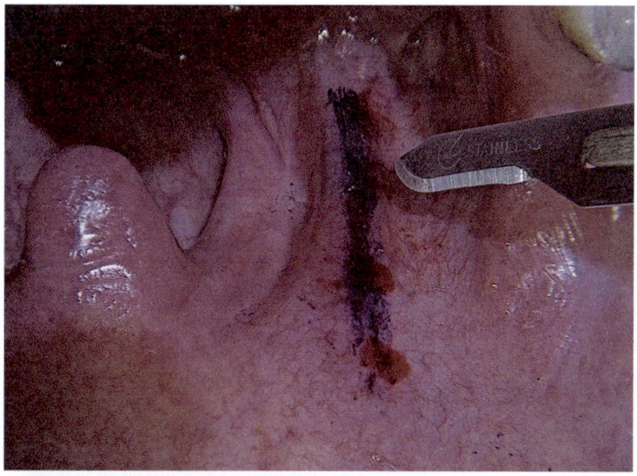

Fig. 19.6 Mucosal incision by cold scalpel

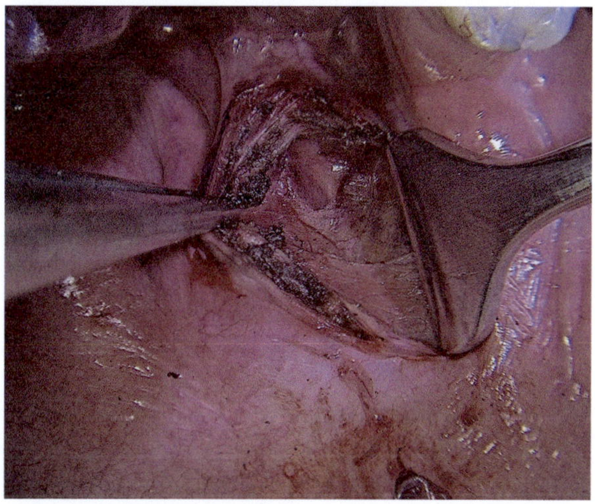

Fig. 19.7 The surgical field, optimally exposed thanks to the use of forceps and a retractor. At this point of the procedure, the styloid process is not yet visible, but only palpable

the styloid, especially when it is still covered by soft tissue and not yet visible within the surgical field. When the styloid is not easily palpable at the beginning, dissection must be carried out in a more "random" way, tends to be more extended and riskier, takes more time, is more bloody, and may fail to find the bony styloid [17, 18] (Fig. 19.7).

A careful evaluation of the 3D imaging before and during the dissection may be of great help to get direct information where to find the styloid in the parapharyngeal space. More recently, surgical navigation was proposed as a possible solution for an easier location of the styloid in transoral as well open approach [26, 27].

After styloid tip identification and exposure (Fig. 19.8), the next step is usually the section of the stylo-hyoid ligament from the styloid tip. This maneuver is always simple, and many different cutting tools may be easily and safely used. The next step is of paramount importance and of variable difficulty according to the patient

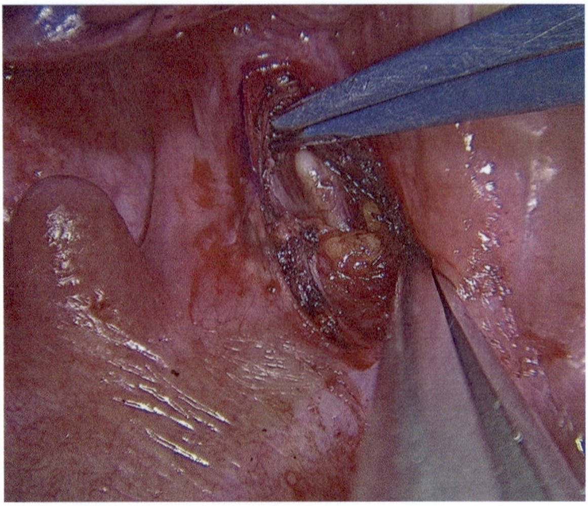

Fig. 19.8 The styloid process is identified. In this frame, we can see hemostasis being achieved using bipolar forceps

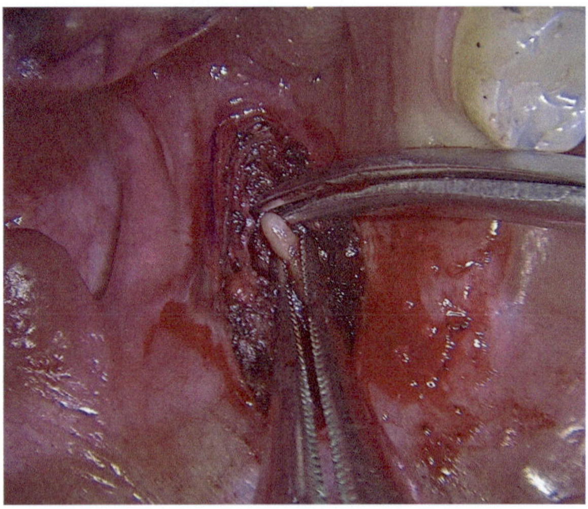

Fig. 19.9 The styloid process is gently retracted using a Kelly clamp, while scissors are used to isolate the process from the surrounding tissues

anatomy. Stripping off all the muscle coming out from the styloid is of great importance to acquire real information about the length of the bone to resect and in order to be able to perform a safe bone cut at the defined level without potential injury of the surrounding structures (Figs. 19.9 and 19.10). A sufficient length of the incision and the gentle traction of the tissues are necessary to keep the styloid under vision during the entire procedure. The key is to keep any chosen instrument really close to the styloid bone periosteum and to gently "scrape" it avoiding any not necessary trauma to the surrounding tissues. Probably, a Freer periosteal elevator or a nasal ring curette may work at the best.

"The use of angled hypophysis ring curette for skeletonization of elongated styloid prevent damage to surrounding neurovascular structure" [28]. We did the same

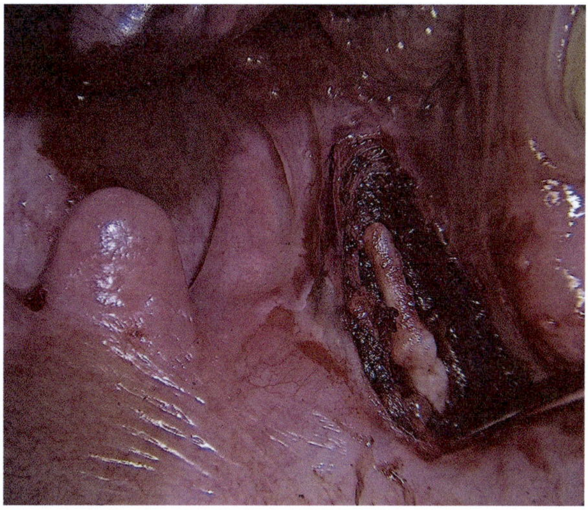

Fig. 19.10 The styloid process is finally exposed in its full length. The most cranial portion is revealed through gentle traction performed with a dissector

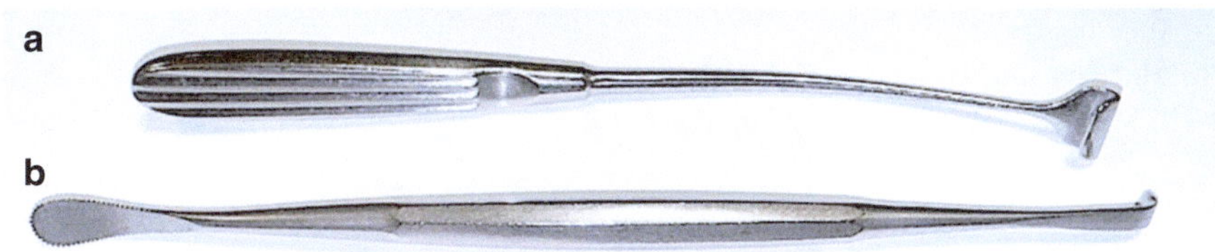

Fig. 19.11 Tonsil pillar retractor (**a**) and dissector (**b**)

in few cases with good results. In our experience, a tonsil pillar retractor and dissector is of paramount importance (Fig. 19.11).

We strongly feel that monopolar cautery is not really recommended for this step for the risk of spreading energy through the surrounding tissues.

The next step is the bone cut in order to remove the excess of styloid bone required for reducing the symptoms. First of all, it is worth to be mentioned that the diameter of the pathological styloid may be widely different in different patients. But even the slimmest one is composed by very dense and hard bone, which requires a proper instrument to be interrupted. Second but not less important issue is the use of a safe instrument, which allows a strong action on the bone but no or minimal potential "collateral damage" on the surrounding structures (e.g., carotid artery). In our opinion, any type of bone rongeurs, even if of proper dimension, are not recommended for safety, even if they are effective in bone cutting. Among the classical options prove to be really efficient in our hands the Citelli nose punch (also called Kerrison punch), strong, effective, and really safe, or an Hajek sphenoid punch (Figs. 19.12 and 19.13).

In case of use of a burr, we strongly advocate the choice of a large ball diamond and not cutting burr. More recently, piezo systems and special lasers were

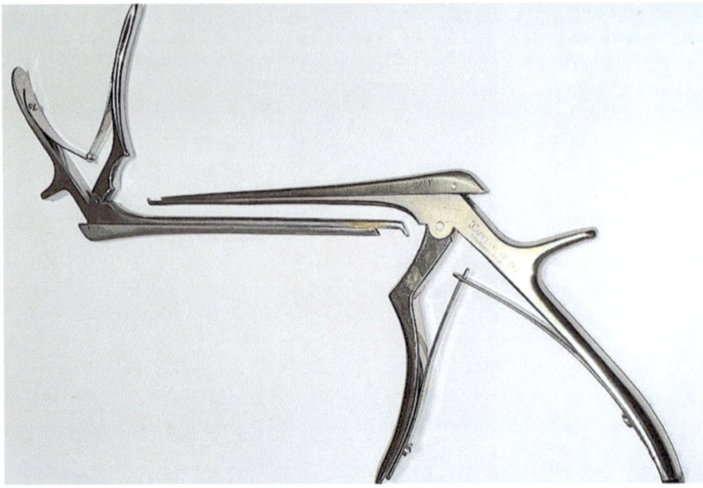

Fig. 19.12 A couple of Citelli (or Kerrison) nose punch

Fig. 19.13 Styloid bone cut by Citelli nose punch

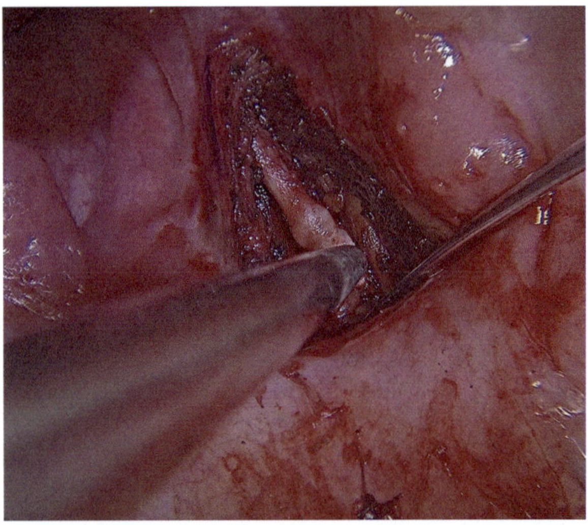

introduced and described [29, 30]. Piezo device use "minimizes the risk of harming other structures in the immediate area" [31]. The styloid stump is usually not really sharp at the tip, but someone claims the need to smooth it before to finalize the procedure [32]. After a final careful hemostasis, the incision is closed with reabsorbable suture (Fig. 19.14). No drain is necessary.

Transoral extra-tonsillar or anterior approach was described in a few papers [33]. After a Xylocaine with adrenaline injection, a 2 cm incision is made in the area of the palatoglossal fold and anterior tonsillar pillar, anteriorly to the palatine tonsil, which is spared. After that, dissection of the superior constrictor muscle and of the

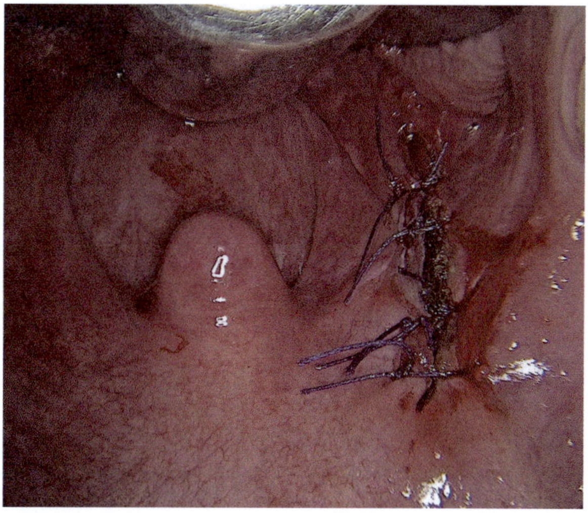

Fig. 19.14 The surgical wound is closed with absorbable single sutures

parapharyngeal fat is the same as previously described. Scheller K et al. described retromolar, paratonsillar approach for styloidectomy, based on a vertical incision of 2–3 cm in the lingual mucosa of the ascending upper jaw [25].

Transoral robotic styloidectomy is described in a separate section of the book.

19.3 Result

We organized the paragraphs reporting our group and literature results in different sections of the book. Our group outcomes with different surgical approaches are discussed at the end of the open surgery chapter. Literature meta-analysis collecting most of the available data about surgical outcomes in worldwide literature is organized as a completely separate chapter. The discussion of the possible complications and complication prevention of the different procedures is included as a separate paragraph inside the relative chapters from a personal and literature perspective.

19.4 Complications and Complication Prevention

The different types of complications of intraoral styloidectomy may be classified according to different criteria, including the time of occurrence. "The intraoral approach presented more than twice as many transient complications as the external approach and with a smaller number of patients involved" [34].

In Table 19.1 are summarized the most important complications based on prevalence or importance according to the timing of occurrence.

The first step of transoral styloidectomy is positioning the patient basically in the tonsillectomy position. All the precautions valid for tonsillectomy are to be applied to styloidectomy [13, 14]. It is worth to mention that in a couple of our cases, TES

Table 19.1 Transoral styloidectomy complications

Intraoperative	Postoperative
Positioning and exposure-related complications:	Pain
Spine problems	Dysphagia
Teeth problems	Trismus
TMJ problems	Rhinolalia
Dissection and styloid visualization difficulties:	Delayed healing
Bleeding	Delayed bleeding
Collateral damages	Infection
Bone cutting-related complications:	Carotid artery thrombosis
Collateral damages	Subcutaneous emphysema
Vessels and nerves	Soft palate paralysis

was associated with Arnold-Chiari syndrome, a well-known risk for intubation and head and neck positioning [35]. A sufficient inter-incisive distance (2.5 cm) will avoid the need of over-stretching the mouth gag blade, with the risk of teeth and/or TMJ damage, which anyway are a potential complication. A step-by-step finger palpation-guided blunt dissection is the key for preventing any significant intraoperative bleeding. "Working in between the internal and external carotid artery, for resection of styloid process is associated with the risk of uncontrolled bleeding and even death on table" [28]. Catastrophic bleeding after carotid artery injury is anyway anecdotal, but it must be put into account. In case of carotid injury, all the possible maneuvers well known in head and neck surgery must be familiar for the surgeon. Minor vessel bleeding from minor vessel and arteries is usually managed by coagulation, ligation, or clipping. Besides bleeding, it is worth of mention that a blind parapharyngeal dissection without the guide of bone palpation may produce a more extended tissue manipulation potentially responsible for prolonged trismus, transient neck emphysema, and definitive one-side palate paralysis [34, 36]. According to the instrument in use, styloid bone cutting may be potentially dangerous for the surrounding anatomical structures. Bleeding or nerve damage may be inadvertently produced by the tip of improperly used bone scissors or by a cutting burr. Protected cutting instruments (Citelli punch forceps—Fig. 19.13) or soft tissue sparing devices (e.g., piezo scalpels) or diamond burr may offer a safe solution with very low probability of collateral damages.

Prolonged postoperative pain is possible especially in case of tonsillectomy performed in the same time. A proper diet and the prescription of NSAID painkillers are usually sufficient. In a few cases, an elastomeric pump with targeted release of morphine proved to be a very effective solution. The intrusion into the parapharyngeal space is an immediate explanation for trouble of speech and swallowing as well as some degree of trismus, which are registered in some cases. The severity of this group of post-op complications is usually minimal, and reassurance and a low dose of steroid was our option. In no case, speech therapy was offered. Delayed healing must be put into account frequently produced by some degree of wound infection (Fig. 19.15). Soft diet, antiseptic mouthwashing, and antibiotics may be the first line of treatment. We did not register any case of wound revision.

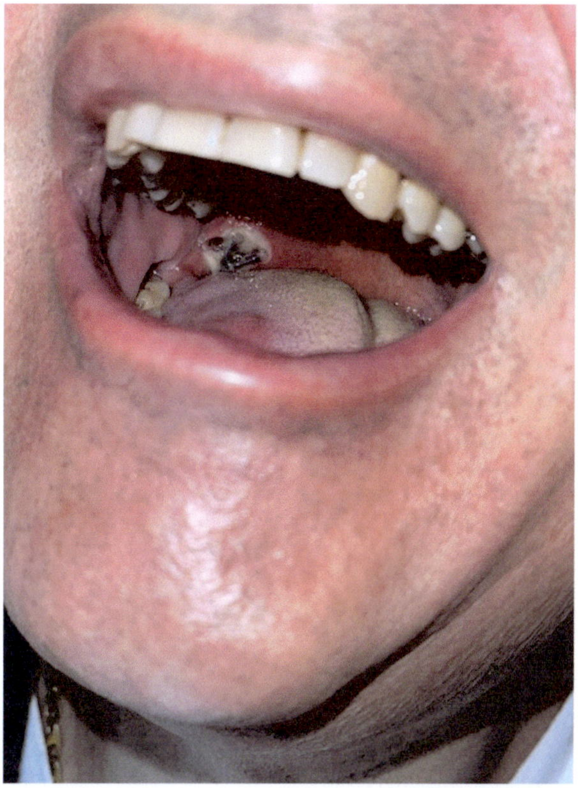

Fig. 19.15 Delayed healing

References

1. Weidenbecher M, Schick B, Iro H. Das Styloidsyndrom und seine Behandlung [Styloid syndrome and its treatment]. Laryngorhinootologie. 2006;85(3):184–90. https://doi.org/10.1055/s-2005-870504. (German).
2. Kaur A, Singh A, Singal R, Gupta S. Is this way: self inflicted fracture of styloid process cures stylalgia. J Med Life. 2013;6(2):202–4.
3. Eagle WW. Elongated styloid process; further observations and a new syndrome. Arch Otolaryngol (1925). 1948;47(5):630–40. https://doi.org/10.1001/archotol.1948.00690030654006.
4. Eagle WW. Elongated styloid process: report of two cases. Arch Otolaryngol. 1937;25:584–7. https://doi.org/10.1001/archotol.1937.00650010656008.
5. Singhania AA, Chauhan NV, George A, Rathwala K. Lidocaine infiltration test: an useful test in the prediction of results of styloidectomy for Eagle's syndrome. Indian J Otolaryngol Head Neck Surg. 2013;65(1):20–3. https://doi.org/10.1007/s12070-012-0577-7.
6. Badhey A, Jategaonkar A, Anglin Kovacs AJ, Kadakia S, De Deyn PP, Ducic Y, Schantz S, Shin E. Eagle syndrome: a comprehensive review. Clin Neurol Neurosurg. 2017;159:34–8. https://doi.org/10.1016/j.clineuro.2017.04.021.
7. Fitzpatrick TH 4th, Lovin BD, Magister MJ, Waltonen JD, Browne JD, Sullivan CA. Surgical management of Eagle syndrome: a 17-year experience with open and transoral robotic styloidectomy. Am J Otolaryngol. 2020;41(2):102324. https://doi.org/10.1016/j.amjoto.2019.102324.

8. Higgins JN, Garnett MR, Pickard JD, Axon PR. An evaluation of styloidectomy as an adjunct or alternative to jugular stenting in idiopathic intracranial hypertension and disturbances of cranial venous outflow. J Neurol Surg B Skull Base. 2017;78(2):158–63. https://doi.org/10.1055/s-0036-1594238.
9. Vigilante N, Khalife J, Badger CA, Shaikh H, Thomas AJ, Swendseid B, Jovin TG, Siegler JE, Tonetti DA. Surgical management of stylocarotid Eagle syndrome in a patient with bilateral internal carotid artery dissection: illustrative case. J Neurosurg Case Lessons. 2024;7(5):CASE23682. https://doi.org/10.3171/CASE23682.
10. DiLosa K, Harding J, Donde N, Silverman D, Heafner T. Symptomatic carotid stenosis in Eagle syndrome managed with traditional endarterectomy and styloidectomy. J Vasc Surg Cases Innov Tech. 2023;10(1):101372. https://doi.org/10.1016/j.jvscit.2023.101372.
11. Breda D, Ferreira S, Colino M, Cerqueira É, Amado I. Recurrent syncope related to carotid compression in Eagle syndrome: a case report. Cureus. 2023;15(9):e45134. https://doi.org/10.7759/cureus.45134.
12. Selvadurai S, Williamson A, Virk JS, Clarke P. Eagle syndrome and carotid artery dissection: a rare skull base cause of stroke. BMJ Case Rep. 2022;15(3):e247954. https://doi.org/10.1136/bcr-2021-247954.
13. Campisi R, Caranti A, Meccariello G, Stringa LM, Bianchini C, Ciorba A, Pelucchi S, Vicini C. Transoral robotic styloidectomy for Eagle syndrome: a systematic review. Clin Otolaryngol. 2024;49(3):293–8. https://doi.org/10.1111/coa.14145.
14. Montevecchi F, Caranti A, Cammaroto G, Meccariello G, Vicini C. Transoral robotic surgery (TORS) for bilateral Eagle syndrome. ORL J Otorhinolaryngol Relat Spec. 2019;81(1):36–40. https://doi.org/10.1159/000493736.
15. Rizzo-Riera E, Rubi-Oña C, García-Wagner M, Costa AA, Miralles J, Enchev E, Rama-López J. Advanced robotic surgery of the parapharyngeal space: transoral robotic styloidectomy in Eagle syndrome. J Craniofac Surg. 2020;31(8):2339–41. https://doi.org/10.1097/SCS.0000000000006804.
16. Kim DH, Lee YH, Cha D, Kim SH. Transoral robotic surgery in Eagle's syndrome: our experience on four patients. Acta Otorhinolaryngol Ital. 2017;37(6):454–7. https://doi.org/10.14639/0392-100X-1502.
17. Prasad KC, Kamath MP, Reddy KJ, Raju K, Agarwal S. Elongated styloid process (Eagle's syndrome): a clinical study. J Oral Maxillofac Surg. 2002;60(2):171–5. https://doi.org/10.1053/joms.2002.29814.
18. Thoenissen P, Bittermann G, Schmelzeisen R, Oshima T, Fretwurst T. Eagle's syndrome—a non-perceived differential diagnosis of temporomandibular disorder. Int J Surg Case Rep. 2015;15:123–6. https://doi.org/10.1016/j.ijscr.2015.08.036.
19. Wang J, Liu Y, Wang ZB, Yan KS. Intraoral and extraoral approach for surgical treatment of Eagle's syndrome: a retrospective study. Eur Arch Otorrinolaringol. 2022;279(3):1481–7. https://doi.org/10.1007/s00405-021-06914-2.
20. Papadiochos I, Papadiochou S, Sarivalasis ES, Goutzanis L, Petsinis V. Treatment of Eagle syndrome with transcervical approach secondary to a failed intraoral attempt: surgical technique and literature review. J Stomatol Oral Maxillofac Surg. 2017;118(6):353–8. https://doi.org/10.1016/j.jormas.2017.06.017.
21. Kent DT, Rath TJ, Snyderman C. Conventional and 3-dimensional computerized tomography in Eagle's syndrome, glossopharyngeal neuralgia, and asymptomatic controls. Otolaryngol Head Neck Surg. 2015;153(1):41–7. https://doi.org/10.1177/0194599815583047.
22. Hamamin OS, Arif AT, Razha AB, Abdul Aziz JM, Rashid MJ, Rasheed MK, Abdullah LL, Abdulrahman Mustafa S, Ghafoor RA, Qutbadeen N, Hamasharif PA. Chronically misdiagnosed Eagle's syndrome, treated through transoral styloidectomy: a rare case report. Ann Med Surg (Lond). 2023;85(7):3611–4. https://doi.org/10.1097/MS9.0000000000000810.
23. Kapoor V, Jindal G, Garg S. Eagle's syndrome: a new surgical technique for styloidectomy. J Maxillofac Oral Surg. 2015;14(Suppl 1):360–5. https://doi.org/10.1007/s12663-013-0597-1.

24. Mevio N, Achena A, Pilolli F, Roncoroni L, Ormellese GL, Placentino A, Dragonetti AG. Eagle syndrome: 3D endoscope-assisted anterior tonsillar fossa approach to styloid process. Am J Otolaryngol. 2021;42(3):102979. https://doi.org/10.1016/j.amjoto.2021.102979.
25. Scheller K, Eckert AW, Scheller C. Transoral, retromolar, para-tonsillar approach to the styloid process in 6 patients with Eagle's syndrome. Med Oral Patol Oral Cir Bucal. 2014;19(1):e61. https://doi.org/10.4317/medoral.18749.
26. Czako L, Hirjak D, Simko K, Thurzo A, Janovszky A, Galis B. 3D navigation in surgery of Eagle syndrome. Bratisl Lek Listy. 2019;120(7):494–7. https://doi.org/10.4149/BLL_2019_078.
27. Czako L, Simko K, Thurzo A, Galis B, Varga I. The syndrome of elongated styloid process, the Eagle's syndrome-from anatomical, evolutionary and embryological backgrounds to 3D printing and personalized surgery planning. Report of five cases. Medicina (Kaunas). 2020;56(9):458. https://doi.org/10.3390/medicina56090458.
28. Walli AK, Thorawade VP, Parelkar K, Nagle S, Kulsange KL. Intraoral styloidectomy in Eagle's syndrome—a risky and infrequently performed approach. J Clin Diagn Res. 2018;12(1):MD01–2. https://doi.org/10.7860/JCDR/2018/27339.11085.
29. Hoffmann E, Räder C, Fuhrmann H, Maurer P. Styloid-carotid artery syndrome treated surgically with Piezosurgery: a case report and literature review. J Craniomaxillofac Surg. 2013;41(2):162–6. https://doi.org/10.1016/j.jcms.2012.07.004.
30. Byun KH, Ahn JH, Lee SJ, Woo SH. A case of Eagle's syndrome treated with carbon dioxide laser. Med Laser. 2020;9:71–5. https://doi.org/10.25289/ML.2020.9.1.71.
31. Hoffmann E, Räder C, Fuhrmann H, Maurer P. Styloid–carotid artery syndrome treated surgically with Piezosurgery: a case report and literature review. J Craniomaxillofac Surg. 2013;2(41):162–6.
32. Zhibin W, Min J. Design and clinical application of the 'styloidectomy' styloid process cutter. J Laryngol Otol. 2006;120(9):753–8. https://doi.org/10.1017/S0022215106002106.
33. Regmi D, Baidhya R, Rajak A, Shrestha S, Bista M. Trans-oral extra tonsillar approach of styloidectomy for treatment of Eagle's syndrome among operated cases of the Department of Otolaryngology-Head and Neck Surgery at a Tertiary Care Hospital: a descriptive cross-sectional study. J Nepal Med Assoc. 2021;59(240):738–40.
34. Ferreira MS, Miranda G, Almeida FT, Gasperini G, Silva BSF, Valladares-Neto J, Santiago Junior JF, Silva MAG. Complications in intraoral versus external approach for surgical treatment of Eagle syndrome: a systematic review and meta-analysis. Cranio. 2024;42(5):570–2. https://doi.org/10.1080/08869634.2021.2020995.
35. Gruffi TR, Peralta FM, Thakkar MS, Arif A, Anderson RF, Orlando B, Coffman JC, Nathan N, McCarthy RJ, Toledo P, Habib AS. Anesthetic management of parturients with Arnold Chiari malformation-I: a multicenter retrospective study. Int J Obstet Anesth. 2019;37:52–6. https://doi.org/10.1016/j.ijoa.2018.10.002.
36. Santini L, Achache M, Gomert R, Mardassi A, Lafont B, Magnan J, Lavieille JP, Devèze A. Transoral surgical treatment of Eagle's syndrome: case report and review of literature. Rev Laryngol Otol Rhinol (Bord). 2012;133(3):141–4.

Open Transcervical Styloidectomy

20

Claudio Vicini, Andrea De Vito, Alberto Caranti,
and Pierfrancesco Bettini

> Despite the popularity of MIS, open surgery is still an indispensable and essential means of accomplishing surgical goals. Surgery is not a means to parade one's skills, and the primary objective should always be the patients' welfare. Only by putting this objective above all can surgeons live up to their responsibilities [1]

20.1 Open Transcervical Styloidectomy (OTS)

This group of surgical techniques was developed and introduced later in the history of Eagle syndrome by Loeser L. and Cardwell E., who in 1942 described the first transcervical approach [2]. Nowadays, they account for a significant number of styloidectomies reported in the worldwide literature. The rationale is similar to that of transoral surgery (TOS), and open transcervical surgery (OTS) should be offered only after the definitive failure of all conservative treatments [3]. The main common features of all open styloidectomy techniques can be summarized as follows:

1. OTS is possible even if the styloid tip is not clearly felt by digital palpation in the oropharynx.
2. OTS may be offered to any patient willing to accept a scar in the neck.
3. Any OTS requires for the surgeon a basic expertise in H&N surgery.
4. Most of the OTS offer to the surgeon a wide and clear vision of the surgical field.
5. It's important in case of bleeding or other complications, because it is easier to manage.

C. Vicini (✉) · A. Caranti · P. Bettini
University of Ferrara, Cona, FE, Italy
e-mail: claudio@claudiovicini.com; pietro.bettini@unife.it

A. De Vito
Morgagni-Pierantoni Hospital, Forlì, FC, Italy

C. Vicini et al. (eds.), *EAGLE Syndrome*,
https://doi.org/10.1007/978-3-031-92829-1_20

6. The average distance of the styloid from the skin is greater than the distance from the pharyngeal wall.
7. The amount of dissected tissue may be bigger than in OTS.
8. OTS may be more time-consuming compared to TOS.
9. The technique may require a drain for the first 24/48 h.

OTS may be carried in “out” or “in” patient setting according to the surgeon preference. General anesthesia is required, usually with orotracheal intubation [4]. Muscle relaxant agent could be avoided in order to allow a nerve monitoring if available (and recommended) [3]. Patient positioning is the conventional one for lateral neck exposure: supine, pillow under the shoulder, and contralateral head rotation. A transparent draping for eyes and mouth may allow a direct inspection during stimulation if neuromonitoring is not available.

In the literature are reported different variations in the surgical technique, according to many parameters. The first distinction is related to the site of skin incision. In a very synthetic way, we may list the following options:

1. *Pre-auricular approach* [5].
2. *Facelift parotidectomy approach* [6].
3. *Submandibular minimally invasive approach* [6].
4. *Classic anterior margin of SCM muscle approach*, very useful in obese patients [7].
5. *Submandibular approach*, which is our preferred in most of the cases [8].
6. *Endoscope-assisted resection of elongated styloid process through a retro-auricular incision* [9].

A second way for classifying OTS is according to the way of visualizing the surgical field and assisting the location of the elongated styloid process.

The use of one or more *ceiling-mounted scialitic surgical lamps* is the most widely way to manage the surgical field illumination. *Head lamp (halogen, LED), magnifying loupe, operative microscope, and 2D or 3D endoscopy-assisted surgery* are alternative available options combining illumination, magnification, and stereoscopy.

CT-based navigation inside the surgical field is one more additional option reported in recent literature [10].

One more way to stratify the different techniques reported in the literature is to define the technology used for cutting the styloid process. As for TOS, the same important issue is the “use of a safe instrument which allows a strong action on the bone but no or minimal ‘collateral damage’ on the surrounding structures (e.g.: carotid artery) [11]. In our opinion any type of bone scissors, even if of proper dimension, are not recommended. Among the classical option prove to be really efficient in our hands the Citelli nose punch, strong, effective and really safe. In case of use of a burr, we strongly advocate the choice of a large ball diamond and not cutting burr. More recently piezo systems and special lasers were introduced and described” [6, 12].

Herein will be described into detail the classic OTS as we routinely perform in our institution experience, with an anterior border of sternocleidomastoid muscle approach (Fig. 20.1).

After skin marking and local vasoconstrictor solution injection, a longitudinal incision of about 1/3 of length of the sternocleidomastoid muscle is deepened at its anterior border (Figs. 20.2 and 20.3).

Skin, subdermal tissue, and platysma are raised with careful identification and sparing of external jugular vein(s) and greater auricular nerve, which are retracted laterally (Figs. 20.4 and 20.5).

The upper limit of the incision is mastoid and SCM tendon. According to the 3D array of styloid that run anteriorly, inferiorly, and medially, this approach intercepts the stylohyoid complex in a more superficial plane, making the surgery easier. On the other hand, this type of incision doesn't run according to the Langer lines, and the final cosmetic result may be less satisfactory than other horizontal incisions. The

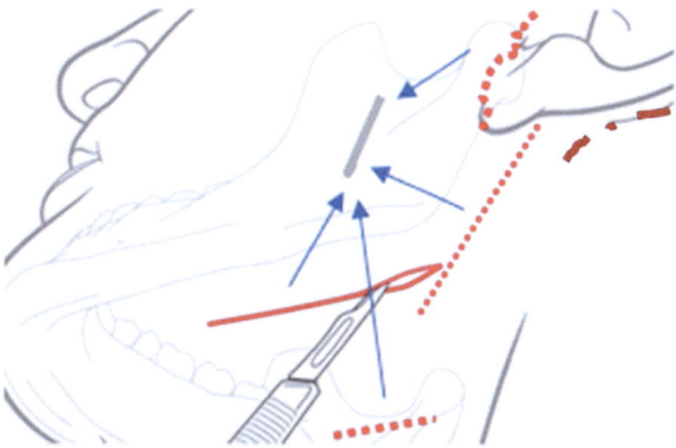

Fig. 20.1 Open styloidectomy incisions

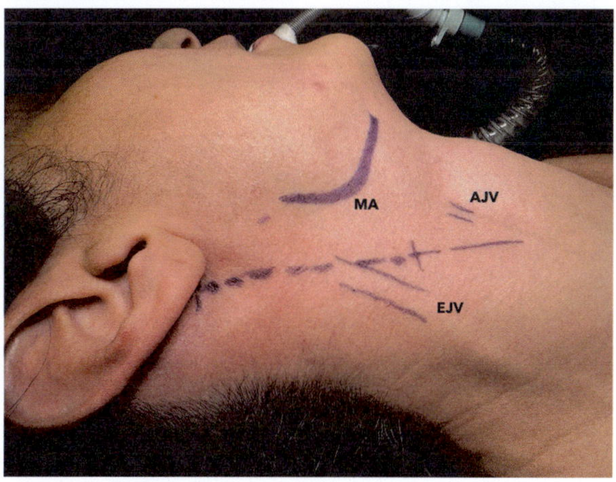

Fig. 20.2 Surgical design at the right lateral cervical level, illustrating the incision line (dashed line), the angle of the mandible (MA), and the course of the external jugular vein (EJV) and anterior jugular vein (AJV)

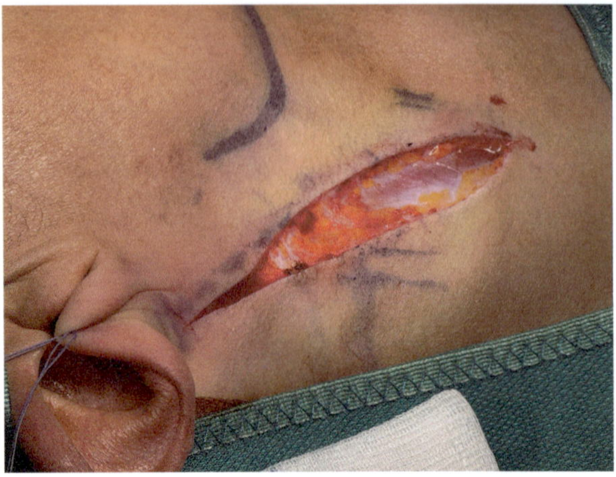

Fig. 20.3 Right lateral cervical incision down to the platysma muscle

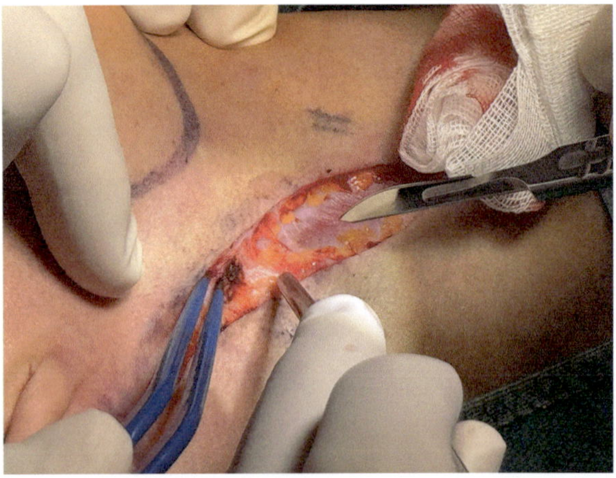

Fig. 20.4 Incision of platysma muscle and careful coagulation of vessels

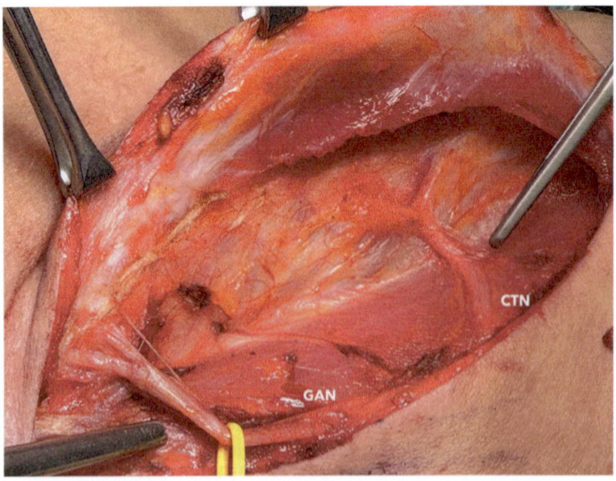

Fig. 20.5 The great auricular nerve (GAN) and the transverse cervical nerve (CTN) are identified and preserved

next key landmark in the depth for styloid approach is the digastric muscle, which is located and widely dissected and exposed (Fig. 20.6).

By means of a strong blue silicone sling, the digastric muscle is gently displaced inferiorly in order to disclose in a deeper plane the styloid muscle bundle (stylohyoid, stylopharyngeal, and styloglossus muscle) including stylohyoid ligament and elongated styloid, which must be identified by careful digital palpation. Occipital artery may be retracted together with the digastric muscle (Fig. 20.7).

The digastric muscle is always spared and not divided. In our practice, a couple of long blade Langenbeck retractors proved to be the best tool in order to displace the styloid muscle bundle superiorly and to disclose the styloid (Fig. 20.8). This type of retractor is sufficiently long to reach the depth of the surgical field also in patients with thick neck. The curved tip proved to be better than a straight one. The

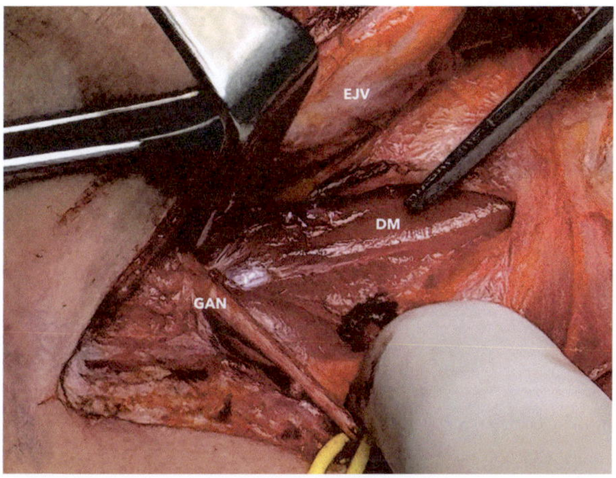

Fig. 20.6 Reaching the posterior belly of the digastric muscle (DM). The great auricular nerve (GAN), displaced inferiorly, and the external jugular vein (EJV), retracted superiorly, can be identified

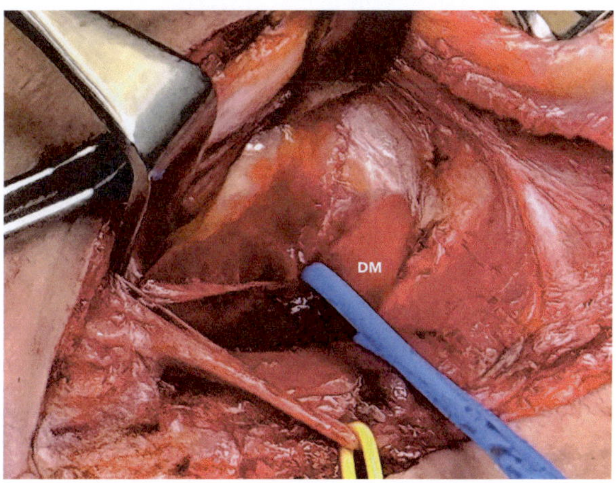

Fig. 20.7 Traction of the digastric muscle (DM)

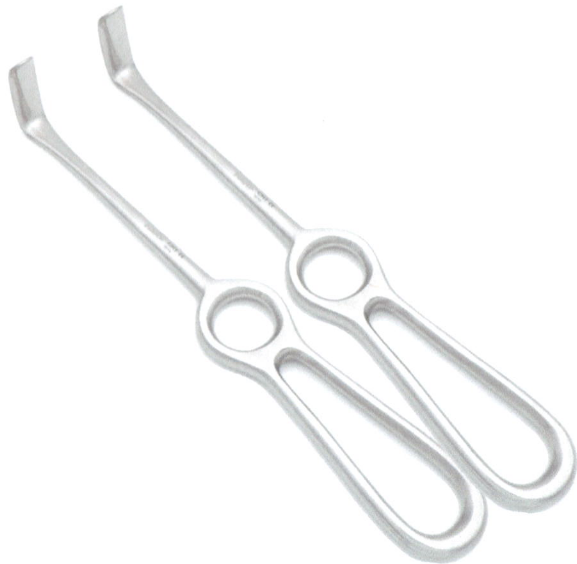

Fig. 20.8 A couple of long blade Langenbeck retractors

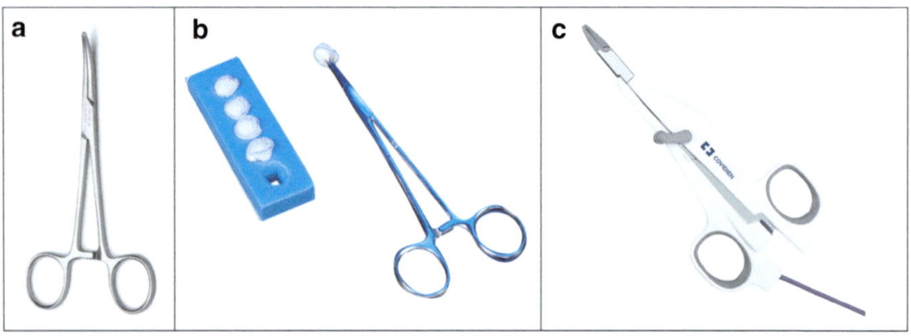

Fig. 20.9 (**a**) A small Kelly forceps. (**b**) A peanut sponge. (**c**) LigaSure Curved, Small Jaw, Open Sealer/Divider

instrument is sufficiently strong and ergonomic for the head assistant in order to help him to displace the tissues as required and in a stable way.

In the literature is also described the possibility of using a navigation technology in order to make easier to find the styloid process [10, 13]. In our experience, a careful progressive blunt dissection is easily guided by a repeated finger palpation of the area where the hard consistence of the styloid is felt. The proper position of the retractor tip is of great importance to keep in sight all the time the estimated position of the styloid. The styloid muscle bundle is progressively spread apart in a blunt way, and the styloid is visualized, usually in the depth and far from the skin surface (4–6 cm). A small Kelly forceps or a Redon dissecting forceps may be the best instrument for this surgical step (Fig. 20.9a). A peanut sponge may be also of interest. We don't recommend the use of scissor or any sharp instrument (scalpel) or monopolar (Fig. 20.9b). If available, a new-generation device like LigaSure Curved, Small Jaw, and Open Sealer/Divider may be helpful (Fig. 20.9c). It is "a bipolar electrosurgical instrument intended for use in open surgical procedures where ligation and division of vessels" is required.

In our experience, it proved to be helpful in tissue manipulation but not really necessary. A head lamp, halogen or LED, and magnification (loupe) made the procedure easier and safer mainly in the final steps in the depth (Fig. 20.10).

During the dissection, bleeding from minor vessels is usually minimal and easily controlled by bipolar coagulation. If a bigger vessel is identified (e.g., posterior auricular artery), it is gently displaced by the Langenbeck retractor. When styloid is under visual control, in the same way as for TOS, the styloid bone is stripped off from all the soft tissues around, superiorly toward the skull base and inferiorly to the tip of styloid at the junction with fibrous ligament (Fig. 20.11).

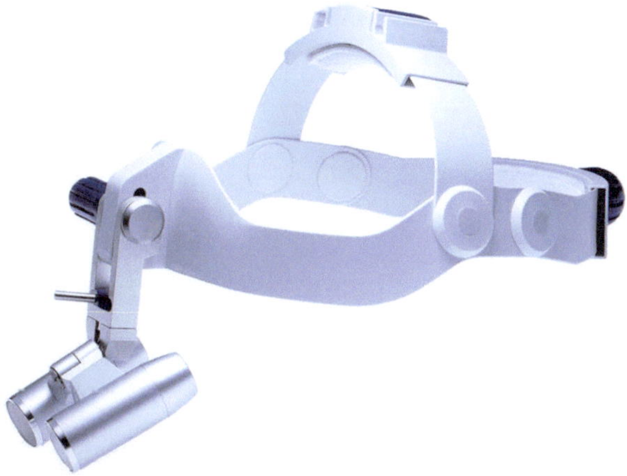

Fig. 20.10 An example of head loupe with LED lamp and 3.5× magnification

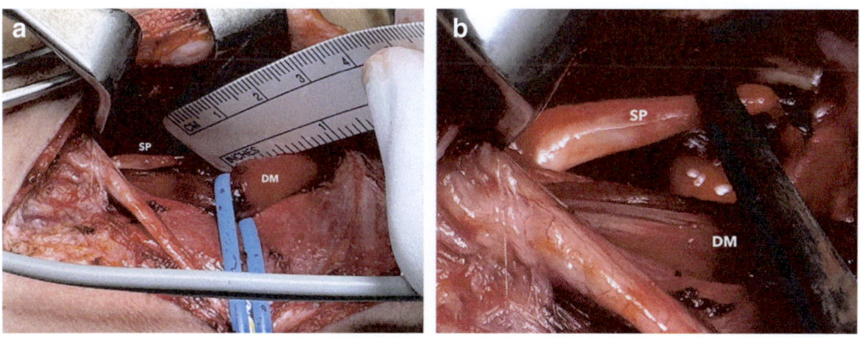

Fig. 20.11 (**a**) Visualization of the styloid process (SP) under digastric muscle (DM); the ruler shows the depth at which it is located in relation to the skin. (**b**) The final exposure of SP is stripped off from all surrounding soft tissues

A couple of easily available instruments proved to be very useful in this surgical step. First of all, a simple freer elevator may be the first choice, using its sharp tip, very effective in scraping the styloid bone periosteum (Fig. 20.12).

A hypophysectomy curette may also be useful but non-necessary. During this step, Langenbeck retractors play a key role in maintaining continuous visual control of the surgical field. In case of extensive superior dissection, don't forget the lateral position of the facial nerve trunk. Inferiorly the separation of the styloid tip from the stylohyoid ligament doesn't imply special risks (Fig. 20.13).

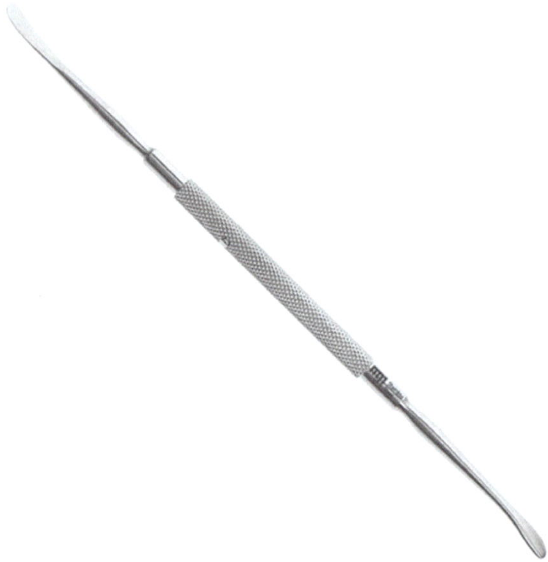

Fig. 20.12 A double-ended freer elevator

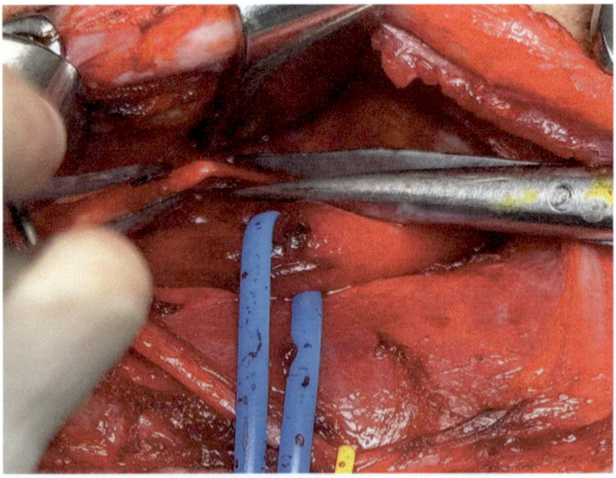

Fig. 20.13 Resection of stylohyoid ligament

The next step is the bone cut at the chosen level. We do emphasize that in our opinion it's useless to perform a total styloidectomy. Keeping in mind the pre-op imaging and the length of the styloid, it's easy to have an idea of the residual bone after removal and measuring of the surgical specimen. A residual bone stump less than 20 mm may be considered sufficient.

The required instrumentation for the osteotomy is already discussed for TOS (Citelli punch) (Fig. 20.14). If required, the bone stump may be smoothed in many ways if sharp after osteotomy, in our setting by a large ball diamond burr.

Usually a mini-drain is inserted before the final suture (Figs. 20.15, 20.16, and 20.17).

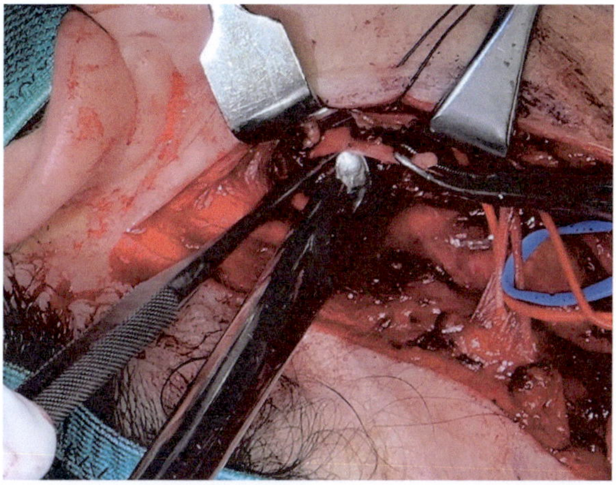

Fig. 20.14 Styloid bone is in interrupted by a Citelli nose punch

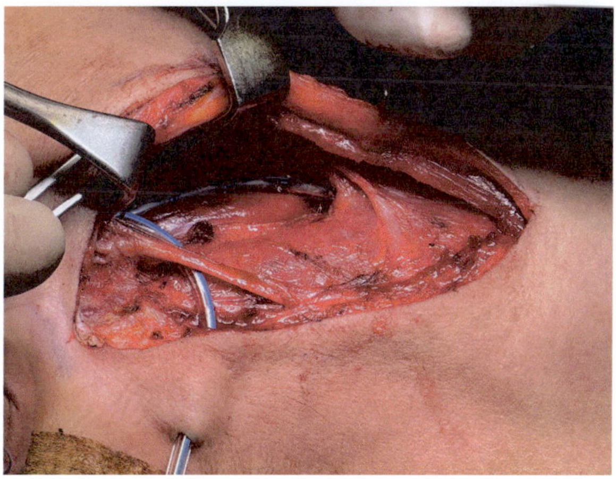

Fig. 20.15 Placement of mini-drain

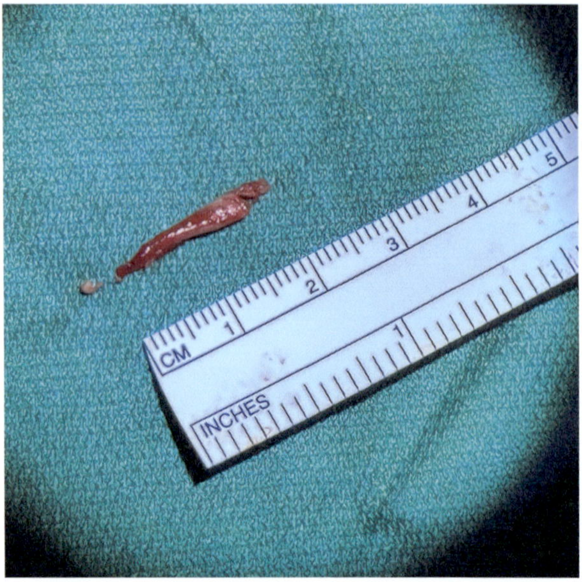

Fig. 20.16 Portion of the styloid process removed

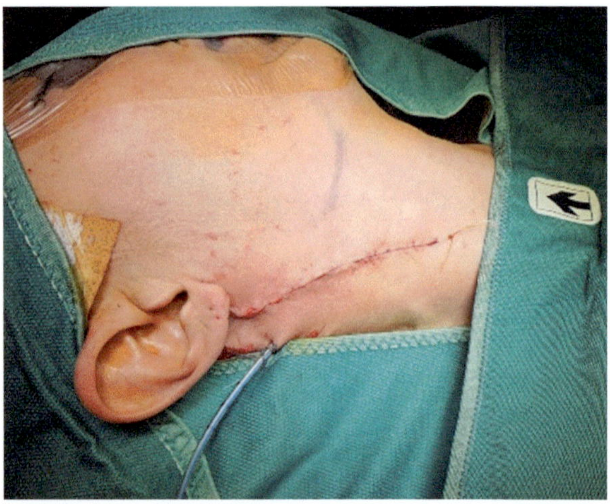

Fig. 20.17 Final suturing and lateral cervical drainage under suction

20.2 Complications

In Table 20.1 are summarized some of the most reported intraoperative and postoperative complications. Bleeding during the dissection is usually minimal and easy to control, and it is not a real complication [3, 14]. In obese patients and

Table 20.1 Open styloidectomy: list of possible complications

Intraoperative	Postoperative
Bleeding Difficult styloid location	Bleeding Facial nerve weakness External ear hypoesthesia Pain Delayed healing Infection Keloid scar First bite syndrome

sometimes also in thin subjects, the stylohyoid bundle may be encountered in the depth of the surgical field and relatively far from the surface [15]. Sometimes the surgery may be really challenging, but patience, adequate tissue retraction, repeated finger palpation of the tissues, and the availability of a sufficient light source and magnification may prevent the failure to find and resect the styloid. In these cases, dissection may require more time than expected, and facial weakness of the lower branch is more probable [3, 8]. A prolonged and strong retraction (with nerve compression/stretching) by the assistant may produce a transient marginal branch dysfunction, which always spontaneously resolved in our experience. A great auricular nerve dysfunction may occur even if the nerve is routinely identified and spared. The simple traction of the nerve required for widening the surgical window is sufficient to produce a tedious hypo−/paresthesia of the earlobe in few cases. Time and reassurance are always helpful. The time course of pain after surgery is not the same for all the patients. More commonly, the pre-op pain that required styloidectomy is not any more perceived immediately after surgery. Sometimes it is described as fluctuating and progressively lower day by day. In a few cases, a transient worsening, always under control by not morphine painkillers, is encountered. A prolonged pain treatment after the discharge and reassurance are the key for the management. As in any kind of neck surgery, delayed healing, sometimes produced by wound infection, is possible, which is the same for keloid. In Fig. 20.18, we reported a normal scar after 6 months from surgery.

Anyway, we didn't register this kind of reported complications in our series. One case of first bite syndrome as described in the literature is included in our OS series [16]. The symptoms appeared a couple of weeks after surgery, and pain was induced by the first bites of every meal, especially induced by dry foods. The patient didn't accept the treatment with carbamazepine and was informed about the possibility of repeated injections of Botox. She was instructed to avoid any type of food that stimulates a massive saliva production and to try chewing on the healthy side of the mouth.

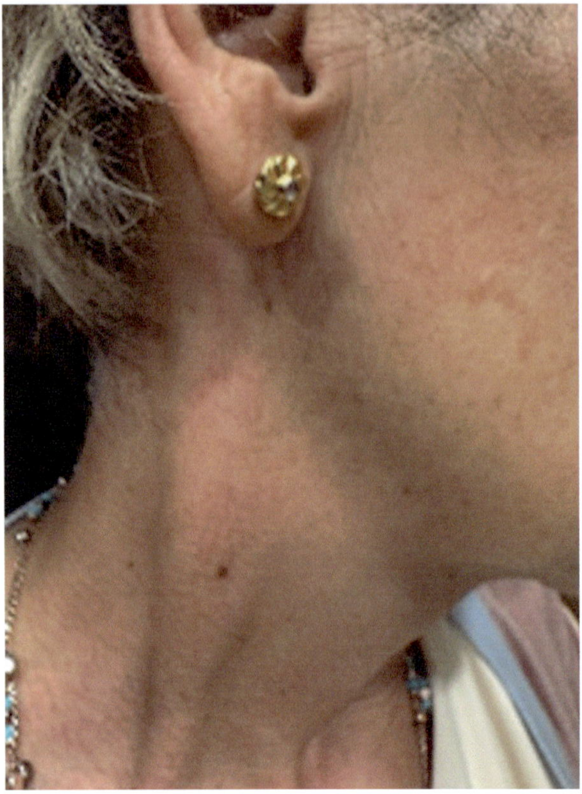

Fig. 20.18 A normal scar after 6 months

20.3 Personal Outcome

In this paragraph are reported the surgical outcomes in a group of TES patients referred to the Department of Otolaryngology—Head and Neck Surgery of Morgagni-Pierantoni Hospital in Forlì to the ENT Department of the University Hospital Sant'Anna in Ferrara and to the San Pier Damiano Hospital, GVM Group, Faenza, from January 2013 to May 2024. We included in this analysis all patients aged between 18 and 65 years who were diagnosed with TES and underwent surgical treatment with styloidectomy, either open or transoral approach, including TORS. For each patient, the following data were collected:

- Age.
- Sex.
- Body mass index (BMI).
- Side (unilateral right or left or bilateral).
- Comorbidities.
- History of tonsillectomy or head trauma.

- Average time between the onset of symptoms and the diagnosis of Eagle syndrome (ES).
- Length of the styloid process.
- Length of the resected styloid segment.
- Surgical time.
- Visual analog scale (VAS) score for symptoms pre- and post-operation.
- Glasgow Benefit Inventory (GBI) score at 3 months post-operation.

Statistical analysis was performed, and graphs were devised, with STATA 12.0 software (StataCorp., College Station, TX, USA) and SPSS for Windows (v.21, SPSS Inc., Armonk, USA).

Fifty patients were identified as affected by typical Eagle syndrome (TES) and operated on. Among these, 13 had bilateral ES, resulting in a total of 63 styloidectomies. Twelve styloidectomies (19% of the total) were performed using transoral robotic surgery (TORS) and 1 (1.6%) via the transoral approach using traditional techniques, while the remaining 50 (79.4%) were conducted via a transcervical approach. Of the 13 bilateral ES cases, 4 were treated using TORS and 9 using a cervicotomy approach. In the open approach, the ES was treated in two stages: first, the more symptomatic side and then the second side at least 6 months later. Conversely, thanks to the minimally invasive approach, the cases treated with TORS were addressed in a single surgical session.

The average age of the treated patients was 46.5 ± 13.1 years (25–72), with a significant predominance of females (64%). The epidemiological data of the patients are summarized in Table 20.2.

Table 20.2 Patient's profile

	Overall	TORS	Cervical	Classical transoral
Number of patients	50	8 (16%)	41 (82%)	1 (2%)
Number of styloidectomy	63	12 (19%)	50 (79.4%)	1 (1.6%)
Number of bilateral ES	13 (26%)	4 (50%)	9 (22%)	0
Age at surgery	46.5 ± 13.14	41.75 ± 10.33	46.83 ± 13.17	71
Female to male ratio	32:18 (64%:26%)	7:1 (87.5%:12.5%)	25:16 (61%:29%)	0:1 (0%:100%)
BMI (kg/m^2)	24.91 ± 4.04	23.38 ± 2.62	25.11 ± 4.22	30.00
Previous tonsillectomy	23 (46%)	2 (25%)	20 (48.8%)	1 (100%)
Previous concussion	13 (26%)	3 (37.50%)	10 (24.4%)	1 (100%)
Previous medical therapy	32 (74%)	7 (87.50%)	29 (70.7%)	1 (100%)
Previous endocrine system disorder	9 (26%)	1 (12.5%)	12 (29.3%)	0 (0%)
Previous TMJ disorder	20 (40%)	5 (62.5%)	14 (34.15%)	0.133
Time to diagnosis (months)	51.96 ± 47.93	52.25 ± 49.17	53.02 ± 48.34	6

In Table 20.3, we have summarized the pre- and postoperative VAS scores for each symptom analyzed. All VAS scores were calculated for each styloidectomy. Therefore, in patients with bilateral ES, they were specifically asked to distinguish the severity of symptoms for the right side and the left side.

The mean preoperative total symptom score (TSS) was 40.18 ± 20.43, while the postoperative TSS, evaluated at 6 months, was 15.42 ± 16.14 ($P < 0.001$). In 100% of the cases treated, some degree of reduction in TSS was achieved. We did not find statistically significant differences in the preoperative and postoperative total symptom score (TSS) between patients with unilateral and bilateral Eagle syndrome (*P*-values of 0.472 and 0.623, respectively).

Regarding the postoperative Glasgow Benefit Inventory (GBI) score, 4 patients reported a total GBI score that was negative (8%), and 1 patient reported a total GBI score of 0 (2%), while 45 patients had a positive total postoperative GBI score (90% of patients). The *P*-value for these results is <0.001. An analysis of the GBI score subcategories—general, social, and physical—showed a success rate of 84% in the general GBI, 62% in the physical GBI, and 44% in the social GBI, all with p-values <0.001. All results related to the GBI score are detailed in Table 20.4. We also

Table 20.3 In this table, we have summarized the mean VAS scores for each symptom and the respective standard deviation, both pre- and postoperative

Symptom	Mean pre ± std. dev	Mean post ± std. dev	Percentage reduction (%)
VAS score neck pain	5.74 ± 2.481	2.36 ± 2.173	58.88
VAS score ear pain	4.32 ± 3.297	1.58 ± 2.021	63.43
VAS score ear fullness	3.66 ± 3.30	1.24 ± 2.015	66.12
VAS score tinnitus	2.82 ± 3.75	1.3 ± 2.270	53.90
VAS score dental pain	2.86 ± 3.344	1.4 ± 2.321	51.05
VAS score painful swallowing	4.06 ± 3.40	1.28 ± 2.138	68.47
VAS score swallowing pain	3.9 ± 3.424	1.8 ± 2.294	53.85
VAS score foreign body sensation in throat	4.48 ± 3.227	1.56 ± 2.130	65.18
VAS score facial pain	4.26 ± 3.312	1.42 ± 2.041	66.67
VAS score headache	4.08 ± 3.096	1.48 ± 2.022	63.73

We have also calculated the average percentage reductions after surgery
std dev Standard deviation, *pre* preoperative, *post* postoperative

Table 20.4 Representation of success rates of the four GBI categories

	Total GBI score (%)	General GBI score (%)	Physical GBI score (%)	Social GBI score (%)
Success rate	86	84	62	44
Result = 0	2	4	18	44
Failure rate	8	8	16	8

Table 20.5 Difference in total symptom score pre- and postoperative and average GBI scores by surgical technique

Surgical approach	Difference in total symptom score	Average total GBI score	Average general GBI score	Average physical GBI score	Average social GBI score
Transcervical	23.49 ($P < 0.001$)	21.63 ($P < 0.001$)	27.13 ($P < 0.001$)	14.96 (0.11.116)	9.87 ($P < 0.001$)
TORS	30.63 ($P < 0.001$)	25.00 ($P < 0.001$)	27.60 ($P < 0.001$)	22.92 ($P < 0.001$)	16.67 ($P < 0.001$)
Classic transoral	30.00	22.20	25.00	50.00	0.00

compared the total GBI score between patients with bilateral and unilateral Eagle syndrome, but once again, we did not find statistically significant differences (*P*-value 0.529).

The separated data for the TSS and GBI score according to the surgical techniques used—cervical, transoral traditional, and TORS—are summarized in Table 20.5. Comparative analysis among the various techniques didn't show a statistically significant difference between TORS and open in terms of TSS and GBI scores. Since only one case was performed using the traditional transoral technique, it is not comparable to the other two techniques.

Moreover, we asked patients whether they would undergo surgical intervention again. The response was affirmative in 80% of the total cases (40 patients). When breaking down the data, 62.5% of patients who underwent the procedure using TORS would choose to do it again, compared to 82.5% of those treated with the transcervical technique ($P = 0.3279$).

We also conducted some correlation analyses to try to identify predictive factors related to the surgical outcome. By creating a correlation matrix among some of the main variables (available in Fig. 20.19), we found that the factor most correlated with the surgical outcome is the preoperative TSS. The higher the TSS, the better the surgical outcome appears to be.

The length of the resected segment, however, does not seem to be significant. Based on the significance of the preoperative TSS, we continued our analysis by conducting a second correlation test between the average preoperative VAS scores for each symptom and the surgical outcome. This highlighted a positive correlation between the preoperative VAS scores of some symptoms, such as odynophagia, swallowing pain, and foreign body sensation, and a better surgical outcome. In particular, the strongest correlation was found for preoperative odynophagia (see Table 20.6 and Fig. 20.20).

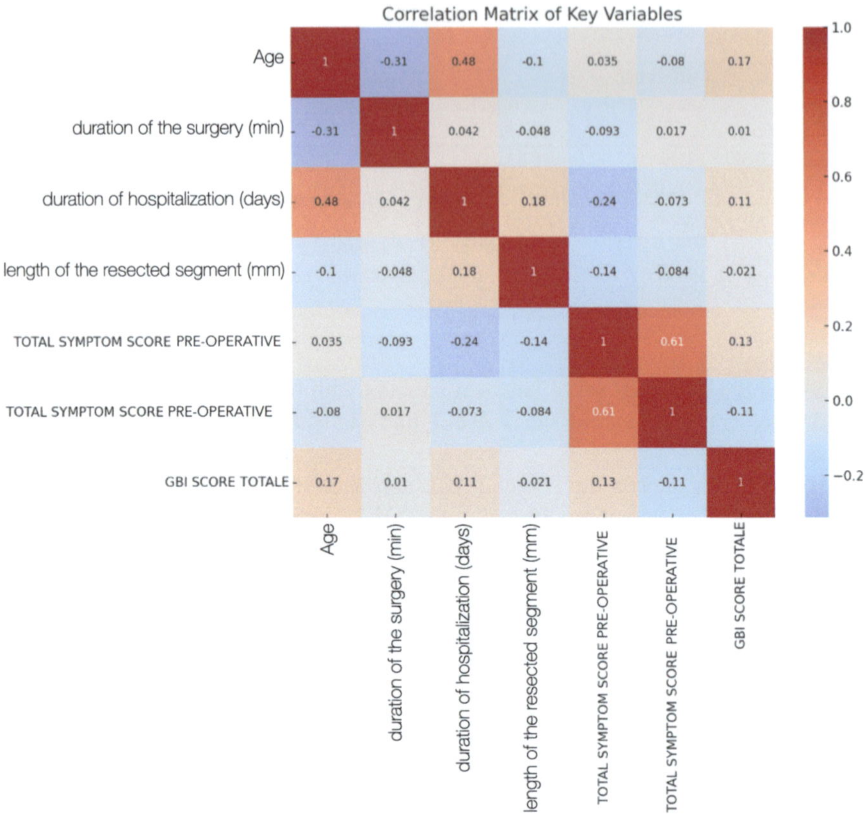

Fig. 20.19 Correlation matrix between the variables: age, duration of the surgery, duration of hospitalization, length of the resected segment, preoperative total symptom score, postoperative total symptom score, and total GBI score

Table 20.6 Correlation test between preoperative VAS score values for each ES symptom and surgical outcome

Pre-op symptom	Correlation with outcome
VAS score Dolore al collo pre-operatorio	0.152
VAS score otalgia pre-operatorio	0.400
VAS score fullness auricolare pre-operatorio	0.318
VAS score Acufene pre-operatorio	0.367
VAS score Dolore dentario pre-operatorio	0.307
VAS score Odinofagia pre-operatorio	0.573
VAS score Dolore alla deglutizione pre-operatorio	0.510
VAS score Sensazione di corpo estraneo a livello faringeo pre-operatorio	0.468
VAS score Dolore facciale pre-operatorio	0.308
VAS score Cefalea pre-operatorio	0.328

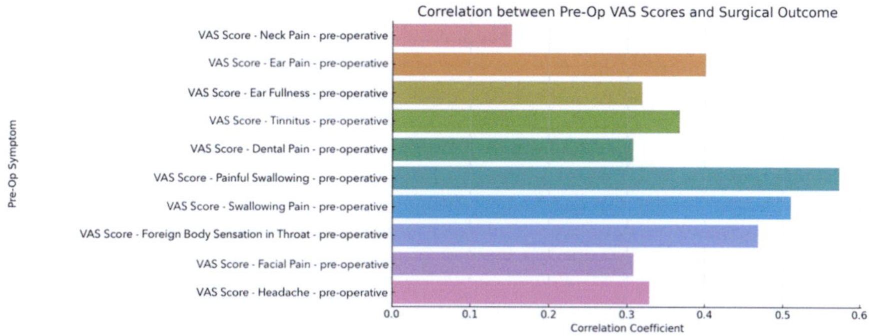

Fig. 20.20 Graphical representation of the correlation coefficients for each preoperative VAS score of ES symptoms and surgical outcome

References

1. Zhao Z, Gu J. Open surgery in the era of minimally invasive surgery. Chin J Cancer Res. 2022;34:63–5. https://doi.org/10.21147/j.issn.1000-9604.2022.01.06.
2. Loeser L, Cardwell E. Elongated styloid process: a cause of glossopharyngeal neuralgia. Arch Otolaryngol. 1942;36:198–202.
3. Müderris T, Bercin S, Sevil E, Beton S, Kırıs M. Surgical management of elongated styloid process: intraoral or transcervical? Eur Arch Otorrinolaringol. 2014;271:1709–13. https://doi.org/10.1007/s00405-013-2664-0.
4. Williams JV, McKearney RM, Revington PJ. Eagle's syndrome: a novel surgical approach to the styloid process using a preauricular incision. J Oral Maxillofac Surg. 2011;69:1617–22. https://doi.org/10.1016/j.joms.2010.11.023.
5. Buono U, Mangone GM, Michelotti A, Longo F, Califano L. Surgical approach to the stylohyoid process in eagle's syndrome. J Oral Maxillofac Surg. 2005;63:714–6. https://doi.org/10.1016/j.joms.2004.10.013.
6. Bargiel J, Gontarz M, Marecik T, Szczurowski P, Gąsiorowski K, Zapała J, Wyszyńska-Pawelec G. Minimally invasive cervical Styloidectomy in stylohyoid syndrome (eagle syndrome). J Clin Med. 2023;12:6763. https://doi.org/10.3390/jcm12216763.
7. Constanzo F, Ramina R, Coelho NM. Modified craniocervical approach for resection of the styloid process in patients with eagle's syndrome. J Neurol Surg B Skull Base. 2021;82(Suppl 3):e179–83. https://doi.org/10.1055/s-0039-3400297.
8. Pigache P, Fontaine C, Ferri J, Raoul G. Transcervical styloidectomy in eagle's syndrome. Eur Ann Otorhinolaryngol Head Neck Dis. 2018;135(6):433–6. https://doi.org/10.1016/j.anorl.2018.05.001.
9. Chen R, Liang F, Han P, Cai Q, Yu S, Huang X. Endoscope-assisted resection of elongated styloid process through a retroauricular incision: a novel surgical approach to eagle syndrome. J Oral Maxillofac Surg. 2017;75(7):1442–8. https://doi.org/10.1016/j.joms.2017.01.016.
10. Thoenissen P, Bittermann G, Schmelzeisen R, Oshima T, Fretwurst T. Eagle's syndrome-a non-perceived differential diagnosis of temporomandibular disorder. Int J Surg Case Rep. 2015;15:123–6. https://doi.org/10.1016/j.ijscr.2015.08.036.
11. Chrcanovic BR, Custódio AL, de Oliveira DR. An intraoral surgical approach to the styloid process in eagle's syndrome. Oral Maxillofac Surg. 2009;13:145–51. https://doi.org/10.1007/s10006-009-0164-6.

12. Ran T, Lin C, Ma T, Qin Y, Li J, Zhang Y, Xu Y, Li C, Wang M. Ultra-pulsed CO_2 laser osteotomy: a new method for the bone preparation of total knee arthroplasty. Front Bioeng Biotechnol. 2022;10:858862. https://doi.org/10.3389/fbioe.2022.858862.
13. Sukegawa S, Kanno T, Yoshimoto A, Matsumoto K, Sukegawa-Takahashi Y, Masui M, Furuki Y. Use of an intraoperative navigation system and piezoelectric surgery for styloidectomy in a patient with eagle's syndrome: a case report. J Med Case Rep. 2017;11(1):322. https://doi.org/10.1186/s13256-017-1464-3.
14. Wang J, Liu Y, Wang ZB, Yan KS. Intraoral and extraoral approach for surgical treatment of eagle's syndrome: a retrospective study. Eur Arch Otorrinolaringol. 2022;279(3):1481–7. https://doi.org/10.1007/s00405-021-06914-2.
15. Katsevman GA, Daffner SD, Brandmeir NJ, Emery SE, France JC, Sedney CL. Complexities of spine surgery in obese patient populations: a narrative review. Spine J. 2020;20(4):501–11. https://doi.org/10.1016/j.spinee.2019.12.011.
16. Cernea CR, Hojaij FC, De Carlucci D Jr, Plopper C, Vanderley F, Guerreiro CA, Viana MS. First-bite syndrome after resection of the styloid process. Laryngoscope. 2007;117(1):181–2. https://doi.org/10.1097/01.mlg.0000245059.40028.

21 Transoral Robotic Styloidectomy for Eagle Syndrome

Andrea Costantino, Filippo Montevecchi, Ruggero Campisi, Alberto Caranti, Claudio Vicini, and J. Scott Magnuson

21.1 Introduction

Eagle syndrome is a rare condition characterized by elongation of the styloid process or calcification of the stylohyoid ligament, resulting in a constellation of symptoms such as throat pain, foreign body sensation, dysphagia, and sometimes even facial pain or tinnitus. While conservative treatments like pain management and steroid injections can alleviate symptoms for some patients, surgical intervention is often required for those with persistent or severe symptoms. Among the surgical options available, transoral robotic styloidectomy has emerged as a minimally invasive and highly effective technique for the resection of the elongated styloid process [1, 2].

This chapter focuses on the transoral robotic approach to styloidectomy, highlighting the indications, surgical technique, outcomes, and potential complications associated with this procedure. To provide a comprehensive understanding, the chapter also discusses the anatomical considerations critical for safe and effective surgery, as well as the preoperative evaluation necessary to identify candidates who would benefit most from this approach. Additionally, it reviews the latest advancements in robotic surgery technology that have enhanced precision and outcomes in

A. Costantino (✉) · J. S. Magnuson
Department of Otolaryngology – Head and Neck Surgery, Advent Health Orlando, Celebration, FL, USA
e-mail: andrea.costantino@adventhealth.com

F. Montevecchi
Otorhinolaryngology Forli Private Hospitals, Forli, Italy

R. Campisi · A. Caranti · C. Vicini
University of Ferrara, Cona, FE, Italy
e-mail: claudio@claudiovicini.com

C. Vicini et al. (eds.), *EAGLE Syndrome*,
https://doi.org/10.1007/978-3-031-92829-1_21

the treatment of Eagle syndrome. Through case studies and clinical experiences, this chapter aims to offer valuable insights for surgeons looking to adopt or refine their use of the transoral robotic approach in managing this complex condition.

21.2 Indications for Transoral Robotic Styloidectomy

21.2.1 When to Consider Surgery

Transoral robotic styloidectomy is indicated for patients with Eagle syndrome who experience significant symptoms that have not responded to conservative treatments. These symptoms typically include persistent throat pain, difficulty swallowing, or a constant sensation of a foreign body in the throat. The decision to proceed with surgery is often based on the severity of symptoms, the degree of elongation of the styloid process as confirmed by imaging, and the impact of the condition on the patient's quality of life.

21.2.2 Patient Selection Criteria

Ideal candidates for transoral robotic styloidectomy are those with a confirmed diagnosis of Eagle syndrome, characterized by an elongated styloid process of more than 2.5–3 cm, visible on imaging studies such as a CT scan. The patient should be in overall good health, with no contraindications to surgery or anesthesia. Additionally, patients who have undergone unsuccessful conservative treatments, including physical therapy, oral anti-inflammatory medications, or corticosteroid injections, are prime candidates for this surgical approach. Transoral exposure is a critical factor in determining the suitability of patients for this procedure. Factors such as body mass index (BMI), inter-incisive distance, Mallampati score, and dental status play essential roles. These factors play a crucial role in ensuring optimal access, visualization, and safety during the procedure.

21.3 Preoperative Planning

Preoperative imaging is crucial for planning a transoral robotic styloidectomy. A detailed CT scan represents the gold standard for identifying an ossified styloid process. A 3D reconstruction allows for precise measurement of the styloid process and identification of its relationship with surrounding structures. MRI may be used to assess soft tissue involvement, particularly if there is suspicion of associated vascular or neural compression.

In addition to imaging, a thorough clinical examination is essential. The physical examination should include a detailed assessment of the oral cavity and oropharynx to evaluate factors for determining the feasibility of transoral exposure. Palpation of the styloid process through the tonsillar fossa may also provide valuable information about the size and orientation of the styloid process, aiding in surgical planning.

Before surgery, patients undergo a comprehensive preoperative assessment, including a review of medical history, physical examination, and any necessary laboratory tests. Patients are counseled on the risks and benefits of the procedure and the expected postoperative course. Anesthesia considerations are discussed, given the specific positioning required for the procedure.

21.4 Surgical Technique: Transoral Robotic Styloidectomy

21.4.1 Robotic System Overview

The transoral robotic styloidectomy procedure is performed using the Da Vinci surgical system (Intuitive Surgical, Sunnyvale, CA), which offers significant advantages over traditional surgical methods. The system provides enhanced precision, dexterity, and high-definition 3D visualization, allowing for accurate and safe dissection in the confined spaces of the oropharynx. Robotic instruments offer a greater range of motion than the human hand, enabling complex maneuvers around delicate structures like nerves and blood vessels. This minimally invasive approach eliminates the need for external incisions, reducing scarring, postoperative pain, and recovery time. Additionally, the ergonomic design of the robotic console reduces surgeon fatigue, ensuring consistent performance throughout the procedure. The system's precision and control improve patient safety by minimizing the risk of injury to surrounding tissues, while its scalability ensures reproducible outcomes across different surgical settings.

While the Da Vinci system is the primary robotic platform used by the authors in their practice, it is important to note that other robotic systems are also available on the market. The choice of system can vary between different countries and institutions, depending on factors such as availability, cost, and surgeon preference. Each system may have its own unique features and capabilities, but they all aim to provide similar benefits in terms of precision, safety, and minimally invasive access to difficult-to-reach areas of the body.

21.4.2 Step-by-Step Surgical Procedure

Positioning and Exposure

For the transoral robotic styloidectomy, patient positioning and the operative setting are crucial for optimizing the surgical approach. Surgery is performed under general anesthesia, and a nasotracheal intubation is preferred. The patient is positioned supine with the head extended, often supported by a headrest to maintain this position. This extension allows for a direct line of sight into the oropharynx and enhances access to the surgical field, facilitating the precise movement of robotic instruments.

The use of the FK-WO (Feyh-Kastenbauer Weinstein-O'Malley) retractor or a Boyle-Davis mouth opener is essential for adequate exposure of the lateral oropharyngeal region. These devices help maintain an open surgical field by retracting the soft tissues and tongue, providing clear visualization of the tonsillar fossae.

Robot Setup

The Da Vinci system (Si, Xi, or SP) is positioned to allow optimal alignment with the patient's oral cavity. The patient-side cart is placed at a 90° (SP and Xi) or a 45° angle (Si) to the surgical bed, at chest level. For the SP system, the robotic head is positioned approximately 10 cm from the mouth, aligning the port cannula with the patient's airway. The flexible endoscope is then introduced through the inferior channel of the cannula and guided into the oropharynx, where it is adjusted into a "Cobra" shape by the surgeon at the console. The two robotic arms, typically equipped with spatula monopolar cautery and Maryland forceps, are inserted through the lateral channels. The "elbows" of these instruments are positioned within the oral cavity, while the "wrists" are maneuvered into the oropharynx, allowing precise dissection and removal of the elongated styloid process. This arrangement not only maximizes the operative space but also minimizes the risk of instrument collisions, ensuring a smooth and effective surgical procedure (Fig. 21.1). The surgical team's familiarity with the setup and careful alignment of the robotic system are important to prevent interference or collisions between robotic arms and to ensure that the instruments have unobstructed access. This careful planning and exposure setup are key to the success of the procedure, minimizing complications and improving surgical outcomes.

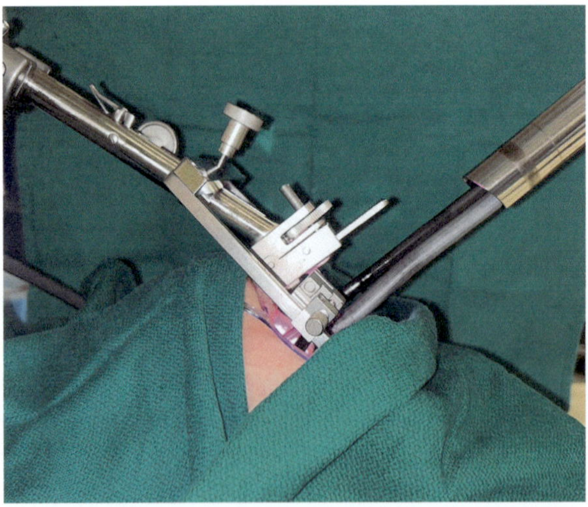

Fig. 21.1 Example of robotic setup with mouth opener to maximize access to the oropharynx, central rigid endoscope, and two robotic arms, typically equipped with spatula monopolar cautery and Maryland forceps

Incision and Access
A mucosal incision is initiated at the pterygomandibular raphe, providing an entry point to the deeper structures. Blunt dissection is then employed to carefully access the parapharyngeal space, minimizing the risk of injury to surrounding tissues. Upon reaching the parapharyngeal fat pad, the incision is extended inferiorly to enhance visibility and create a wider access area (Fig. 21.2). This approach facilitates a clear and controlled pathway for the subsequent surgical steps, ensuring safe and efficient maneuvering within the confined surgical field.

Exposure and Dissection
Due to the lack of tactile feedback from the robotic arms, finger palpation is employed to accurately localize the styloid process. Once identified, the surgeon uses the robotic instruments to meticulously dissect the soft tissues surrounding the styloid process (Fig. 21.3). While blunt dissection is advantageous for gently

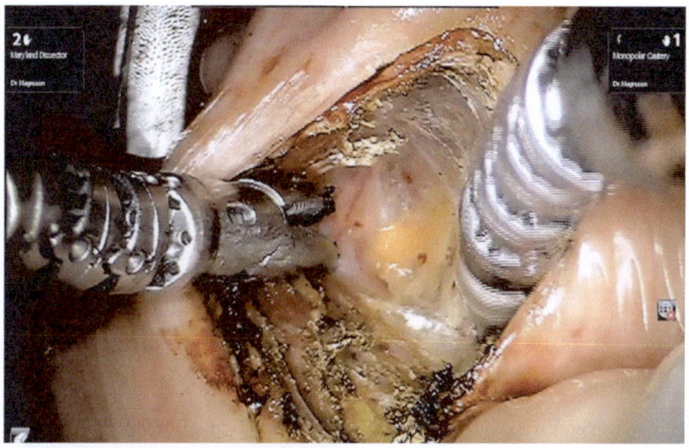

Fig. 21.2 Incision of the oral mucosa at the level of the pterygomandibular raphe, providing an entry point to the deeper structures

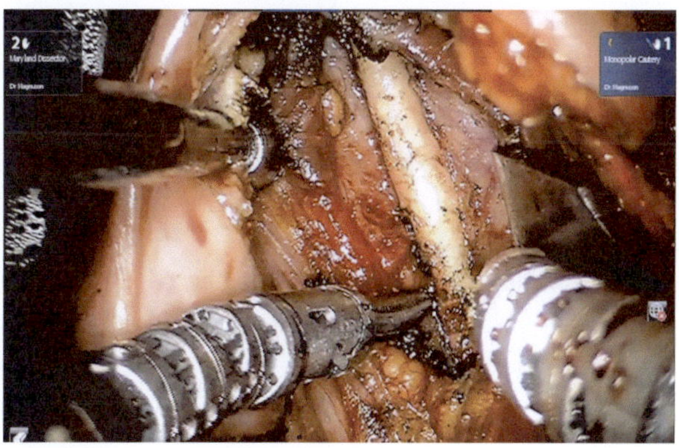

Fig. 21.3 Frame documenting the careful dissection of the soft tissues surrounding the styloid process

separating tissues, electrocautery is used judiciously, primarily above the bone, to minimize the risk of injuring surrounding vessels. The advanced 3D visualization offered by the robotic system allows for precise identification and protection of vital structures, such as the carotid artery and cranial nerves, throughout the dissection process.

Resection

After achieving adequate exposure, the styloid process is resected in a caudo-cranial direction. The distal portions are carefully removed first, with the proximal limit of resection determined by the extent of surgical exposure. A bedside assistant plays a crucial role in this process, utilizing a Kerrison rongeur forceps to excise the hard bone (Fig. 21.4). The length of the styloid process to be removed is guided by preoperative imaging as well as intraoperative findings, ensuring that the resection is both thorough and safe.

Hemostasis and Closure

The surgical field is irrigated with a saline solution, and hemostasis is achieved using bipolar cautery or other hemostatic agents as necessary (Fig. 21.5). Once

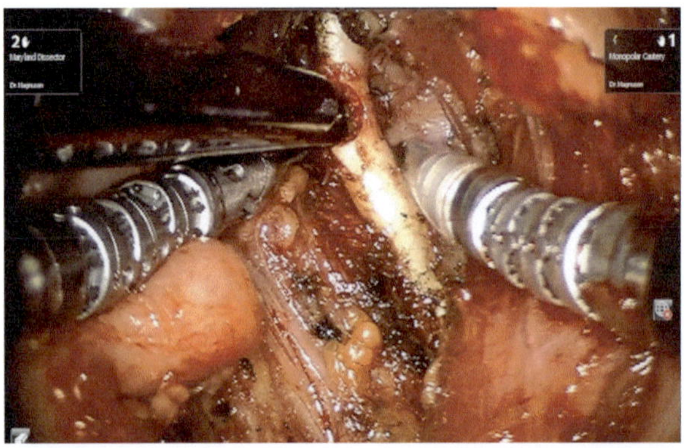

Fig. 21.4 Frame showing the coordinated action of the two robotic arms and the Kerrison rongeur forceps used by the bedside assistant

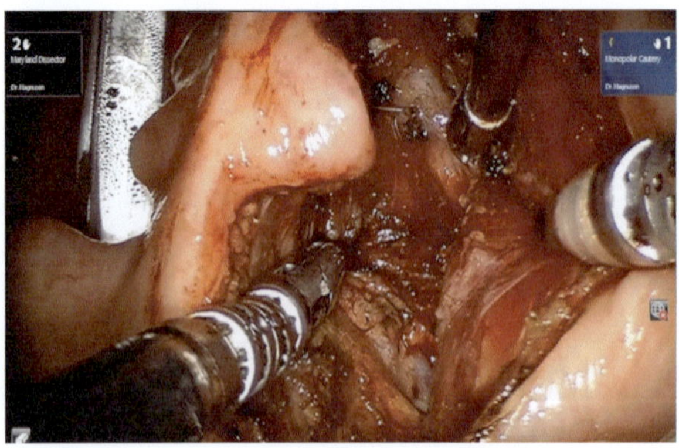

Fig. 21.5 In this image, the surgical field is observed, completely bloodless after the removal of the styloid process

hemostasis is confirmed, the mucosal incision is closed with absorbable sutures, securing the surgical site and minimizing the risk of postoperative bleeding or infection.

21.5 Postoperative Care and Recovery

21.5.1 Immediate Postoperative Management

Following surgery, patients are monitored in the recovery room for any immediate complications, such as bleeding or airway obstruction. Pain management is tailored to the patient's needs, with oral analgesics typically sufficient to control postoperative discomfort. Patients are usually discharged on the same day or after an overnight observation, depending on the complexity of the surgery and the patient's overall health.

21.5.2 Long-Term Recovery

Patients are advised to follow a soft diet for the first few days after surgery to minimize irritation of the surgical site. Swallowing exercises may be recommended to help restore normal function more quickly. Follow-up visits are scheduled to assess healing, remove any non-absorbable sutures if used, and evaluate symptom resolution. Most patients experience significant symptom relief within a few weeks, with full recovery expected within 4–6 weeks.

21.6 Complications

As with any surgical procedure, there are potential risks and complications associated with transoral robotic styloidectomy. By understanding and preparing for these potential complications, the surgical team can take proactive measures to reduce risks and enhance patient safety and outcomes during transoral robotic styloidectomy. These may include:

- *Nerve Injury*: Although rare, there is a risk of damage to the glossopharyngeal or hypoglossal nerves during dissection, which could result in dysphagia or altered sensation.
- *Infection*: The oral cavity is a naturally contaminated environment, so there is a risk of postoperative infection, though this is minimized with proper surgical technique and postoperative care.
- *Bleeding*: Intraoperative or postoperative bleeding can occur, particularly given the proximity to major blood vessels. This is usually well-controlled with robotic precision and appropriate hemostatic measures.

- *Dental Injury*: The use of a transoral approach, especially with robotic instruments, poses a risk of dental injury. This can include damage to teeth, particularly in patients with poor dental health, or dislodgment of dental work. Protective measures, such as using dental guards, are recommended to minimize the risk of injury.
- *Anesthesia-Related Complications*: Given the specific positioning required for this procedure, there is a risk of anesthesia-related complications. Care must be taken to secure the endotracheal tube firmly to prevent accidental extubation during the surgery, particularly if nasotracheal intubation is performed. Continuous monitoring of the patient's airway is essential, and any signs of respiratory distress or other anesthesia-related issues should be addressed promptly to ensure patient safety.

21.7 Comparison with Other Surgical Approaches

Traditionally, the transoral approach has been associated with poor visualization of the surgical field, leading to a higher risk of injury to neurovascular structures and an increased likelihood of deep neck infections. Because of these challenges, the external approach has long been considered the gold standard. However, the external approach also has significant drawbacks, including the presence of visible scars on the neck or face and a longer operative time compared to transoral methods.

The transoral approach to styloidectomy offers several advantages over the traditional external approach, including the avoidance of external scars, reduced risk of nerve injury, and shorter recovery times. While the external approach may still be necessary in cases with extensive styloid process elongation or complicated anatomy, the transoral robotic method is increasingly favored for its minimally invasive nature and excellent outcomes.

Robotic surgery provides enhanced visualization, greater precision, and the ability to perform complex dissections in confined spaces, making it an ideal choice for styloidectomy. The use of robotic instruments also reduces surgeon fatigue and allows for more ergonomic surgical maneuvers, contributing to the overall success of the procedure.

21.8 Clinical Outcomes

Transoral robotic styloidectomy has shown excellent outcomes in terms of symptom relief and patient satisfaction. The minimally invasive nature of the procedure results in reduced postoperative pain, faster recovery times, and minimal scarring. Most patients report a significant reduction or complete resolution of their Eagle syndrome symptoms following surgery. Only 5 studies have been conducted on the use of TORS for Eagle syndrome treatment, with a total of 20 TORS procedures described [3–7].

21.8.1 Key Findings

The average age of patients undergoing TORS was 53.2 years, with a majority being female (65%).

The average operation time was 68.8 min, and 95% of patients resumed an oral diet on the first postoperative day.

The average hospital stay was 1.9 days, with half of the patients discharged after 1 day.

Complications were minimal, with only one reported case of suture dehiscence.

Most patients (80%) experienced complete symptom relief, while others reported significant but not complete improvement.

TORS is a safe and effective surgical option for ES, comparable to both traditional transoral and transcervical approaches. It offers advantages such as reduced hospitalization time and quicker recovery. However, the cost of TORS remains a potential limitation depending on the healthcare context.

21.9 Future Directions and Innovations

As robotic technology continues to evolve, future developments may include smaller, more versatile robotic instruments and improved imaging systems that enhance the surgeon's ability to perform delicate procedures in the oropharyngeal region. These advancements could further improve the safety and efficacy of transoral robotic styloidectomy. Ongoing research into the long-term outcomes of transoral robotic styloidectomy, as well as comparisons with other surgical techniques, will help refine patient selection criteria and optimize surgical protocols.

21.10 Conclusion

Transoral robotic styloidectomy represents a significant advancement in the surgical management of Eagle syndrome. By offering a minimally invasive alternative to traditional surgery, this technique provides excellent outcomes with reduced risk of complications and faster recovery times. As robotic technology continues to evolve, the future of this approach looks promising, with the potential to benefit even more patients suffering from Eagle syndrome.

References

1. Campisi R, Caranti A, Meccariello G, et al. Transoral robotic styloidectomy for eagle syndrome: a systematic review. Clin Otolaryngol. 2024;49(3):293–8. https://doi.org/10.1111/coa.14145.
2. Keirns D, Asarkar A, Entezami P, Ware E, Nagel TH, Chang BA. Transoral robotic surgery for eagle syndrome: a systematic review. Ear Nose Throat J. Published online April 10, 2024. 2024;10:1455613241246587. https://doi.org/10.1177/01455613241246587.

3. Fitzpatrick TH, Lovin BD, Magister MJ, Waltonen JD, Browne JD, Sullivan CA. Surgical management of eagle syndrome: a 17-year experience with open and transoral robotic styloidectomy. Am J Otolaryngol. 2020;41(2):102324. https://doi.org/10.1016/j.amjoto.2019.102324.
4. Kim DH, Lee YH, Cha D, Kim SH. Transoral robotic surgery in eagle's syndrome: our experience on four patients. Acta Otorhinolaryngol Ital. 2017;37(6):454–7. https://doi.org/10.14639/0392-100X-1502.
5. Montevecchi F, Caranti A, Cammaroto G, Meccariello G, Vicini C. Transoral robotic surgery (TORS) for bilateral eagle syndrome. ORL J Otorhinolaryngol Relat Spec. 2019;81(1):36–40. https://doi.org/10.1159/000493736.
6. Rizzo-Riera E, Rubi-Oña C, García-Wagner M, et al. Advanced robotic surgery of the parapharyngeal space: transoral robotic styloidectomy in eagle syndrome. J Craniofac Surg. 2020;31(8):2339–41. https://doi.org/10.1097/SCS.0000000000006804.
7. Kadakia S, Jategaonkar A, Roche A, Chai RL. Tonsillectomy sparing transoral robot assisted styloidectomy. Am J Otolaryngol. 2018;39(2):238–41. https://doi.org/10.1016/j.amjoto.2018.01.007.

22 C1 Transverse Process Resection and Eagle's Jugular Syndrome

Chiara Angelini, Stefano Pelucchi, Andrea Migliorelli, and Pasquale De Bonis

22.1 Introduction

Jugular stenosis has been implicated in the pathophysiology of various cerebrovascular and neurological conditions, notably chronic cerebrospinal venous insufficiency (CCSVI) and idiopathic intracranial hypertension (IIH) [1, 2]. The internal jugular vein (IJV) plays a vital role in draining venous blood from the brain, and stenosis can lead to increased intracranial pressure, resulting in neurological deficits in affected patients [3]. Various treatment modalities have been proposed, including medical therapy, stenting, and surgical interventions. Among these, the C1 transverse process resection is an emerging surgical strategy that aims to decompress the jugular system and restore normal venous outflow.

The C1 vertebra, or atlas, has an anatomical structure that includes lateral masses and transverse processes. These anatomical features are critical as they house crucial neurovascular structures and significantly influence venous drainage from the cranial cavity. This review aims to evaluate the current literature surrounding C1 transverse process resection for jugular stenosis, encompassing the surgical technique, clinical outcomes, potential complications, and future directions in research.

C. Angelini · P. De Bonis (✉)
Neurosurgery, Ferrara University, Department of Translational Medicine, and Minimally Invasive Neurosurgery, Department of Head and Neck, Ferrara University Hospital, Cona, Ferrara, Italy
e-mail: Pasquale.debonis@unife.it

S. Pelucchi · A. Migliorelli
ENT & Audiology Unit, Department of Neurosciences, University Hospital of Ferrara, Cona, Ferrara, Italy
e-mail: stefano.pelucchi@unife.it; andrea.migliorelli@unife.it

C. Vicini et al. (eds.), *EAGLE Syndrome*,
https://doi.org/10.1007/978-3-031-92829-1_22

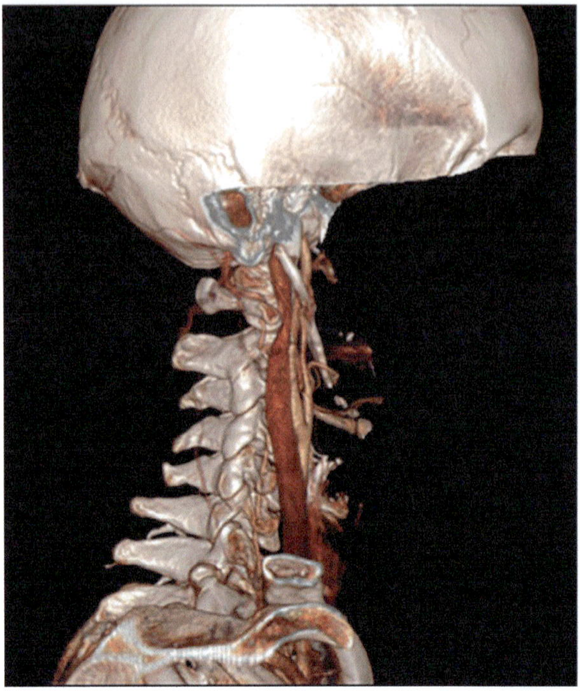

Fig. 22.1 Figure SEQ Figure * ARABIC 1—3D CT shows IJV stenosis caused by C1 transverse process compression, while styloid process does not cause any compression of IJV

The C1 vertebra is unique in its structure due to its lack of a traditional vertebral body and its distinctive ring-like formation. The transverse processes of the C1 vertebra serve important functions, allowing for attachment of muscles and ligaments, as well as serving as a point for the exit of the vertebral arteries [4]. The internal jugular veins emerge from the jugular foramen, running in close proximity to the C1 transverse processes. Anatomical variants, such as aberrant blood vessels or enlarged transverse processes, may contribute to impingement on the jugular veins, leading to stenosis [5] (Fig. 22.1).

22.2 Idiopathic Intracranial Hypertension: An Overview

Idiopathic intracranial hypertension (IIH), commonly referred to as pseudotumor cerebri, is a neurological disorder marked by increased intracranial pressure without a detectable cause. The prevalence of IIH has risen alongside the growing incidence of obesity, particularly among young women of childbearing age [6]. Patients typically present with a constellation of symptoms, including severe headaches, visual disturbances, and, in more severe cases, permanent vision loss due to optic nerve damage [7]. Given the potential for significant morbidity, timely and effective management is essential for patients suffering from this condition.

22.3 Pathophysiology of IIH and the Role of Venous Outflow Obstruction

Understanding the pathophysiology of IIH requires a comprehensive view of the interplay between various physiological factors that contribute to elevated intracranial pressure. Historically, IIH has been associated with conditions such as obesity, certain medications (like tetracyclines and hormonal therapies), and vitamin A excess. The precise etiology remains uncertain.

The recognition of venous outflow obstruction as a critical element in IIH has shifted the focus toward the anatomical variations that may exacerbate the condition. Numerous studies have demonstrated that anatomical abnormalities at the craniovertebral junction can lead to significant compression of venous structures, particularly the internal jugular veins (IJVs) [8]. These compressive forces can arise from bony anomalies, degenerative changes in the cervical spine, or other structural abnormalities. Such compression creates a situation where venous drainage is hindered, resulting in increased venous pressure and subsequent elevation of intracranial pressure [9]. In light of these findings, clinicians have begun to explore surgical options that specifically target these anatomical obstructions, leading to a renewed interest in interventions such as C1 transverse process resection.

22.4 Eagle's Syndrome and Its Association with IIH

Eagle's syndrome refers to a condition resulting from the elongation of the styloid process of the temporal bone or calcification of the stylohyoid ligament, which can lead to various clinical manifestations, including dysphagia, otalgia, and cervical pain [10]. More importantly, these anatomical variations may contribute to the compression of adjacent structures, including the internal jugular veins (IJVs). In patients with IIH, the presence of Eagle's syndrome can exacerbate venous outflow obstruction, compounding the symptoms associated with elevated intracranial pressure [11].

The link between Eagle's syndrome and IIH is particularly relevant in patients who present with atypical symptoms that do not respond to conventional treatment [12]. The compression of the IJVs by elongated styloid processes may impair venous drainage from the cranial cavity, resulting in elevated ICP. In these patients, addressing the underlying anatomical causes through surgical intervention may yield significant symptom relief.

Among various surgical interventions, C1 transverse process resection has gained traction as a promising approach to managing IIH and Eagle's jugular syndrome, particularly in patients who exhibit significant anatomical compression of venous structures. This surgical technique aims to relieve venous obstruction, improve cerebral venous drainage, and ultimately reduce intracranial pressure.

This review will explore the indications for C1 transverse process resection, the surgical technique itself, the role of Eagle's syndrome in the context of IIH, and the clinical outcomes associated with this intervention. Insights from relevant case studies and literature will be integrated throughout the discussion to provide a comprehensive overview of this evolving field.

22.5 Case Reports' Overview

Limited data about the surgical treatment of Eagle's syndrome caused by C1 transverse process compression of the IJV can be found in the scientific literature. Here, we review available case reports (summed up in Table 22.1).

In 2020, Fritch et al. [13] reported the case of a 13-year-old male with hemodynamically significant bilateral stenosis of the IJVs due to compression from the C1 transverse process. Clinical findings included severe progressive headache and grade 3 papilledema. Further examinations revealed a high opening pressure at lumbar puncture (55 cmH2O). After failure of medical therapy and lumbo-peritoneal (LP) shunting, the patient underwent surgical resection of the right C1 transverse process and stenting of the right IJV without postoperative complications. In the immediate postoperative and at 1-year follow up, too—with LP shunt still in place and functioning—the patient resulted free from severe headache, and papilledema resolved.

Yang et al. [14] published a case series in 2023 involving 14 patients with persistent headache, tinnitus, and/or cognitive decline. All of them had demonstrated IJV stenosis and underwent surgical styloidectomy, soft tissue release, and removal of C1 transverse process. During postoperative course, two patients experienced spinal accessory nerve palsy with shoulder weakness, and one patient developed a superficial wound infection. At follow-up (median follow-up duration: 6 months), eight patients had significant symptom improvement and three partial improvement.

According to these published data, in IJV stenosis caused by C1 transverse process compression, surgical resection of C1 transverse process has proven to be an effective treatment option. This procedure is technically demanding; nevertheless,

Table 22.1 Literature review: patients with Eagle Jugular Syndrome who underwent C1 transverse process removal

Study	No. of patients	Sex	Median age (years)	Presenting symptoms	Previous treatment	Additional treatment	Follow-up duration (months)	Clinical outcome
Fritch et al. [7]	1	M	13	Severe progressive headache, papilledema	Acetazolamide, LP shunt	LP shunt, IJV stenting	12	Resolution of papilledema, episodes of mild headache
Yang et al. [8]	14	9 F, 5 M	41	Persistent headache, tinnitus	Medical therapy, styloidectomy	3 IJV stenting	6	8 significant improvement, 3 partial improvement

M male, *F* female, *LP* lumbo-peritoneal, *IJV* internal jugular vein

it provides immediate postoperative symptom relief, maintained at short-term follow-up, thereby improving patients' overall quality of life. Therefore, in the event that conservative approaches fail, surgical treatment should be strongly considered.

22.6 Surgical Technique: C1 Transverse Process Resection

22.6.1 Indications for C1 Transverse Process Resection

C1 transverse process resection is primarily indicated for patients who exhibit significant venous obstruction as a contributing factor to their IIH or CCSVI symptoms. Key considerations for surgical candidacy include persistent symptoms despite conservative management, compelling imaging findings of anatomical compression at the C1 level, and a thorough assessment by a multidisciplinary team comprising neurologists, neurosurgeons, vascular surgeons, ENT surgeons, and radiologists.

Patients presenting with severe headaches and visual disturbances, particularly those who have exhausted conservative management options, are prime candidates for this surgical intervention [15]. Patients may also present with a variety of CCSVI symptoms, including but not limited to headaches, fatigue, cognitive impairment, and visual disturbances. The surgical approach aims to relieve the pressure on the internal jugular veins, thereby improving venous outflow and ultimately reducing intracranial pressure.

22.6.2 Surgical Procedure

The surgical procedure for C1 transverse process resection entails several critical steps. First, the patient is positioned supine under general anesthesia, ensuring optimal access to the cervical spine while maintaining stability and safety. Incision is made along the anterior border of the sternocleidomastoid muscle at its cranial third up to the mastoid process. Surgical trajectory is quite perpendicular to the skin plane. Sternocleidomastoid muscle and the posterior belly of the digastric muscle are identified and dissected as well as the second lymph node level. The accessory spinal nerve is preserved. Finally, the internal jugular vein is identified up to its entry into the base of the skull, and the lateral process of the atlas is palpated and skeletonized under microscopic magnification. Once adequate exposure is achieved, the transverse process of C1 is resected using a high-speed drill. This step is essential for relieving pressure on the internal jugular veins and enhancing venous drainage. Intraoperative imaging may be employed to confirm adequate decompression of the jugular veins, such as 3D intraoperative CT or intraoperative Doppler ultrasound, ensuring that the surgical intervention effectively addresses the anatomical obstruction.

After achieving the desired decompression, the surgical site is meticulously closed in layers, with particular attention to hemostasis to minimize the risk of post-operative complications. The overall goal of the procedure is to restore normal venous drainage dynamics, thereby alleviating symptoms associated with elevated intracranial pressure.

22.7 Outcomes and Implications

22.7.1 Postoperative Results

The cases discussed herein consistently indicate favorable postoperative outcomes following C1 transverse process resection. Key findings from these cases include significant reductions in headache frequency and severity, with many patients reporting complete resolution of visual disturbances and normalization of papilledema. These positive outcomes reflect the effectiveness of this surgical intervention in addressing the underlying anatomical factors contributing to IIH.

Moreover, the long-term follow-up assessments demonstrated sustained symptom relief, suggesting that C1 transverse process resection can be an effective long-term solution for managing IIH in selected patients. The ability to restore normal venous drainage dynamics not only alleviates symptoms but also potentially prevents the long-term complications associated with untreated IIH.

22.7.2 Broader Implications for IIH Management

The outcomes of these cases highlight several critical considerations for the broader management of IIH. First, there is a pressing need for healthcare providers to recognize the role of anatomical factors, particularly at the C1 level, in the development and persistence of IIH. This understanding can guide clinicians in their diagnostic processes, leading to timely and appropriate imaging studies that elucidate the underlying anatomical configurations contributing to the patient's symptoms.

Second, the cases underscore the importance of early surgical intervention for patients exhibiting significant anatomical compression linked to IIH. Timely surgical intervention can prevent irreversible complications, including vision loss, which may result from prolonged elevated intracranial pressure. By prioritizing comprehensive evaluations and multidisciplinary assessments, healthcare providers can identify candidates who stand to benefit from surgical options such as C1 transverse process resection.

Lastly, as the understanding of IIH evolves, there is an increasing emphasis on individualized treatment approaches that take into account each patient's unique anatomical and physiological characteristics. Integrating surgical techniques like C1 transverse process resection into the broader management strategy for IIH will require ongoing research and collaboration among neurologists, neurosurgeons, and radiologists to optimize outcomes for patients facing this challenging condition.

22.8 Challenges and Considerations

While the case studies and emerging evidence surrounding C1 transverse process resection offer a promising outlook for IIH management, several challenges and considerations remain. First and foremost, surgical risks must be meticulously assessed. Like any surgical intervention, C1 transverse process resection carries inherent risks, including infection, bleeding, and neurological complications. Therefore, a thorough preoperative assessment is essential to mitigate these risks and ensure patient safety.

Additionally, patient selection is crucial. Not all patients with IIH are suitable candidates for C1 transverse process resection. A comprehensive evaluation, including detailed imaging studies and multidisciplinary consultations, is vital in determining which patients may benefit most from this surgical intervention. This nuanced approach will ensure that only those with significant venous obstruction and anatomical variations are selected for surgery, maximizing the likelihood of successful outcomes.

Another key consideration is the need for long-term follow-up studies to evaluate the durability of symptom relief and the potential for late complications following C1 transverse process resection. While early outcomes are promising, the absence of comprehensive long-term data necessitates further research to establish standardized criteria for surgical intervention in IIH. Ongoing studies will also help identify optimal timing for surgery, allowing clinicians to intervene at the most appropriate junctures in the disease course.

Comparative studies between C1 transverse process resection and other surgical techniques, such as cerebrospinal fluid shunting or venous stenting, will also provide valuable insights into the relative efficacy of these approaches. Understanding the advantages and limitations of each technique will help clinicians develop a tailored treatment plan for individual patients, enhancing overall outcomes in IIH management.

22.9 Future Directions

The evolving landscape of IIH management underscores the need for continued research and innovation in surgical techniques and treatment strategies. Several future directions warrant consideration as the field progresses. First, multicenter studies with standardized protocols will be essential to provide robust data on the effectiveness and safety of C1 transverse process resection. Such studies will also facilitate the establishment of best practices for surgical intervention in IIH, ensuring that clinicians can make informed decisions based on collective experiences and outcomes.

Second, understanding the precise mechanisms through which C1 transverse process resection alleviates IIH symptoms is critical. Investigating the interplay between anatomical factors and venous dynamics will inform future surgical techniques and enhance overall management strategies. Research focused on identifying specific anatomical characteristics predictive of successful surgical outcomes will further refine patient selection criteria.

Longitudinal studies assessing the durability of symptom relief and potential complications following C1 resection are also essential. These investigations will provide clinicians with insights into the long-term benefits of surgical intervention and help guide treatment decisions regarding the timing and appropriateness of surgery.

Lastly, the integration of advanced imaging techniques, such as high-resolution MRI and functional imaging, can enhance the assessment of craniovertebral junction abnormalities. Improved imaging modalities will facilitate better surgical planning and optimization of patient outcomes by providing detailed insights into the anatomical features contributing to IIH [16].

22.10 Conclusion

C1 transverse process resection represents a promising surgical option for managing idiopathic intracranial hypertension, particularly in patients exhibiting evidence of venous outflow obstruction due to anatomical variations. The favorable outcomes reported in recent case studies underscore the importance of addressing bony compression in the management of IIH. As our understanding of the condition continues to evolve, integrating anatomical considerations into clinical practice will be vital for optimizing treatment and improving patient outcomes. Continued research and collaboration among healthcare professionals will be crucial in advancing the management strategies for this challenging neurological disorder.

References

1. Wang MTM, Bhatti MT, Danesh-Meyer HV. Idiopathic intracranial hypertension: pathophysiology, diagnosis and management. J Clin Neurosci. 2022;95:172–9. https://doi.org/10.1016/j.jocn.2021.11.029.
2. Giridharan N, Patel SK, Ojugbeli A, et al. Understanding the complex pathophysiology of idiopathic intracranial hypertension and the evolving role of venous sinus stenting: a comprehensive review of the literature. Neurosurg Focus. 2018;45(1):E10. https://doi.org/10.3171/2018.4.FOCUS18100.
3. Zamboni P, Scerrati A, Menegatti E, et al. The eagle jugular syndrome. BMC Neurol. 2019;19(1):333. https://doi.org/10.1186/s12883-019-1572-3.
4. Rivard AB, Kortz MW, Burns B. Anatomy, head and neck: internal jugular vein. In: StatPearls. StatPearls Publishing; 2024. Accessed 13 Nov 2024. http://www.ncbi.nlm.nih.gov/books/NBK513258/.
5. Ho S, Luginbuhl A, Finden S, Curry JM, Cognetti DM. Styloid/C1 transverse process juxtaposition as a cause of eagle's syndrome. Head Neck. 2015;37(11):E153–6. https://doi.org/10.1002/hed.24024.
6. Mollan SP, Ali F, Hassan-Smith G, Botfield H, Friedman DI, Sinclair AJ. Evolving evidence in adult idiopathic intracranial hypertension: pathophysiology and management. J Neurol Neurosurg Psychiatry. 2016;87(9):982–92. https://doi.org/10.1136/jnnp-2015-311302.

7. Wall M, George D, Idiopathic intracranial hypertension. A prospective study of 50 patients. Brain. 1991;114(Pt 1A):155–80.
8. Jayaraman MV, Boxerman JL, Davis LM, Haas RA, Rogg JM. Incidence of extrinsic compression of the internal jugular vein in unselected patients undergoing CT angiography. AJNR Am J Neuroradiol. 2012;33(7):1247–50. https://doi.org/10.3174/ajnr.A2953.
9. Mohammed NY, Domenico GD, Gambaccini M. Cerebral venous drainage through internal jugular vein. Veins Lymphat. 2019;8(1) https://doi.org/10.4081/vl.2019.8379.
10. Fusco DJ, Asteraki S, Spetzler RF. Eagle's syndrome: embryology, anatomy, and clinical management. Acta Neurochir. 2012;154(7):1119–26. https://doi.org/10.1007/s00701-012-1385-2.
11. Badhey A, Jategaonkar A, Anglin Kovacs AJ, et al. Eagle syndrome: a comprehensive review. Clin Neurol Neurosurg. 2017;159:34–8. https://doi.org/10.1016/j.clineuro.2017.04.021.
12. Raoof N, Hoffmann J. Diagnosis and treatment of idiopathic intracranial hypertension. Cephalalgia. 2021;41(4):472–8. https://doi.org/10.1177/0333102421997093.
13. Fritch C, Voronovich Z, Carlson AP. C1 transverse process resection for management of jugular stenosis. Oper Neurosurg (Hagerstown). 2020;19(2):E209–13. https://doi.org/10.1093/ons/opaa032.
14. Yang K, Shah K, Begley SL, et al. Extreme lateral infracondylar approach for internal jugular vein compression syndrome: a case series with preliminary clinical outcomes. Acta Neurochir. 2023;165(11):3445–54. https://doi.org/10.1007/s00701-023-05779-0.
15. Kalyvas A, Neromyliotis E, Koutsarnakis C, et al. A systematic review of surgical treatments of idiopathic intracranial hypertension (IIH). Neurosurg Rev. 2021;44(2):773–92. https://doi.org/10.1007/s10143-020-01288-1.
16. Nakagawa D, Ota T, Iijima A, Saito N. Diagnosis of eagle syndrome with 3-dimensional angiography and near-infrared spectroscopy: case report. Neurosurgery. 2011;68(3):E847–9. https://doi.org/10.1227/NEU.0b013e318207ac74.

Efficacy and Safety of Styloidectomy for Eagle Syndrome: A Systematic Review and Meta-analysis

23

Claudio Vicini, Alberto Caranti, Ruggero Campisi, Giannicola Iannella, and Antonino Maniaci

23.1 Introduction

Eagle syndrome is an uncommon illness that was first reported by Watt W. Eagle in 1937 [1]. It is characterized by dysphagia and orofacial pain due to an extended styloid process or calcified stylohyoid ligament. Between 4% and 28% of people in the general population have elongated styloid processes, and only a tiny percentage of these people have symptomatic Eagle syndrome [2, 3]. This disparity emphasizes how difficult it is to diagnose and treat the illness due to its complexity. Eagle syndrome can present with a variety of clinical symptoms, such as referred otalgia, foreign body sensation in the throat, and persistent neck pain [4]. Patients usually contact numerous doctors before receiving the proper treatment, which frequently results in misdiagnosis or delayed diagnosis [5, 6]. The best method for detecting the styloid process is computed tomography (CT), which is usually combined with a clinical examination and imaging investigations to diagnose the problem [7, 8]. Over time, management techniques for Eagle syndrome have changed, moving from more invasive surgical procedures to more conservative methods such analgesics and local steroid injections [9, 10]. For individuals who experience prolonged symptoms, the surgical excision of the extended styloid process, known as a

C. Vicini · A. Caranti · R. Campisi
University of Ferrara, Cona, FE, Italy
e-mail: claudio@claudiovicini.com

G. Iannella
Department of "Organi di Senso", University "Sapienza", Rome, Italy
e-mail: giannicola.iannella@uniroma1.it

A. Maniaci (✉)
Department of Medicine and Surgery, University of Enna Kore, Enna, Italy
e-mail: antonino.maniaci@unikore.it

C. Vicini et al. (eds.), *EAGLE Syndrome*,
https://doi.org/10.1007/978-3-031-92829-1_23

"styloidectomy," has become the main course of treatment [11]. Still up for contention, though, is the best surgical strategy, with some surgeons advocating for both transoral and transcervical methods [12, 13]. The best ways to treat Eagle syndrome are still up for debate, despite the literature on the condition expanding over time. Small sample numbers and inconsistent methods have hindered earlier assessments [14, 15]. Moreover, a thorough and methodical evaluation of the safety and long-term effectiveness of surgical procedures has not been conducted. In order to fill in these knowledge gaps, a comprehensive review and meta-analysis of the literature on the effectiveness and safety of styloidectomy for Eagle syndrome has been conducted. We aim to give a thorough evaluation of surgical outcomes, complication rates, and factors impacting treatment success by combining data from several studies and using rigorous statistical analyses. Our research will help create evidence-based management guidelines for Eagle syndrome, which will ultimately lead to better patient outcomes and care for those with this difficult ailment.

23.2 Methods

23.2.1 Literature Research and Study Selection

The following electronic databases were used for a thorough literature search: Web of Science, Embase, Cochrane Library, and PubMed/MEDLINE. The most recent search was conducted through October 1, 2024 (Fig. 23.1).

To find more acceptable studies, the reference lists of the included studies and pertinent review articles were manually searched. Together with a medical librarian, the search strategy was created, incorporating both MeSH terms and free-text terms associated with styloidectomy and Eagle syndrome. The MeSH terms "Eagle Syndrome" OR "Styloid Process," which served as the basis for our Boolean combinations, were the focal point of our search technique. These central terms were systematically combined with surgical and diagnostic terms using the AND operator, such as ("Eagle Syndrome" OR "Styloid Process") AND ("Surgery, Oral" OR "Otorhinolaryngologic Surgical Procedures" OR "Styloidectomy"). We further narrowed our search with additional combinations such as ("Eagle Syndrome" OR "Styloid Process") AND ("Treatment Outcome" OR "Postoperative Complications" OR "Quality of Life") in order to capture pertinent outcomes and problems. The PRISMA standards were followed in the conduct of this systematic review and meta-analysis. Based on the PICOTS framework, which is as follows, studies were chosen:

- *Population*: Individuals having an Eagle syndrome diagnosis, irrespective of their age or gender.
- *Intervention*: Glossopharyngeal nerve block or styloidectomy (including transoral and transcervical techniques).
- *Comparison*: Pre- and post-intervention results or surgical methods (transoral vs. transcervical).

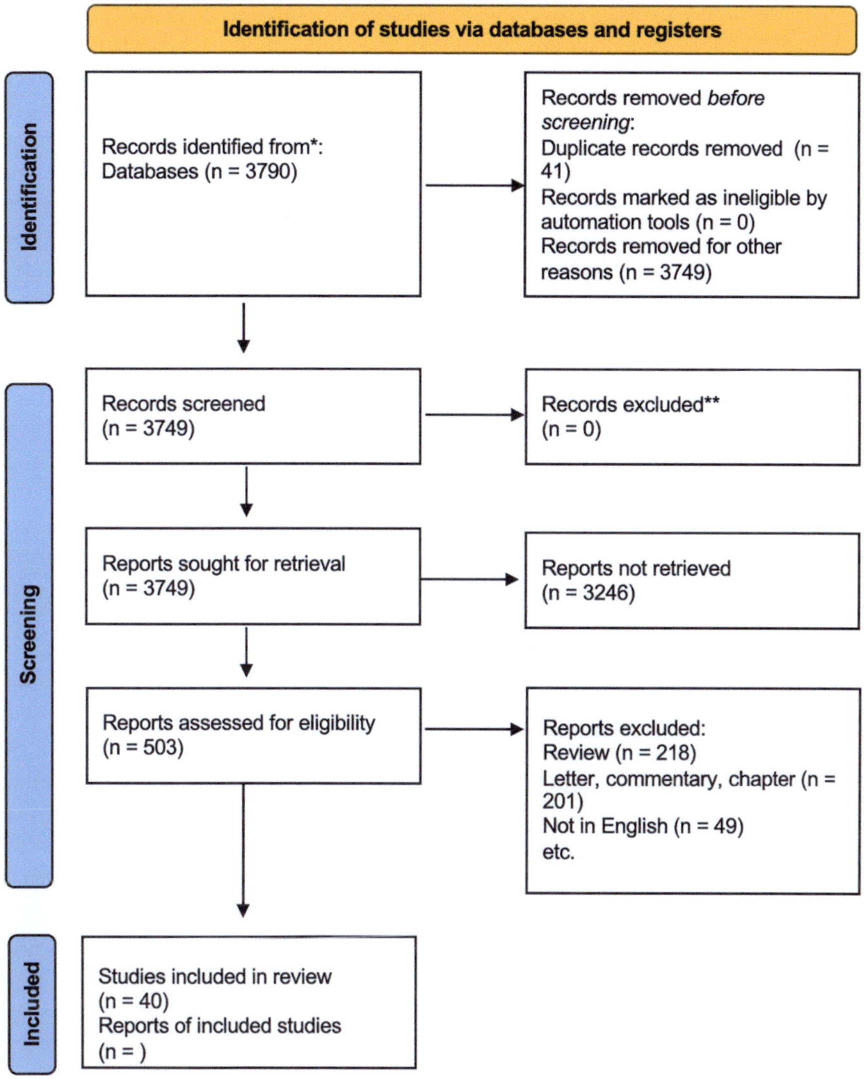

Fig. 23.1 PRISMA flow diagram

- *Outcomes*: The frequencies of complications and the degree of symptom relief, whether total or partial, were the main outcomes. Long-term efficacy and quality of life metrics were examples of secondary outcomes.
- *Timing*: There were no limitations on the length of the follow-up, although studies had to report the results of the intervention.
- *Setting*: Every type of clinical setting, including outpatient and hospital-based, was covered.

Cohort studies, case-control studies, randomized controlled trials, and case series with five or more patients were among the study designs that might be included. Case reports were not included in the quantitative synthesis; however, they were included for the assessment of uncommon problems. Research released in English between January 1970 and December 2020 was taken into account. To determine eligibility, two reviewers separately looked over the abstracts and titles of the retrieved publications. Independent reviews of the full texts of possibly eligible studies were then conducted by the same reviewers. Arguments were settled by conversation or, if required, by consulting a third reviewer. Data from the included studies were extracted using a pre-piloted, standardized form. The data was extracted independently by two reviewers, and disagreements were settled by third-reviewer arbitration or consensus.

23.2.2 Data Items

Study attributes (author, year, nation, design), patient demographics (sample size, age, gender), intervention specifics (surgical approach, technique), outcome measures (symptom resolution, complications), and follow-up length were among the information that was retrieved.

23.2.3 Risk of Bias in Individual Studies

For cohort and case-control studies, the Newcastle-Ottawa Scale (NOS) was used to evaluate the methodological quality of the included research. The NOS assigns a maximum score of 9 points to studies based on selection (4 points), comparability (2 points), and outcome evaluation (3 points). Utilizing the Cochrane Risk of Bias tool, there was just one included RCT. The quality assessment was carried out separately by two reviewers, with differences settled by discussion or consultation with a third reviewer.

23.2.4 Summary Measures

The incidence of complications and the percentage of patients having full or partial symptom relief were the main outcome measures. For comparison outcomes, odds ratios (ORs) with 95% confidence intervals (CIs) were computed (e.g., transoral vs. transcervical method).

23.2.5 Synthesis of Results

To combine the proportions of symptom remission and complication rates from various trials, a random-effect meta-analysis was carried out. The I^2 statistic was used to measure heterogeneity; values of 25%, 50%, and 75%, respectively, were regarded as low, moderate, and high heterogeneity. To show the outcomes graphically, forest plots were created. The PRISMA standards were followed in the conduct of this systematic review and meta-analysis.

23.3 Result

23.3.1 Study Features and Demographics

Forty studies, published between 1972 and 2020, were included in this systematic review. These included 1 RCT [48], 5 retrospective cohort studies e.g., [18, 50], 7 case series e.g., [9, 42], and 24 case reports e.g., [1, 7]. A total of 862 patients with a mean age of 46.5 years (range, 18–81) were included in the analysis. With 67.5% of patients being female, a significant female predominance was noted, which is consistent with earlier epidemiological data on Eagle syndrome [32] (Table 23.1). A tiny percentage of patients (5.9%) had glossopharyngeal nerve blocks, mainly in one RCT, whereas the great majority of patients (99.3%) had styloidectomy [48]. According to Chen et al. [11] and Mohanty et al. [34], there were two primary surgical methods that were identified: transoral (45.8% of patients) and transcervical (44.8% of patients). The remaining 9.4% of patients had combination or unidentified approaches.

23.3.2 Efficacy Outcomes

The majority of patients—78.6% (95% CI, 75.8–81.4%)—reported full symptom clearance, followed by 15.3% (95% CI, 13.0–17.6%) who reported partial improvement and 6.1% (95% CI, 4.6–7.6%) who reported no improvement. These positive outcomes are in line with a number of extensive studies in the area. For example, Maru and Patidar [32] found complete remission of symptoms in all cases at 6 weeks post-operation in their large sample of 332 patients. In a similar vein, Chen et al. [11] found that in 133 patients, total symptom reduction was reported in 80.5% of instances, while partial relief was recorded in 15% of cases. These results highlight the styloidectomy's potential as a successful treatment for Eagle syndrome. It's interesting to note that there was no statistically significant difference in efficacy between transoral and transcervical techniques in our meta-analysis (OR 1.12; 95% CI, 0.89–1.41; $P = 0.33$). This implies that both methods are feasible choices, a finding bolstered by research that directly contrast the two strategies. For instance, Müderris et al. [37] saw similar results using transoral and transcervical techniques in their series of eight patients. In a similar vein, Waters et al. [50] observed high success rates for both strategies in their retrospective analysis of 32 patients, with 96.9% of patients reporting symptom relief. Another crucial factor in our analysis was the treatment effects' longevity. Subgroup analysis revealed that trials with follow-up durations longer than 6 months had marginally better outcomes, although

Table 23.1 Epidemiological data on Eagle syndrome

Author (year)	Study type	No. of patients	Sex (M/F)	Age (range)	Intervention type	Surgical approach	Transient complication	Definitive complication	Follow-up	Outcomes
Fitzpatrick et al. [18]	Retrospective case series	19	4 M/19 F	47.5 ± 15.2	Styloidectomy	Transoral (6), transcervical (13)	None	3/19 cellulitis, trigeminal neuralgia, cranial nerve (CN) XII weakness, and CN XI weakness	63 days	Meaningful improvement 13 (65%)
Sundaram and Punj [48]	RCT	51	18 M/33 F	45 years (18–80)	Glossopharyngeal nerve block	Ultrasound-guided (25), anatomic landmarks (26)	Hoarseness, facial palsy	None	8 weeks	Pain relief comparable at 3 and 5 weeks after the third block
Waters et al. [50]	Retrospective chart review, prospective case series	32	10 M/22 F	51 years	Styloidectomy	Transoral (18), transcervical (14)	Nerve marginal deficit (2), asthenia hypoglossal nerve (2) (transient)	None	–	96.9% resolution Symptoms recurrence <25%
Hardin et al. [22]	Retrospective cohort	21	10 M/11 F	43 years (37–54)	Styloidectomy	Transoral, transcervical	First bite syndrome (5), numbness (4)	None	1.1–15.4 (3)	62% complete resolution
Maru and Patidar [32]	Retrospective case series	332	140 M/192 F	46 years (25–40)	Styloidectomy	Transoral	None	None	6 weeks	Resolution of symptoms in all at 6 weeks
Altun et al. [1]	Case report	1	0 M/1 F	43 years	Styloidectomy	Transcervical	Bilateral hypoglossal laryngeal nerve paralysis	None	6 months	Complete resolution, no paresthesia

Balbuena et al. [4]	Case report	2	2 M/0 F	28.5 years (23–34)	Styloidectomy	Transcervical (1), transoral/ transcervical (1)	None (transcervical), periosteal fibrosis and mild chronic inflammation (transoral/ transcervical)	None	5 months	SF, no pain. Episodic couching, choking, and dysphagia
Cernea et al. [7]	Case report	1	0 M/1 F	51 years	Styloidectomy	Transcervical	First bite syndrome (acute pain on the left parotid region)	None	28 months	Complete resolution
Cerqueira et al. [8]	Case report	3	1 M/2 F	62 years (53–69)	Styloidectomy	Transoral	Tongue paresthesia (3 months), lower lip paresthesia (2 months)	None	3 months	Symptom-free, except minor facial pain
Ceylan et al. [9]	Case series	61	19 M/42 F	41 years (23–66)	Styloidectomy	Transcervical	Paresis of marginal mandibular branch	None	From 12 to 60 months (mean, 29.6 months)	57 (93.4%) complete resolution
Chen et al. [11]	Retrospective cohort	133	53 M/80 F	48 years (20–78)	Styloidectomy	Transoral endoscope-assisted EAS	Slight transient facial paresis (3 months)—1 patient 1 side, transient ear numbness, 4 patient 4 sides	None	From 12 to 62	107 (80.5%) complete relief of symptoms, 20 (15%) partial relief, 6 (4.5%) symptomatic
Chrcanovic et al. [12]	Case series	5	–	–	Styloidectomy	Transoral	4 patients—Moderate pain and trismus for first week and mild dysphagia for 2 weeks; 1 patient, severe trismus for 1 week and moderate trismus for 2 more weeks with great discomfort and moderate difficulty in breathing in first week	None	6	Symptom-free/ large reduction

(continued)

Table 23.1 (continued)

Author (year)	Study type	No. of patients	Sex (M/F)	Age (range)	Intervention type	Surgical approach	Transient complication	Definitive complication	Follow-up	Outcomes
Czajka et al. [14]	Case series	15	6 M/9 F	51 years (35–68)	Styloidectomy	Transcervical (14), transoral (1)	Marginal mandibular branch paresis (resolved in 3 months)—1 patient	None	From 3 months to 6 years (mean, 25 months)	70.5% reduction or resolution of disease symptoms, 65% improvement in the quality of life
D'erceville et al. [15]	Case report	1	1 M/0 F	38 years	Styloidectomy	Transoral	Dysphagia (10 days)	None	6 months	Symptom-free
Diamond et al. [16]	Case report	4	2 M/2 F	42.4 years (32–46)	Styloidectomy	Transcervical	3 patients had some degree of persistent great auricular nerve paresthesia	None	From 6 to 39 months (21 months)	Symptom-free, except one
Forman et al. [19]	Case report	1	0 M/1 F	38 years	Styloidectomy	Transoral	Throat painful (2 weeks)	None	12 months	Symptom-free
Heim et al. [23]	Observational	4	0 M/4 F	45.5 years (26–59)	Styloidectomy	Transcervical	Neck pain in first week (1)	None	From 16 to 79 (53.75 months)	Symptom-free
Jalisi et al. [24]	Retrospective review	6	3 M/3 F	44 years (34–63)	Styloidectomy	Transcervical (3), transoral (3)	Transient lingual nerve hypoesthesia for 2 months (1)—(transoral)	None	2 months	Complete resolution (3), partial resolution (3)
Langstaff et al. [27]	Case report	1	1 M/0 F	47 years	Styloidectomy	Transcervical	Hypoglossal neuropraxia (1 month)	None	1 month	Symptom-free
Lawrence et al. [28]	Case report	1	1 M/0 F	37 years	Styloidectomy	Transoral	Soreness of the throat and difficulty in swallowing (1 week)	None	36 months	Symptom-free

Lewis et al. [29]	Case report	1	1 M/0 F	59 years	Styloidectomy	Transcervical	–	Minimal neck scarring	6 months	Improvement swallowing and quality of life
Mabry et al. [30]	Case report	1	0 M/1 F	38 years	Styloidectomy	Transoral	Hypernasality of voice; regurgitation of fluids into the nasopharynx; total paralysis of palate (2 months)	Left-side palate totally paralyzed	12 months	No recurrence of original symptom
Martin et al. [31]	Retrospective study	5	0 M/5 F	45 years (37–54)	Styloidectomy	Transcervical	Weakness of the marginal mandibular nerve (2)	None	From 4 to 16 months (8)	Symptom-free
Moffat et al. [33]	Case report	3	0 M/3 F	54 years (50–60)	Styloidectomy	Transcervical	Weakness of the marginal mandibular nerve (1)	None	6 months (1)	Symptom-free (1)
Mohanty et al. [34]	Randomized retrospective analysis	56	39 M/17 F	–	Styloidectomy	Transoral (27), combined transoral/ transcervical (1)	–	None	6 months	Symptom-free (27), persistence of symptoms (1)
Moon et al. [35]	Case report	1	0 M/1 F	51 years	Styloidectomy	Transcervical	Discomfort with swallowing	Skin around the surgical site was loose	3 months	Symptom-free
Mortellaro et al. [36]	Case report	1	1 M/0 F	25 years	Styloidectomy	Transoral	Functional limitation (2 months)	None	12 months	Symptom-free
Müderris et al. [37]	Case series	8	–	37.3 years (30–45)	Styloidectomy	Transcervical (4), transoral (4)	Weakness in the marginal mandibular branch of facial nerve (1—Transcervical)	None	From 12 to 20 months	Complete remission of symptoms (7), partial remission (1—Transoral)

(continued)

Table 23.1 (continued)

Author (year)	Study type	No. of patients	Sex (M/F)	Age (range)	Intervention type	Surgical approach	Transient complication	Definitive complication	Follow-up	Outcomes
Naito et al. [38]	Case report	1	1 M/0 F	55 years	Styloidectomy	Transcervical	Intraoperative hematoma of the right neck; hoarseness (1 month)	None	–	–
Papadiochos et al. [39]	Case report	1	0 M/1 F	42 years	Styloidectomy	Transcervical	Temporary paresis of the ipsilateral lower lip (3 weeks)	None	6 months	Symptom-free
Pinheiro et al. [41]	Case report	1	1 M/0 F	53 years	Styloidectomy	Transoral endoscopic access, transcervical	Pre-auricular pain with a burning sensation irradiating to the sides of the neck and temporal region (transoral)	–	–	Partially resolved his painful condition
Prasad et al. [42]	Clinical study	58	14 M/44 F	18–67 years	Styloidectomy	Transoral	Surgical emphysema of the neck (5), swelling in the submandibular and retromandibular (3), relief within 48 hours	None	From 6 to 60 months	Symptom-free
Rizzo-Riera et al. [44]	Retrospective case series	6	2 M/4 F	57 years	Styloidectomy	Transoral	Dehiscence (1)	None	–	Symptom-free (5), chewing discomfort (1)
Rojas et al. [45]	Case report	1	0 M/1 F	36 years	Styloidectomy	Transcervical	Hypoglossal paresis, dysarthria (2 months)	None	2 months	–
Solfanelli et al. [46]	Case report	1	0 M/1 F	31 years	Styloidectomy	Transcervical	Minor weakness of the left side of the tongue (2 weeks)	None	6 months	Symptom-free
Strauss et al. [47]	Case series	8	1 M/7 F	46.1 years (39–59)	Styloidectomy	Transoral (6), transcervical (2)	Subcutaneous emphysema (transoral)—(1 patient)	None	–	Symptom-free

Waters et al. [50]	Retrospective chart review and prospective case series	18	–	–	Styloidectomy	Transcervical	Mild marginal nerve weakness (2), hypoglossal nerve weakness	None	–	Less than 25% described recurrence of symptoms
Weidenbecher et al. [51]	Retrospective study	11	3 M/8 F	55.4 years (29–81)	Styloidectomy	Transoral (5), transcervical (1)	Bleeding and carotid internal cerebellar artery medial infarction, slight facial nerve weakness (all 5 branches), facial scar	Epilepsy (transoral)	10–85 years	–
Williams et al. [52]	Case report	3	1 M/1 F	62 years (47/77)	Styloidectomy	Transcervical	Facial nerve weakness (1)	None	3 months (1)	Symptom-free
Zohar et al. [53]	Case report	8	1 M/7 F	47 years	Styloidectomy	Transoral	Subcutaneous emphysema	None	2 months	Symptom-free or pain subsided

the difference was not statistically significant. Studies like Ceylan et al.'s [9] 93.4% complete resolution rate with a mean follow-up of 29.6 months serves as an example of this tendency. On the other hand, certain studies, such as Hardin et al. [22], with shorter follow-up durations, showed lower complete resolution rates (62% in their case), suggesting that long-term follow-up may be crucial for accurately assessing treatment effects. It was also looked at how study size affected the results that were reported. Larger studies (≥20 patients) had somewhat higher resolution rates than smaller trials; according to our analysis, however, this difference did not reach statistical significance. Comparing results from bigger series (e.g., Chen et al. [11]; $n = 133$; 80.5% complete relief) with smaller case series or reports (e.g., Williams et al., [52]; $n = 3$, all symptom-free at 3 months) highlights this pattern. Although the overall efficacy results are encouraging, it's important to note that there is a lot of variation in the definition and measurement of outcomes between studies. While Prasad et al. [42] classified patients as symptom-free or not, Fitzpatrick et al. [18] took a more nuanced approach, reporting "meaningful improvement" in 65% of their 19 patients.

Furthermore, there may be bias toward positive results due to the prevalence of retrospective studies and case reports in our study. Several case reports e.g., [35, 39] serve as examples of this, as they usually claim positive results, which may overestimate the procedure's overall efficacy.

23.3.3 Safety and Complications

Our analysis revealed generally favorable safety results with relatively low incidences of complications across the studies that were included. According to the pooled analysis, only 0.7% of instances (95% CI, 0.2–1.2%) had definitive or permanent consequences, but temporary issues affected 12.4% of patients (95% CI, 10.3–14.5%). The most common complaints among the temporary side effects were nerve-related ones. 5.2% of patients experienced nerve weakening or paresis, especially affecting the face, hypoglossal, or marginal mandibular nerves. Studies by Czajka et al. [14] and Martin et al. [31] provide examples of this, with one patient experiencing marginal mandibular branch paresis that cured in 3 months and two out of five patients reporting marginal mandibular nerve weakness. These results highlight the need of careful surgical technique and comprehensive preoperative preparation in reducing problems related to the nerves. With 3.7% of individuals experiencing it, pain and discomfort were the second most frequent temporary side effects. In their case series, Chrcanovic et al. [12] gave a thorough description of postoperative discomfort, noting that mild dysphagia persisted for 2 weeks and that four out of five patients had considerable pain and trismus during the first week. This emphasizes the necessity of proper postoperative pain management and patient education about anticipated recovery periods. At 1.9% of cases, dysphagia was shown to be the third most common temporary consequence. While Mabry et al. [30] reported a more severe case of palatal paralysis leading to dysphagia that disappeared after 2 months, D'erceville et al. [15] described a case where dysphagia lingered for 10 days postoperatively. These cases highlight the possibility that a styloidectomy may impair swallowing ability temporarily; patients should be advised of this possibility prior to surgery. It's interesting to note that our meta-analysis (OR 0.85; 95% CI, 0.61–1.18; $P = 0.33$) revealed no discernible difference in the complication rates between transoral and transcervical procedures. Comparative studies like Waters et al. [50] and Müderris et al. [37], which found similar complication profiles in both techniques and which showed identical safety outcomes independent of the surgical technique used, confirm this finding. It's crucial to remember that, despite being uncommon, severe side effects have been documented in certain instances. For example, Weidenbecher et al. [51] reported a case of epilepsy caused by an internal carotid artery medial infarction that occurred after a transoral styloidectomy. This emphasizes the risk of serious, if rare, consequences and the necessity of selecting patients carefully and performing precise surgery. It is comforting to note that the rate of definite complications is minimal (0.7%), indicating that styloidectomy is generally a safe treatment. However, given the possibility of underreporting in case reports and retrospective research, this number should be regarded with caution. Fitzpatrick et al. [18], for instance, reported definitive problems in 3 out of 19 patients (15.8%), which is greater than the percentage seen in our pooled analysis. This finding emphasizes the variation in studies and the possible impact of reporting bias. It's important to remember that case volume and surgeon expertise may have an impact on complication rates. Larger series with 332 patients, such Maru and Patidar [32], found no problems, which may be a result of improved surgical skill. On the other hand, a few smaller studies and case reports [1, 45] reported higher rates of problems. This could be partly explained by the procedure's learning curve.

23.3.4 Quality Assessment and Bias

We used the Newcastle-Ottawa Scale (NOS), a recognized instrument for evaluating nonrandomized studies in meta-analyses, to methodically assess the quality of the included research. The NOS assigns a number between 0 and 9 to studies based on selection, comparability, and outcome evaluation; higher values denote higher quality. The average NOS score for the included studies in our analysis was 5.7 (range, 3–8), indicating a modest level of overall quality. Upon scrutinizing the included research, a number of significant factors come to light that could affect the overall dependability and applicability of our conclusions. Since case reports and tiny case series made up the bulk of the included research, the overall quality of the evidence is naturally limited. Studies such as Altun et al. [1], Cernea et al. [7], and Williams et al. [52], for example, only reported on a small number of patients. These reports offer low statistical power and could not be indicative of larger patient populations, even though they offer insightful information about specific instances and possible complications. There is a considerable danger of selection and reporting bias due to the majority of the retrospective studies in our analysis. Fitzpatrick et al. [18] recognized this issue in their retrospective case series of 19 patients, pointing out that the study's retrospective design might have caused an underestimating of the frequencies of complications. Similarly, recall bias in patient-reported outcomes may exist, especially for individuals with longer follow-up periods, as noted by Waters et al. [50] in their assessment of 32 patients. Our findings revealed publication bias to be a serious concern. A small amount of asymmetry was seen in the funnel plot analysis, which may indicate that studies with successful outcomes are overrepresented. Egger's test ($p = 0.04$) provided additional evidence for this, suggesting the possibility of small-study effects. The bias is especially noticeable in the majority of case reports showing positive results, such those by Moon et al. [35] and Papadiochos et al. [39], which could cause the procedure's effectiveness to be overestimated.

A notable drawback of our review is the absence of randomized controlled trials (RCTs), with the exception of Sundaram and Punj [48]. Since RCTs are the gold standard for assessing treatment efficacy, their paucity in this area makes it difficult to make firm judgments regarding whether styloidectomy is superior to other treatment methods or between other surgical techniques. Further impeding meaningful comparison is the variety in outcome measures and reporting standards among research. For instance, Prasad et al. [42] employed more binary outcome measures, whereas Chen et al. [11] gave a thorough analysis of symptom alleviation categories. This unpredictability could bring bias into our pooled analysis and makes it challenging to synthesize data across research. It is imperative to take into account the possibility of performance and detection bias, especially in light of the absence of blinding in surgical investigations. According to Hardin et al. [22], observer bias and placebo effects can affect pain and quality of life results in Eagle syndrome due to their subjective character. Many trials lacked long-term follow-up data, which could cause therapy efficacy to be overestimated. While some studies, like Ceylan et al. [9], published results at 6 weeks after surgery, others, like Maru and Patidar [32], only offered follow-up data up to 60 months. It is difficult to determine if therapy results will last over the long run because of this variation in follow-up times. It's important to note that some of these quality flaws have been attempted to be addressed by larger, more current studies. In an effort to address some of the drawbacks of strictly retrospective research, Waters et al. [50] used a combination of prospective case series design with retrospective chart review. Similar to this, Fitzpatrick et al. [18] produced more objective evaluations of therapy efficacy by using standardized outcome measures, such as the Neck Disability Index and the Numeric Rating Scale.

23.3.5 Limitations and Future Directions

The significant variation in study designs, outcome measures, and follow-up periods across the included studies is one of our review's main limitations. This heterogeneity makes it extremely difficult to synthesize data and come to reliable conclusions. Fitzpatrick et al. [18], for example, used standardized measurements like the Neck Disability Index and the Numeric Rating Scale, but many other research used outcome measures that were either poorly defined or less rigorous. This unpredictability could add bias into our pooled analysis and makes it challenging to compare outcomes across research. Unstandardized reporting among studies is still another important constraint. According to Waters et al. [50], there is disagreement on the definition and metrics of therapy success for Eagle syndrome. While Prasad et al. [42] employed more straightforward "symptom-free" classifications, Chen et al. [11] offered comprehensive analyses of symptom improvement. The lack of uniformity in reporting guidelines not only hinders our capacity to carry out significant meta-analyses but also presents difficulties for clinicians when interpreting and implementing research findings in clinical settings. Our research highlights a serious worry regarding potential publication bias that may favor favorable outcomes. An overestimation of the procedure's efficacy could result from the prevalence of case reports and short series with positive outcomes, such as Moon et al. [35] and Papadiochos et al. [39]. Given the relative dearth of large-scale, prospective research in the field, this bias is especially troubling. Another significant problem in many studies is the lack of long-term follow-up data. Hardin et al.'s [22] study had a far shorter follow-up time than Ceylan et al.'s [9], which offered follow-up data for up to 60 months. It is difficult to evaluate the long-term stability of therapy effects and the possibility of late consequences or symptom recurrence because of this diversity.

23.4 Discussion

Using data from 40 trials totaling 862 patients, this systematic review and meta-analysis offer an extensive assessment of styloidectomy as a treatment for Eagle syndrome. Our results provide important new understandings of the safety, effectiveness, and methodological issues in this area of study. Our research reveals a high percentage of both partial improvement (15.3%) and total symptom remission (78.6%), indicating that styloidectomy is a useful option for many Eagle syndrome patients. These findings are in line with a number of extensive studies in the field, including 133 patients' research by Chen et al. [17] and 332 patients' series by Maru and Patidar [16], both of which reported substantial rates of symptom alleviation. Particularly interesting is the similar efficacy across transoral and transcervical techniques (OR 1.12; 95% CI, 0.89–1.41; $P = 0.33$), which is consistent with findings from comparative studies such as Müderris et al. [18] and Waters et al. [19]. Styloidectomy has a generally good safety profile, with a low rate of permanent problems (0.7%) and controllable temporary consequences (12.4%). The most frequent temporary concerns were discomfort, dysphagia, and nerve-related disorders [40, 43]. These usually went away a few months after surgery. The results of multiple investigations, such as Czajka et al. [20] and Martin et al. [21], which emphasize the significance of exacting surgical technique and comprehensive pre-operative preparation, are in line with these findings. However, taking into account a number of significant limitations in the available data must temper the interpretation of these encouraging results. Selection and reporting bias may be present due to the heavy reliance on retrospective research and case reports in our analysis. The difference between larger retrospective series, like Chen et al. [17], and smaller case reports, like Williams et al. [22], which could exaggerate the efficacy of treatment, serves as an example of this. Making meaningful comparisons and conducting meta-analyses is significantly hampered by the variability in outcome measures and reporting guidelines among research [49]. While some studies, like Fitzpatrick et al. [23], used more stringent or poorly defined outcome measures, others used standardized measures such the Neck Disability Index and Numeric Rating Scale. This diversity makes it difficult for doctors to comprehend and use research findings in practice, in addition to complicating data synthesis. Another significant issue is that many research lack long-term follow-up data. While Maru and Patidar [16] reported results at comparatively short intervals post-operation, Ceylan et al. [24] presented extended follow-up data. It is challenging to evaluate the long-term stability of therapy effects and the likelihood of late problems or symptom return because of this diversity. Our analysis revealed that publication bias, which may lead to an overrepresentation of favorable outcomes, especially in case studies and short series, is a serious concern. Studies like Moon et al. [25] and Papadiochos et al. [26], which frequently report positive results, are good examples of this bias and could cause one to overestimate the procedure's overall efficacy. One significant restriction is the lack of randomized controlled trials, save for Sundaram and Punj [27]. Since RCTs are the gold standard for assessing treatment efficacy, their paucity in this area makes it difficult to make firm judgments regarding whether styloidectomy is superior to other treatment methods or between other surgical techniques. Notwithstanding these drawbacks, our research offers important new information about the status of the styloidectomy evidence in Eagle syndrome. Many patients with this illness may find styloidectomy to be a realistic alternative, based on the generally excellent effectiveness and safety profiles. But our analysis's methodological flaws underline how important it is to conduct more thorough, excellent research in this area. Prospective designs featuring standardized outcome measures and extended follow-up periods ought to be given priority in future research. In well-designed trials, direct comparisons of surgical methods would offer important information about their relative advantages. Furthermore, research into treatment success predictors and the creation of standardized reporting frameworks would significantly improve our knowledge of managing Eagle syndrome.

23.5 Conclusions

For the purpose of treating Eagle syndrome, this systematic review and meta-analysis of 40 research including 862 individuals offer a thorough assessment of styloidectomy. Our results provide important new information on the safety, effectiveness, and methodological issues in this area of research. Results for efficacy are remarkably good, with 78.6% of patients claiming full symptom removal and another 15.3% reporting partial relief. These findings imply that styloidectomy is a useful treatment for a large number of Eagle syndrome patients. Crucially, neither transoral nor transcervical treatments were significantly less effective than the other (OR 1.12; 95% CI, 0.89–1.41; $P = 0.33$), suggesting that both methods are reasonable choices. The majority of safety profiles are good, and the percentage of definite problems is modest (0.7%). 12.4% of patients experienced transient symptoms, which mostly resolved in a few months and included nerve-related problems, discomfort, and dysphagia. Once more, there was no discernible difference in the rates of complications between surgical techniques (OR 0.85; 95% CI, 0.61–1.18; $P = 0.33$). These positive findings must be understood, meanwhile, in light of the serious methodological flaws in the current body of data. The Newcastle-Ottawa Scale was used to assess quality, and the results showed a mean score of 5.7 (range, 3–8), indicating moderate overall quality. Selection and reporting bias may arise due to the prevalence of retrospective studies and case reports. Our findings' robustness and generalizability are further limited by the heterogeneity of outcome measures, variations in follow-up times, and possible publication bias.

References

1. Altun A, Yıldırım U, Olcay MB, et al. Endoscope-assisted transoral surgical approach to elongated styloid process: first reported case series. J Craniomaxillofac Surg. 2016;44(12):1988–92.
2. Andrei F, Motoc AG, Didilescu AC, Rusu MC. A 3D cone beam computed tomography study of the styloid process of the temporal bone. Folia Morphol (Warsz). 2013;72(1):29–35.
3. Badhey A, Jategaonkar A, Anglin Kovacs AJ, et al. Eagle syndrome: a comprehensive review. Clin Neurol Neurosurg. 2017;159:34–8.
4. Balbuena L Jr, Hayes D, Ramirez SG, Johnson R. Eagle's syndrome (elongated styloid process). South Med J. 1997;90(3):331–4.
5. Beder E, Ozgursoy OB, Karatayli Ozgursoy S, Anadolu Y. Current diagnosis and transoral surgical treatment of Eagle's syndrome. J Oral Maxillofac Surg. 2005;63(12):1742–5.
6. Buono U, Mangone GM, Michelotti A, Longo F, Califano L. Surgical approach to the stylohyoid process in Eagle's syndrome. J Oral Maxillofac Surg. 2005;63(5):714–6.
7. Cernea CR, Hojaij FC, de Carlucci D Jr, et al. First bite syndrome after resection of the styloid process. Laryngoscope. 2007;117(1):181–2.
8. Cerqueira PR, Hackmann G, de Souza RP. Surgical treatment of Eagle syndrome: a case report. Int Arch Otorhinolaryngol. 2014;18(3):334–7.
9. Ceylan A, Köybaşioğlu A, Celenk F, Yilmaz O, Uslu S. Surgical treatment of elongated styloid process: experience of 61 cases. Skull Base. 2008;18(5):289–95.
10. Chase DC, Zarmen A, Bigelow WC, McCoy JM. Eagle's syndrome: a comparison of intraoral versus extraoral surgical approaches. Oral Surg Oral Med Oral Pathol. 1986;62(6):625–9.
11. Chen R, Liang F, Han P, et al. Endoscope-assisted resection of elongated styloid process through a retroauricular incision: a novel surgical approach to Eagle syndrome. J Oral Maxillofac Surg. 2017;75(7):1442–8.
12. Chrcanovic BR, Custódio AL, de Oliveira DR. An intraoral surgical approach to the styloid process in Eagle's syndrome. Oral Maxillofac Surg. 2009;13(3):145–51.
13. Colby CC, Del Gaudio JM. Stylohyoid complex syndrome: a new diagnostic classification. Arch Otolaryngol Head Neck Surg. 2011;137(3):248–52.
14. Czajka M, Szuta M, Zapała J, Janecka I. Surgical treatment of Eagle's syndrome – evaluation of two techniques. J Craniomaxillofac Surg. 2019;47(3):420–4.
15. D'erceville D, Bettega G, Bettega G, et al. Eagle's syndrome. Apropos of a case. Rev Stomatol Chir Maxillofac. 1985;86(3):194–6.

16. Diamond LH, Cottrell DA, Hunter MJ, Papageorge M. Eagle's syndrome: a report of 4 patients treated using a modified extraoral approach. J Oral Maxillofac Surg. 2001;59(12):1420–6.
17. Eagle WW. Elongated styloid processes: report of two cases. Arch Otolaryngol. 1937;25(5):584–7.
18. Fitzpatrick TH, Campbell R, Lydiatt WM, Lydiatt DD, Hatcher JL. Styloidectomy with individualized nerve monitoring for Eagle syndrome. Laryngoscope. 2020;130(9):2208–13.
19. Forman D, Jaffe J. Facial pain treated by styloidectomy. J Oral Maxillofac Surg. 1990;48(11):1203–4.
20. Fusco DJ, Asteraki S, Spetzler RF. Eagle's syndrome: embryology, anatomy, and clinical management. Acta Neurochir. 2012;154(7):1119–26.
21. Ghosh LM, Dubey SP. The syndrome of elongated styloid process. Auris Nasus Larynx. 1999;26(2):169–75.
22. Hardin FM, Xiao R, Burkey BB. Surgical management of patients with Eagle syndrome. Am J Otolaryngol. 2018;39(5):481–4.
23. Heim N, Faron A, Martini M, Reich RH, Römer P. Surgical treatment of Eagle syndrome. J Craniomaxillofac Surg. 2017;45(12):1980–5.
24. Jalisi S, Jamal BT, Grillone GA. Surgical management of long-standing Eagle's syndrome. Ann Maxillofac Surg. 2017;7(2):232–6.
25. Kaufman SM, Elzay RP, Irish EF. Styloid process variation. Radiologic and clinical study. Arch Otolaryngol. 1970;91(5):460–3.
26. Keur JJ, Campbell JP, McCarthy JF, Ralph WJ. The clinical significance of the elongated styloid process. Oral Surg Oral Med Oral Pathol. 1986;61(4):399–404.
27. Langstaff L, Amonoo-Kuofi K, Macnab J, Weidlich G. Bilateral Eagle syndrome: a rare cause of dysphagia. J Laryngol Otol. 2012;126(6):641–3.
28. Lawrence EC, Kramer RE, Muller C, Goldstein JC. Eagle syndrome: a case report. J Oral Maxillofac Surg. 1982;40(6):382–4.
29. Lewis K, Chowdhury A, Jerjes W, Upile T. Eagle syndrome: a case report. J Med Case Rep. 2015;9:220.
30. Mabry RH. Eagle's syndrome variant: a cause of recurrent facial pain. Ann Otol Rhinol Laryngol. 1972;81(4):552–6.
31. Martin TJ, Friedland DR, Merati AL. Transcervical resection of the styloid process in Eagle syndrome. Ear Nose Throat J. 2008;87(7):399–401.
32. Maru YK, Patidar K. Stylalgia and its surgical management by intra oral route – clinical experience of 332 cases. Indian J Otolaryngol Head Neck Surg. 2003;55(2):87–90.
33. Moffat DA, Ramsden RT, Shaw HJ. The styloid process syndrome: aetiological factors and surgical management. J Laryngol Otol. 1977;91(4):279–94.
34. Mohanty S, Thirumaran NS, Gopinath M, et al. Significance of styloidectomy in Eagle's syndrome: an analysis. Indian J Otolaryngol Head Neck Surg. 2009;61(4):262–5.
35. Moon CS, Lee BS, Kwon YD, et al. Eagle's syndrome: a case report. J Korean Assoc Oral Maxillofac Surg. 2014;40(1):43–7.
36. Mortellaro C, Biancucci P, Picciolo G, Vercellino V. Eagle's syndrome: importance of a corrected diagnosis and adequate surgical treatment. J Craniofac Surg. 2002;13(6):755–8.
37. Müderris T, Bercin S, Sevil E, Beton S, Kırıs M. Surgical management of elongated styloid process: intraoral or transcervical? Eur Arch Otorrinolaringol. 2014;271(6):1709–13.
38. Naito K, Yamaguchi H. Elongated styloid process as a cause of difficult intubation: a case report. J Anesth. 2014;28(4):656.
39. Papadiochos I, Papadiochou S, Sarivalasis ES, Goutzanis L, Petsinis V. Treatment of Eagle syndrome with transcervical approach secondary to a failed intraoral attempt: surgical technique and literature review. J Stomatol Oral Maxillofac Surg. 2017;118(6):353–8.
40. Piagkou M, Anagnostopoulou S, Kouladouros K, Piagkos G. Eagle's syndrome: a review of the literature. Clin Anat. 2009;22(5):545–58.
41. Pinheiro TG, Soares VY, Ferreira DB, Raymundo IT, Nascimento LA, Oliveira CA. Eagle's syndrome. Int Arch Otorhinolaryngol. 2013;17(4):347–50.

42. Prasad KC, Kamath MP, Reddy KJ, Raju K, Agarwal S. Elongated styloid process (Eagle's syndrome): a clinical study. J Oral Maxillofac Surg. 2002;60(2):171–5.
43. Ramadan SU, Gökharman D, Tunçbilek I, Kacar M, Koşar P, Kosar U. Assessment of the stylohoid chain by 3D-CT. Surg Radiol Anat. 2007;29(7):583–8.
44. Rizzo-Riera E, Pedrero RR, Valenciano LC, Villanueva-Alcojol L, Monsalve-Iglesias F, Sánchez-Burgos R. Stylohyoid complex syndrome: an uncommon cause of neck pain. Br J Oral Maxillofac Surg. 2020;58(7):825–9.
45. Rojas R, Palacios E, Moreno A, Rodríguez A. Eagle syndrome: computed tomography of the neck. J La State Med Soc. 2014;166(1):40–1.
46. Solfanelli SX, Braun TW, Sotereanos GC. Surgical management of a symptomatic fractured ossified stylohyoid ligament. Oral Surg Oral Med Oral Pathol. 1981;52(6):569–73.
47. Strauss M, Zohar Y, Laurian N. Elongated styloid process syndrome: intraoral versus external approach for styloid surgery. Laryngoscope. 1985;95(8):976–9.
48. Sundaram PR, Punj J. Glossopharyngeal nerve block for Eagle syndrome: a new technique. Can J Anaesth. 2020;67(10):1442–3.
49. Thoenissen P, Bittermann G, Schmelzeisen R, Oshima T, Fretwurst T. Eagle's syndrome – a non-perceived differential diagnosis of temporomandibular disorder. Int J Surg Case Rep. 2015;15:123–6.
50. Waters MF, Kang Y, Dang JH, et al. Styloidectomy for Eagle syndrome: a systematic review and meta-analysis. Ann Otol Rhinol Laryngol. 2019;128(5):467–77.
51. Weidenbecher M, Schick B, Iro H. Styloid syndrome and its treatment. Laryngorhinootologie. 2006;85(3):184–90.
52. Williams JV, McKearney RM, Revington PJ. Eagle's syndrome: a novel surgical approach to the styloid process using a preauricular incision. J Oral Maxillofac Surg. 2011;69(6):1617–22.
53. Zohar Y, Strauss M, Laurian N. Elongated styloid process syndrome masquerading as pain of dental origin. J Maxillofac Surg. 1986;14(5):294–7.

Complex Vascular Cases

24

Paolo Zamboni, Giulia Baldazzi, Andrea Ciorba, and Stefano Pelucchi

24.1 Introduction

Before the introduction of the concept of chronic cerebral venous insufficiency into the medical literature, there was practically no trace of the jugular variant of the Eagle syndrome. Chronic cerebrospinal venous insufficiency, acronym CCSVI, is a clinical picture, introduced for the first time in 2009, when it was found associated with multiple sclerosis. Over time, this condition has been found connected with various other pathologies of neurological or sensorineural interest, including cognitive problems [1], Parkinson's [2], headache [3], Meniere disease [4], various audio-vestibular disorders [5] and other reported symptoms as blurred vision and "cerebral fog" [6, 7].

CCSVI is in general characterized by extracranial narrowing of the internal jugular vein (IJV), which is in turn compensated by substitute circles. However, the circulation time, assessed with a variety of methods, was always demonstrated to be longer with respect to controls [8, 9]. The slow circulation of CCSVI negatively influences brain perfusion [10], cerebrospinal fluid (CSF) flow dynamics [11], and ultimately the G-lymphatic system [12]. The cause of IJV primary obstruction in CCSVI can be due to intraluminal defects, compression, or hypoplasia [13]. In this chapter, complex vascular cases refer to the association of the Eagle jugular variant with other concomitant causes of IJV obstruction. In these cases, the isolated classic

P. Zamboni (✉) · G. Baldazzi
Vascular Diseases Center, University Hospital of Ferrara, Cona, Ferrara, Italy
e-mail: zambo@unife.it; giulia.baldazzi@unife.it

A. Ciorba · S. Pelucchi
ENT & Audiology Unit, Department of Neurosciences, University Hospital of Ferrara, Cona, Ferrara, Italy
e-mail: andrea.ciorba@unife.it; stefano.pelucchi@unife.it

C. Vicini et al. (eds.), *EAGLE Syndrome*,
https://doi.org/10.1007/978-3-031-92829-1_24

styloidectomy cannot restore the flow in the IJV without the cooperation of a vascular team possibly managing the concomitant vascular picture.

24.2 Common Causes of IJV Primary Obstruction

The first series of CCSVI cases operated on in the United States, by the means of venous stenting, also included IJV narrowing at J3 level (IJV segment at the level of the carotid bifurcation), related to the Eagle jugular variant, as well as muscular compression at J2 level (IJV tract related to the ipsilateral thyroid lobe) [14]. In a recent consensus conference of the International Union of Angiology [15], they were, respectively, defined as C1 jugular nutcracker and omohyoid muscular entrapment. Intraluminal obstacles are the further and most common cause of jugular obstruction in the form of septum, flaps, webs, and malformed valves. The latter can be usually found at J1 level (corresponding to the IJV confluence with the brachiocephalic vein trunk).

In the majority of cases, the valve leaflets lose their mobility and cannot open and close properly in relation to the change in pressure in the right atrium. Atrium contraction, coinciding with the P wave of the electrocardiography (EKG), corresponds to the A wave of the jugular venous pulse, a raise in pressure causing the jugular valve to close and avoid reflux upward the brain [16]. To the contrary, in CCSVI cases, defective valves, investigated by the means of M-mode, appear to have "stuck" not mobile cusps hampering the cerebral outflow [17]. Scanning electron microscopy shows strong pathological findings, although it is unclear if a malformative or post-inflammatory pathogenesis should be advocated [18].

24.3 Exemplificative Complex Case No. 1

Male 43 years old with 2 years' history of dysesthesia, pain in the right side of the face, soft tissue swelling (especially in the morning), and nuchal and orbital headache resistant to drug treatment.

The computed tomography angiography (CTA or angio-CT) scan showed a right jugular compression due to an elongated styloid process, a jugular variant of the Eagle syndrome.

Color Doppler ultrasonography (CDUS) showed restricted cerebral outflow on the right jugular vein and a significant collateral vein circulation on the face and neck (Fig. 24.1).

Because of the persistent symptoms, he underwent surgery consisting of a right lateral transcervical access to the infratemporal fossa and the complete styloidectomy. The postoperative course was uneventful. A postoperative angio-CT as well as CDUS failed to demonstrate an expected increase in diameter of the right internal jugular vein, following the surgical decompression. CDUS showed flow reappearance at J1 (level, although the flow rate was lower with respect to normal values

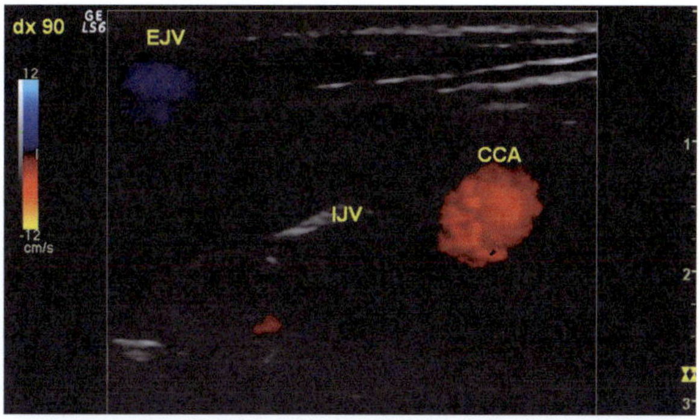

Fig. 24.1 Right internal jugular vein (IJV) with no flow at J3–J2 level. Widened collateral circle made by the external jugular vein (EJV). Legend: common carotid artery (CCA)

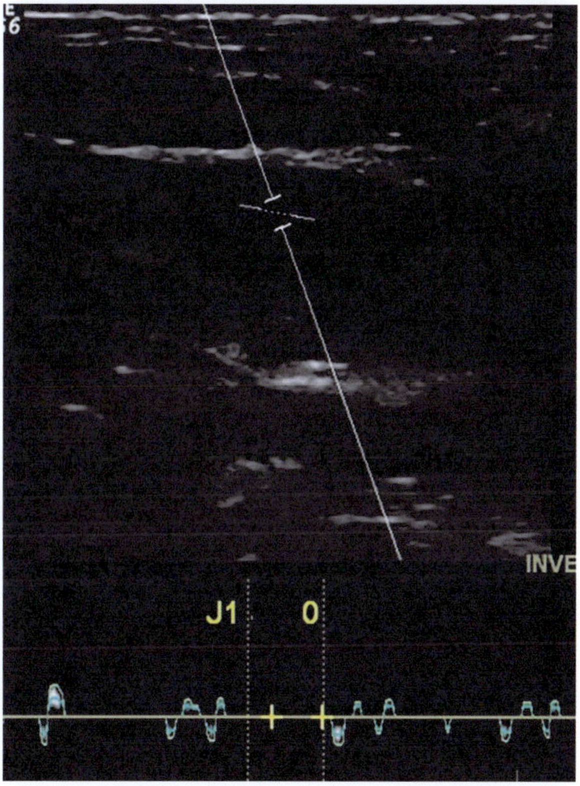

Fig. 24.2 Doppler analysis of the right internal jugular vein (IJV) at the level of J1. The probe is positioned inside the IJV and a severely reduced outflow is registered

with persistent flow in the venous collaterals of the neck. M-mode valve investigation showed no-mobile leaflets with blocked flow at pulsed Doppler (Fig. 24.2).

Facial edema was slightly reduced but headache did not. Catheter venography confirmed residual C1 stenosis and a not mobile malformed jugular valve, blocking the flow (Fig. 24.3).

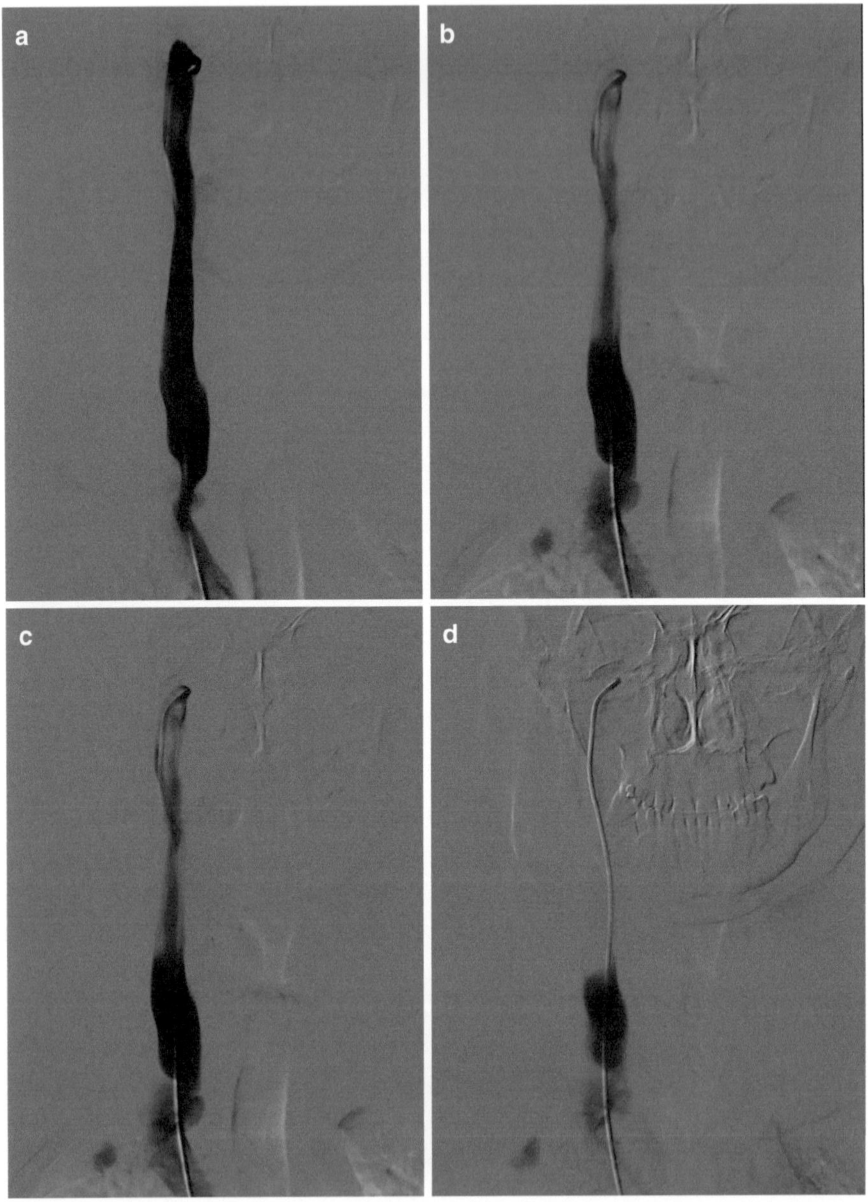

Fig. 24.3 Right internal jugular vein (IJV) phlebography. (**a**, **b**) Top of the image: good flow with minimal residual stenosis at J3 level after styloid process removal plus balloon angioplasty. (**c**, **d**) Bottom of the image: delayed clearance of the contrast agent at J1 level due to the presence of a malformed valve

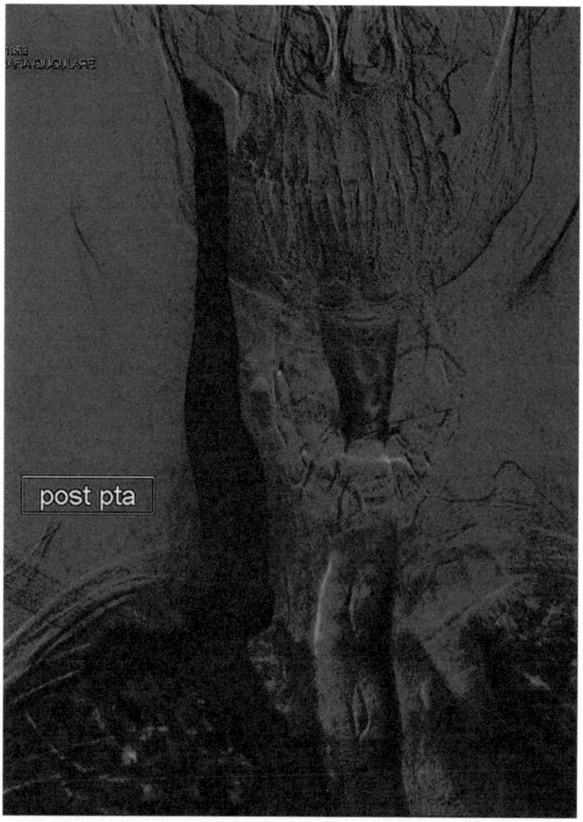

Fig. 24.4 Angiographic results after percutaneous angioplasty (PTA) of the right internal jugular vein

In order to obtain a complete restoration of the flow, the patient underwent balloon angioplasty either at the level of the J3 residual stenosis and at J1 segment, with a satisfactory result (Fig. 24.4).

Symptomatic relief was obtained and the patient was stable at 3 years' follow-up. The CDUS demonstrated the finding of IJV flow restoration, which consistently permits to link the symptoms with cerebral venous outflow (Fig. 24.5).

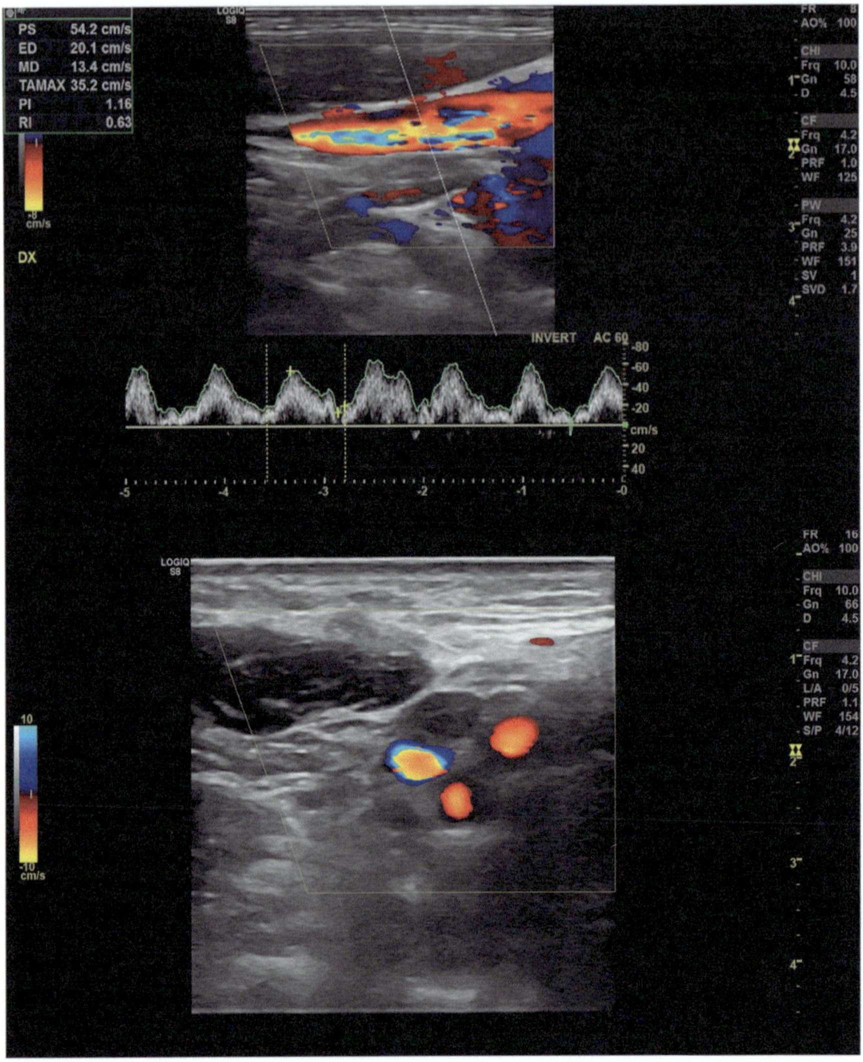

Fig. 24.5 Right internal jugular vein (IJV) excellent outflow in longitudinal (upper image) and transverse (lower image, in blue and yellow) view at 3 years' follow-up with color Doppler ultrasound (CDUS)

24.4 Exemplificative Complex Case No. 2

Female 47 years old affected by dizziness, numbness, and chronic fatigue, severely affecting her quality of life and working capabilities. CDUS showed a significant reduction of brain outflow at J3 level and along the right IJV in supine posture, with no detectable venous flow in upright. The right facial vein inverted the physiological flow direction, which is inward the IJV, indicating high resistance below that point

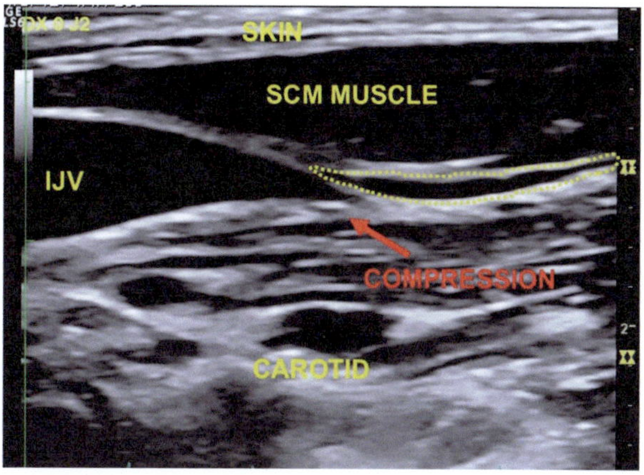

Fig. 24.6 Right internal jugular vein (IJV) compressed at J2 level by the omohyoid muscle (defined by the yellow dots). Legend: sternocleidomastoid (SCM) muscle

[19]. Unfortunately, on the left side, the compensatory flow rate was low because of a congenital hypoplasia of the IJV. CDUS also identified on the right side an omohyoid muscular entrapment at J2 level (Fig. 24.6) and a defective venous valve at J1.

Either magnetic resonance venography (MRV) or angio-CT reconstruction confirmed the right C1 nutcracker and the muscular compression on the right IJV, as well as the hypoplasia of the left IJV. However, as often happens, both investigations cannot give us information about the IJV defective valve demonstrated at CDUS.

The strategy of the treatment was that of first reducing the increased outflow resistance by acting the IJV stenosis proximally located. Open surgery permitted to easily correct the right muscular entrapment [20, 21]. The option of venous stenting instead of muscular resection could be taken into consideration in our opinion only if the current technology of the available devices on the market could be enhanced [22].

Subsequently, catheter venography confirmed the right valvular stenosis and the left hypoplasia, as well. This allowed us to successfully treat in the same session both the malformed valve and the hypoplasia by the means of balloon angioplasty.

Finally, the catheter was unable to cross the right C1 nutcracker giving a definitive indication to open surgery. Symptoms began to improve only after the conclusion of all the procedures used to fix the IJV flow. Chronic fatigue was the first symptom to improve, approximately within the first week, confirming the link between this symptom and brain perfusion [14, 23, 24]. Numbness and dizziness significantly improved over a couple of months, maybe because fluid redistribution in the brain requires a longer time.

24.5 Conclusions

The proximal compression of the internal jugular vessels in Eagle syndrome may often not be the sole cause of narrowing of these vessels. In the absence of an in-depth diagnostic study, which must necessarily start from an accurate noninvasive

CDUS study, the surgical treatment of the styloid process in case of the Eagle jugular variant could result in a complete failure. For this reason, it is recommended to address these pathologies at an interdisciplinary level with groups that can mutually give their contribution to making the indications, choosing the therapeutic strategy, and instrumentally following up these complex patients.

References

1. Beggs CB, Magnano C, Shepherd SJ, Marr K, Valnarov V, Hojnacki D, Bergsland N, Belov P, Grisafi S, Dwyer MG, Carl E, Weinstock-Guttman B, Zivadinov R. Aqueductal cerebrospinal fluid pulsatility in healthy individuals is affected by impaired cerebral venous outflow. J Magn Reson Imaging. 2014;40(5):1215–22. https://doi.org/10.1002/jmri.24468.
2. Liu M, Xu H, Wang Y, Zhong Y, Xia S, Utriainen D, Wang T, Haacke EM. Patterns of chronic venous insufficiency in the dural sinuses and extracranial draining veins and their relationship with white matter hyperintensities for patients with Parkinson's disease. J Vasc Surg. 2015;61(6):1511–20.e1. https://doi.org/10.1016/j.jvs.2014.02.021.
3. Beggs CB, Giaquinta A, Veroux M, De Marco E, Mociskyte D, et al. Mid-term sustained relief from headaches after balloon angioplasty of the internal jugular veins in patients with multiple sclerosis. PLoS One. 2018;13(1):e0191534. https://doi.org/10.1371/journal.pone.0191534.
4. Bruno A, Califano L, Mastrangelo D, De Vizia M, Bernardo B, Salafia F. Chronic cerebrospinal venous insufficiency in Ménière's disease: diagnosis and treatment. Veins Lymphat. 2014;3(1) https://doi.org/10.4081/vl.2014.3854.
5. Migliorelli A, Ciorba A. Cerebral venous outflow abnormalities and inner ear: an underestimated piece of the puzzle? Veins Lymphat. 2023;12(1) https://doi.org/10.4081/vl.2023.11585.
6. Zhou D, Meng R, Zhang X, Guo L, Li S, Wu W, et al. Intracranial hypertension induced by internal jugular vein stenosis can be resolved by stenting. Eur J Neurol. 2018 Feb;25(2):365-e13. doi: 10.1111/ene.13512.
7. Zhou D, Ding JY, Ya JY, Pan LQ, Yan F, Yang Q, et al. Understanding jugular venous outflow disturbance. CNS Neurosci Ther. 2018 Jun;24(6):473-482. doi: 10.1111/cns.12859
8. Veroux P, Giaquinta A, Perricone D, Lupo L, Gentile F, Virgilio C, Carbonaro A, De Pasquale C, Veroux M. Internal jugular veins out flow in patients with multiple sclerosis: a catheter venography study. J Vasc Interv Radiol. 2013;24(12):1790–7. https://doi.org/10.1016/j.jvir.2013.08.024.
9. Zamboni P, Menegatti E, Conforti P, Shepherd S, Tessari M, Beggs C. Assessment of cerebral venous return by a novel plethysmography method. J Vasc Surg. 2012;56(3):677–85.e1. https://doi.org/10.1016/j.jvs.2012.01.074.
10. Zamboni P, Sisini F, Menegatti E, Taibi A, Malagoni AM, Morovic S, Gambaccini M. An ultrasound model to calculate the brain blood outflow through collateral vessels: a pilot study. BMC Neurol. 2013;13:81. https://doi.org/10.1186/1471-2377-13-81.
11. Zivadinov R, Magnano C, Galeotti R, Schirda C, Menegatti E, Weinstock-Guttman B, Marr K, Bartolomei I, Hagemeier J, Malagoni AM, Hojnacki D, Kennedy C, Carl E, Beggs C, Salvi F, Zamboni P. Changes of cine cerebrospinal fluid dynamics in patients with multiple sclerosis treated with percutaneous transluminal angioplasty: a case-control study. J Vasc Interv Radiol. 2013;24(6):829–38. https://doi.org/10.1016/j.jvir.2013.01.490.
12. Zamboni P. Chapter 29 – the contribution of extra cranial venous drainage to neuro-inflammation in multiple sclerosis. In: Minagar A, editor. Neuroinflammation. 2nd ed. Academic Press; 2018. p. 579–99., ISBN 9780128117095. https://doi.org/10.1016/B978-0-12-811709-5.00036-3.
13. Giaquinta A, Beggs CB, Veroux M, De Marco E, Sanzone A, Virgilio C, Veroux P. Factors influencing the hemodynamic response to balloon angioplasty in the treatment of outflow

anomalies of internal jugular veins. J Vasc Surg Venous Lymphat Disord. 2017;5(6):777–88. https://doi.org/10.1016/j.jvsv.2017.06.015.
14. Dake MD, Dantzker N, Bennett WL, Cooke JP. Endovascular correction of cerebrovenous anomalies in multiple sclerosis: a retrospective review of an uncontrolled case series. Vasc Med. 2012;17(3):131–7. https://doi.org/10.1177/1358863X12440125.
15. D'Oria M, Zlatanovic P, Anthony A, Dua A, Flores AM, Tanious A, Rodríguez Morata A, Scerrati A, Baccellieri D, Biscetti F, Baldazzi G, Mantovani G, Sen I, Peinado Cebrian J, Rocha-Neves J, Sousa J, Davidovic L, Juszynski M, Markovic M, Oller Grau M, Tessari M, Hynes N, Gloviczki P, Shaw P, Zamboni P, Hinchliffe R, Ricci R, Sultan S, Acharya Y, Troisi N, Antignani PL, Mansilha A, Komlos PP. International Union of Angiology consensus document on vascular compression syndromes. Int Angiol. 2023;42(4):282–309.
16. Mohammed NY, Di Domenico G, Gambaccini M. Cerebral venous drainage through internal jugular vein. Veins Lymphat. 2019;8(1) https://doi.org/10.4081/vl.2019.8379.
17. Zivadinov R, Bastianello S, Dake MD, Ferral H, Haacke EM, Haskal ZJ, Hubbard D, Liasis N, Mandato K, Sclafani S, Siddiqui AH, Simka M, Zamboni P, International Society for Neurovascular Disease. Recommendations for multimodal noninvasive and invasive screening for detection of extracranial venous abnormalities indicative of chronic cerebrospinal venous insufficiency: a position statement of the International Society for Neurovascular Disease. J Vasc Interv Radiol. 2014;25(11):1785–94.e17. https://doi.org/10.1016/j.jvir.2014.07.024.
18. Zamboni P, Tisato V, Menegatti E, Mascoli F, Gianesini S, Salvi F, Secchiero P. Ultrastructure of internal jugular vein defective valves. Phlebology. 2015;30(9):644–7. https://doi.org/10.1177/0268355514541980.
19. Jakimovski D, Bergsland N, Dwyer MG, Choedun K, Marr K, Weinstock-Guttman B, Zivadinov R. Cerebral blood flow dependency on systemic arterial circulation in progressive multiple sclerosis. Veins Lymphat. 2022;11(1) https://doi.org/10.4081/vl.2022.10953.
20. Zamboni P, Menegatti E, Cittanti C, Sisini F, Gianesini S, Salvi F, Mascoli F. Fixing the jugular flow reduces ventricle volume and improves brain perfusion. J Vasc Surg Venous Lymphat Disord. 2016;4:434–45. https://doi.org/10.1016/j.jvsv.2016.06.006.
21. De Bonis P, Menegatti E, Cavallo MA, Sisini F, Trapella G, Scerrati A, Zamboni P. JEDI (jugular entrapment, dilated ventricles, intracranial hypertension) syndrome: a new clinical entity? A case report. Acta Neurochir. 2019;161(7):1367–70. https://doi.org/10.1007/s00701-019-03908-2.
22. Massi I, Zamboni P. What are the ideal characteristics of a venous stent? Veins Lymphat. 2021;10(1) https://doi.org/10.4081/vl.2021.9739.
23. Malagoni AM, Galeotti R, Menegatti E, Manfredini F, Basaglia N, Salvi F, Zamboni P. Is chronic fatigue the symptom of venous insufficiency associated with multiple sclerosis? A longitudinal pilot study. Int Angiol. 2010;29(2):176–82.
24. Zamboni P, Menegatti E, Weinstock-Guttman B, Dwyer MG, Schirda CV, Malagoni AM, Hojnacki D, Kennedy C, Carl E, Bergsland N, Magnano C, Bartolomei I, Salvi F, Zivadinov R. Hypoperfusion of brain parenchyma is associated with the severity of chronic cerebrospinal venous insufficiency in patients with multiple sclerosis: a cross-sectional preliminary report. BMC Med. 2011;9:22. https://doi.org/10.1186/1741-7015-9-22.

MIX
Papier aus verantwortungsvollen Quellen
Paper from responsible sources
FSC® C105338

FSC
www.fsc.org

If you have any concerns about our products,
you can contact us on
ProductSafety@springernature.com

In case Publisher is established outside the EU,
the EU authorized representative is:
Springer Nature Customer Service Center GmbH
Europaplatz 3, 69115 Heidelberg, Germany

Printed by Libri Plureos GmbH
in Hamburg, Germany